'This is a book not afraid to plunge into the dangerously overwhelming depth and breadth of the global agenda for social work. Its editors are right to have confidence in the empowering impact of their international compendium – the exhilaration of the boldly global sweep of some chapters alongside the fascination of the intricate national detailing of others. Every chapter reinforces that social work's historic failings, its contemporary challenges and its future possibilitieshave to be understood in a global context. This is a rich addition to the library of a self-reflexive global social work.'

John Pinkerton, Professor of Child & Family Social Work,
Queen's University Belfast

'The editors of this useful text on social work in an international context have brought together not only informative descriptive material from a number of countries and social work specialisms, but also insightful analysis and reflections. These illustrate both the differences and the similarities in the practices and concepts of social work. The book makes a valuable contribution to the growing literature on local practice in a global environment.'

David N. Jones, Past President, IFSW, Switzerland

'*Social Work in a Global Context: Issues and challenges* offers diverse perspectives on social work in a globalized context. Chapters span countries where social work has recently emerged and those with a long-established professional tradition, adding to the richness of the discussion. These carefully chosen examples demonstrate the central premise of the volume – that social work is both a global profession and one that is heavily influenced by local context. Readers will gain a sophisticated understanding of the complex impacts of global forces on social work. The volume is a most welcome addition to the professional literature.'

Lynne M. Healy, Ph.D., Board of Trustees Distinguished
Professor, University of Connecticut School of Social Work, USA

T0187666

Social Work in a Global Context

Social Work in a Global Context engages with, and critically explores, key issues that inform social work practice around the world.

Social work can take many forms, and is differently understood in different parts of the world. However, at base, it can be seen as a profession which strives to advance the causes of the vulnerable and marginalised with the aim of promoting social justice, equality and human rights. This text provides examples of social work in a wide range of countries, informing our understanding of what social work is. It looks at how practice changes or stays the same, and at the impact of policy, as experienced by service users as well as by practitioners working in challenging circumstances. It also meaningfully reflects on the strengths and challenges that are enabled by diversity.

Divided into four parts, this wide-ranging text discusses:

- what social work means in four different countries;
- some examples of the impact social and political context can have on social work practice;
- how social workers see and work with the vulnerable;
- the future for social work, from disaster work to involving service users.

Social Work in a Global Context is the first truly international book for social work students, practitioners and academics interested in comparative and cross-cultural understandings of social work.

George Palattiyil, PhD is a Lecturer in Social Work at the School of Social and Political Science, and Deputy Director of the Edinburgh India Institute at the University of Edinburgh. He is a qualified social worker and began his academic career in India. He later pursued a PhD in social work at the University of Strathclyde, Glasgow. His main research and teaching interests are in the area of individuals and families affected by HIV and AIDS, human rights, refugees and asylum seekers, older people and international social work and social development, along with a growing interest in the area of cross-border reproductive services.

Dina Sidhva, PhD is an Honorary Fellow at the Edinburgh India Institute at the University of Edinburgh and a freelance researcher. She qualified as a social worker in India and obtained a PhD in social work from the University of Edinburgh. She has taught and practised social work both in India and in Scotland. Her research interests span HIV/AIDS, women and children, asylum seekers and refugees, migration and human rights issues and commercial surrogacy, and focus on giving voice to the voiceless.

Mono Chakrabarti (1942–2015) was Emeritus Professor in Social Policy in the Department of Social Work and Social Policy at the University of Strathclyde, Glasgow. He was a qualified social worker and studied at the University of Edinburgh and the London School of Economics, University of London. Before joining Strathclyde, he was a Lecturer in Social Work and Social Policy at the University of Glasgow. His research interests were migration and ethnicity, mental health, comparative social policy and vocational education. His publications have appeared in various refereed journals, both national and international, and he has written a number of books.

Routledge Advances in Social Work

New titles

Analysing Social Work Communication
Discourse in practice
Edited by Christopher Hall, Kirsi Juhila, Maureen Matarese and Carolus van Nijnatten

Feminisms in Social Work Research
Promise and possibilities for justice-based knowledge
Edited by Stéphanie Wahab, Ben Anderson-Nathe and Christina Gringeri

Chronic Illness, Vulnerability and Social Work
Autoimmunity and the contemporary disease experience
Liz Walker and Elizabeth Price

Social Work in a Global Context
Issues and challenges
Edited by George Palattiyil, Dina Sidhva and Mono Chakrabarti

Forthcoming titles

Contemporary Feminisms in Social Work Practice
Edited by Nicole Moulding and Sarah Wendt

Domestic Violence Perpetrators
Evidence-informed responses
John Devaney, Anne Lazenbatt and Maurice Mahon

Social Work in a Global Context

Issues and challenges

Edited by
George Palattiyil
University of Edinburgh
Dina Sidhva
University of Edinburgh
Mono Chakrabarti
University of Strathclyde

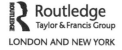

LONDON AND NEW YORK

First published 2016
by Routledge
2 Park Square, Milton Park, Abingdon, Oxon OX14 4RN

and by Routledge
711 Third Avenue, New York, NY 10017

Routledge is an imprint of the Taylor & Francis Group, an informa business

© 2016 G. Palattiyil, D. Sidhva and M. Chakrabarti

British Library Cataloguing in Publication Data
A catalogue record for this book is available from the British Library

Library of Congress Cataloguing in Publication data
  Social work in a global context : issues and challenges / edited by
  George Palattiyil, Dina Sidhva, and Mono Chakrabarti.
    pages   cm. – (Routledge advances in social work)
  Includes bibliographical references and index.
  1. Social service–Cross-cultural studies.   2. Social service–Practice–
  Cross-cultural studies.   I. Palattiyil, George, editor.   II. Sidhva, Dina,
  editor.   III. Chakrabarti, Mono, editor.   IV. Series: Routledge
  advances in social work.
  [DNLM: 1. Social Work.   2. Global Health.   3. Internationality. HV 40]
  HV40.S61786 2016
  361.3–dc23   2015007519

ISBN: 978-0-415-53607-3 (hbk)
ISBN: 978-0-203-11188-8 (ebk)

Typeset in Sabon
by Out of House Publishing

To Mono Chakrabarti (21.02.1942–21.05.2015), who co-edited this book with us. Mono made a significant contribution to the field of social work and social policy in Scotland and beyond. He was a pioneer in promoting anti-racist practice in social work and taught generations of social workers. His writing, research and teaching encapsulated his vision of a society that upheld equality, social justice, human rights and inclusiveness; his commitment to championing the cause of black and minority ethnic community was exemplary. He was a social work academic of great vision and foresight and always promoted a social work perspective that transcended beyond the local to embrace the global.

&

To Pavel Romanov (22.05.1964–09.06.2014), who contributed to this book. He was a truly local and global individual, who believed in the transformative power of knowledge and was unconditionally committed to the values of equality, social justice, diversity and human rights for all.

Contents

Figures

Tables

Contributors

Editor biographies

George Palattiyil, PhD is a Lecturer in Social Work at the School of Social and Political Science and Deputy Director of the Edinburgh India Institute at the University of Edinburgh. He is a qualified social worker and began his academic career in India. He later pursued a PhD in social work at the University of Strathclyde, Glasgow. His main research and teaching interests are in the area of individuals and families affected by HIV and AIDS, human rights, refugees and asylum seekers, older people and international social work and social development, along with a growing interest in the area of cross-border reproductive services.

Dina Sidhva, PhD is an Honorary Fellow at the Edinburgh India Institute at the University of Edinburgh and a freelance researcher. She qualified as a social worker in India and obtained a PhD in social work from the University of Edinburgh. She has taught and practised social work both in India and in Scotland. Her research and teaching interests include HIV/AIDS, women and children, asylum seekers and refugees, migration and human rights issues, commercial surrogacy and domestic abuse, with a focus on helping marginalised, disadvantaged and voiceless people to express their 'voice' and agency.

Mono Chakrabarti (1942–2015) was Emeritus Professor in Social Policy in the Department of Social Work and Social Policy at the University of Strathclyde, Glasgow. He was a qualified social worker and studied at the University of Edinburgh and the London School of Economics, University of London. Before joining Strathclyde, he was a lecturer in Social Work and Social Policy at the University of Glasgow. His research interests were migration and ethnicity, mental health, comparative social policy and vocational education. His publications have appeared in various refereed journals, both national and international, and he has written a number of books.

Contributor biographies

Barbara Fawcett is Professor of Social Work (Adults and Communities) at the University of Birmingham. Previously she spent ten years as the Professor of Social Work and Policy Studies at the University of Sydney, Australia. Prior to moving to Australia she was Head of the Department of Applied Social Sciences at the University of Bradford. She spent thirteen years in the field before entering academia. She has produced nine books and a large number of journal articles focusing on mental health, 'disability', postmodern feminism and research methodologies.

Liz Beddoe is an Associate Professor of Social Work in the School of Counselling, Human Services and Social Work at the University of Auckland. Liz's research interests include critical perspectives on social work education, professional supervision and the professionalisation project of social work.

Phil Harington was Head of the School of Counselling, Human Services and Social Work 2011–2013 at the University of Auckland. Phil's research interests include community advocacy, practitioner research and models of professionalism in the social professions.

Mark J. Macgowan, PhD is Professor and Coordinator of the Social Work Doctoral Program at Florida International University, Miami. His scholarship area is the effective practice and teaching of group work. He authored *A Guide to Evidence-Based Group Work* (Oxford) and was co-editor of *Evidence-Based Group Work in Community Settings* (Taylor & Francis) and *IASWG Standards for Social Work with Groups* (Taylor & Francis). He held the Fulbright-Scotland Visiting Professorship at the University of Edinburgh, where he taught and completed research about evidence-based group work. His clinical experience has been with persons with substance use problems and those affected by disasters.

Sheila P. Vakharia is an Assistant Professor at LIU Brooklyn where she is also the Coordinator for the Substance Abuse Counselling Concentration in the Social Work Department. She earned her doctorate at Florida International University, her Master's in Social Work from Binghamton University, and a Post-Master's Certificate in the Addictions from New York University. Her clinical experiences were within substance use treatment settings. Her research interests include harm reduction, social work practice, social work education, drug policy and drug user stigma.

Michael A. Hart is a citizen of Fisher River Cree Nation residing in Winnipeg, Canada. He is the Canada Research Chair in Indigenous Knowledges and Social Work and Associate Professor at the Faculty of Social Work, University of Manitoba. He also has been the Director of Manitoba First

Nations Centre for Aboriginal Health Research, Faculty of Medicine, University of Manitoba. His research includes the areas of Indigenous peoples' knowledge of helping, cultural continuity and the well-being of Indigenous youth and Indigenous approaches to research.

Denis C. Bracken is Professor of Social Work and Associate Dean at the University of Manitoba. He has also been Director of the Inner City Social Work Program and Rector of St. Paul's College. Recent research has been on desistance from urban gangs by Aboriginal offenders, and probation practice with ethnic minorities and members of the Travelling Community in Ireland. Dr Bracken has held visiting academic posts at DeMontfort University, the Glasgow School of Social Work, the School of Social Work and Social Policy at Trinity College Dublin and the Institute of Criminology at University College Dublin.

Edward Kruk, PhD is Associate Professor of Social Work at the University of British Columbia. He has over 30 years' experience specialising in practice with children and families, having worked in the fields of child protection, school social work, children's hospital social work, family therapy and family mediation. He was recently awarded the Queen Elizabeth II Diamond Jubilee medal, in recognition of his research and service contributions on the best interests of children. His fifth book, *The Equal Parenting Presumption: Social Justice in the Legal Determination of Parenting after Divorce*, was recently published by McGill-Queen's University Press. He is President of the International Council on Shared Parenting.

Kenneth McLaughlin, PhD is a Senior Lecturer in Social Work at Manchester Metropolitan University where he contributes to modules on sociology, social policy and mental health. He has over twenty years' experience in social work and social care, joining MMU in 2001 and prior to this working as an administrator in a social service training department, a support worker for homeless families, and an Approved Social Worker/Team Manager within a social services mental health team.

Hilary Brown, PhD (Social Work) is Emeritus Professor of Social Care at Canterbury Christ Church University. She has specialised over many years in issues of adult safeguarding and abuse. She teaches and consults to health and social care agencies over complex cases and carries out safeguarding adults reviews. She is also a psychotherapist and supervisor practising in the UK and in India.

Susan Hunter was a Senior Lecturer in Social Work at the University of Edinburgh before her retirement four years ago. She had particular teaching and research responsibilities in community care, ageing, learning disabilities and adult protection. She developed and led the first post-qualifying MSc in Adult Support and Protection (AS&P) in Scotland following the introduction of its pioneering legislation in 2007. She continues to act as Independent Vice Chair of the Perth & Kinross AS&P Committee. Her recent publications have focused on self-directed support and learning disabilities as well as adult safeguarding.

Amelia Seraphia Derr, PhD, MSW is an Assistant Professor at Seattle University in the Department of Anthropology, Sociology and Social Work. Her scholarship, dedicated to promoting immigrant well-being and reducing health disparities, is informed by over ten years of social work practice with immigrant and refugee communities in the United States and abroad. Her research examines how experiences of institutionalised discrimination and societal exclusion influence immigrant health and mental health and how social service providers can play a more active role in creating healthy contexts of reception for immigrants.

Biren (Ratnesh) A. Nagda, PhD, MSW, MA is an educational consultant, former Professor of Social Work at the University of Washington, and the Founding Director of the Intergroup Dialogue, Education and Action (IDEA) Center. He is of Indian descent, born and raised in Kenya, East Africa. Dr. Nagda's research, practice and teaching interests focus on cultural diversity and social justice, intergroup dialogue, and empowerment-oriented social work practice and education. His current theoretical, empirical and practice work is based on re-theorizing intergroup contact and intergroup relations through a social justice perspective.

Mekada J. Graham is Director/Chair and Professor in the Graduate Department of Social Work at California State University Dominguez Hills, in Los Angeles, California, USA. Dr Graham's scholarly works focus on social work theory, childhood, oppression and migration studies. She has published numerous scholarly articles, essays and book chapters, many of which appear in major international academic journals, including the *British Journal of Social Work* and the *European Journal of Social Work*. Dr Graham's recent publications include *European Social Work* (Routledge, London, 2012, co-authored with Professor Charlotte Williams).

Tapologo Maundeni is a Professor in the Department of Social Work at the University of Botswana. She holds a Master's in Social Work from the University of Wisconsin Madison, and a PhD from the University of Glasgow. She has published extensively on issues such as children's rights, child and family welfare, sexual and reproductive health, gender, as well as HIV and AIDS. She also chairs the committee that reviews the University of Botswana's Sexual Harassment Policy as well as the research sub-committee of the University of Botswana's Gender Policy and Programme Committee (GPPC). Prof. Maundeni serves as a reviewer of manuscripts submitted for publication in various internationally renowned journals.

Poloko Nuggert Ntshwarang, BSW, MSW (Major Social Work) is a Lecturer in the Social Work Department at the University of Botswana. Her areas of interest are child welfare, gender issues, HIV and AIDS, especially adolescents' research, as well as hospital social work. She has published several articles related to HIV and AIDS in Botswana.

Vimla V. Nadkarni, PhD is President of the International Association of Schools of Social Work (2012 to 2016) and Vice-President of the Bombay Association of Trained Social Workers (BATSW). She was the Founder Dean of the School of Social Work and Professor in the Centre for Health and Mental Health, Tata Institute of Social Sciences. She headed the erstwhile Department of Medical and Psychiatric Social Work at TISS for twenty years through which she initiated the Cell for AIDS Research Action and Training (CARAT) in 1993. Based on the experience in research and capacity building, the CARAT team was instrumental in getting TISS to become the Principal Recipient of the Global Fund Round 7 Project on Capacity Building of Higher Institutions of Learning in HIV/AIDS Counselling.

Anita Rego, PhD, Head, Health Programs, Effective Intervention, has two and a half decades of experience in work on public health issues and more specifically on maternal and child health, HIV, nutrition and mental health. She has directed large state-level programmes for prevention of HIV and for maternal and child survival in the State of Andhra Pradesh.

Gillian MacIntyre, PhD is a Senior Lecturer in Social Work in the School of Social Work and Social Policy at the University of Strathclyde. She is currently Course Leader on the BA (Hons) in Social Work and also coordinates the service user and carer network in the School in partnership with colleagues at Glasgow Caledonian University. Her research and teaching interests lie primarily in the field of learning disability and mental health.

Pearse McCusker is a Senior Lecturer in Social Work at Glasgow Caledonian University. He is Programme Lead for the BA (Hons) Social Work Degree. Pearse's research interests are the social determinants of mental distress, the use of compulsory legal measures with adults, harnessing practitioner and student experiences to develop new approaches to social work practice and education and the potential of mindfulness for social work.

Elena Iarskaia-Smirnova, Dr of Sociology, PhD in Social Work, is Professor at the Department of Sociology, Editor-in-Chief of the *Journal of Social Policy Studies* and Senior Research Fellow at the Institute for Social Development Studies, National Research University 'Higher School of Economics', Moscow, Russia

Pavel Romanov (1964–2014) was Dr of Sociology, Professor and the Editor-in-Chief of the *Journal of Social Policy* at the National Research

University 'Higher School of Economics', Moscow, Russia in 2007–2014. He also worked at the Department of Social Anthropology and Social Work at Saratov State Technical University (2000–2011) and was a director of a non-governmental independent research organisation, the Center for Social Policy and Gender Studies (2003–2014). This organisation was hounded and closed down during the recent campaign of the Russian government, under the implementation of the so-called 'Foreign Agents Act'.

Wai-Fong Ting PhD has been an Associate Professor at the Department of Applied Social Sciences, the Hong Kong Polytechnic University since 1988 and has been engaged in social work education and research in Hong Kong, Mainland China and Macau for nearly three decades. Over the years, Dr Ting has initiated community-based asset-building projects and social capital development projects in disadvantaged communities and among the various social and economically disadvantaged groups. In Mainland China, she has also launched community-based social capital development project in Jinan, Shandong and post-disaster (earthquake) re-development project in Qingping, Sichuan.

Eric Blyth began his social work career with Kent County Council Social Services Department in 1971. He undertook his social work training at Brunel University and joined the social work teaching staff of the University of Huddersfield in 1983, becoming Professor of Social Work in 2000. He was a visiting professor at the Hong Kong Polytechnic University between 2008 and 2011 and at the National University of Singapore in 2012. Between 2004 and 2010 he was joint editor of the *British Journal of Social Work* and is currently an international editorial advisor for the *China Journal of Social Work*.

Habib Aghabakhshi is Associate Professor of Social Work and Dean of the Social Science Department at Rudehen Islamic Azad University, Tehran, Iran. He was formerly on the faculty at the Department of Social Work at the University of Social Welfare and Rehabilitation in Tehran.

Bill Whyte CBE is Professor of Social Work Studies in Criminal and Youth Justice at the University of Edinburgh. He was Director of the Criminal Justice Social Work Development Centre for Scotland, a Scottish Government funded unit, from 2000 to 2013. Prior to taking up his university post, he was a social worker and a social work manager with a particular interest in criminal and youth justice social work. His teaching, research and publications focus mainly on youth justice and the Children's Hearing system in Scotland, and social work in the criminal justice system. His most recent research has focused on young people involved in serious crime, particularly violent and sexual offending, and the resettlement of adult short-term prisoners. His current research involves young people involved in organised crime and restorative intervention in serious crime (RISC).

Bob Lonne, PhD is a social worker with twenty years' experience in statutory child protection and juvenile justice in rural Queensland and Western Australia. In 2008 he was appointed as the foundation Professor of Social Work at Queensland University of Technology, Brisbane, Australia. He has researched, written and presented widely on contemporary workforce issues in the human services, including work stress and staff turnover. Bob has been involved in national and state health and human services workforce policy forums. Professor Lonne was the National President of the Australian Association of Social Workers from 2005 until 2011.

Foreword 1

The day I am writing this foreword happens to be World Day of Social Justice,[1] reminding us all that we are living in an unjust world, often without really being fully aware of it, and that there is a dire need for us to work towards eradicating poverty and unemployment, indecent work and exploitation, gender inequality and discrimination, and inequitable or minimal distribution of basic social services to those who need them most. This is the global and local context, though the extent of it may differ from one country to another and from one context to another. In the midst of prosperity, wealth and abundant resources, why have we created such a world? It is important to pause and ponder this question, and further ask: what was the world like in the past? What was our previous global context? What are the global and local contexts today? How and why has our current situation evolved in such contexts? What kind of future contexts are we creating? Where do we want to go? What kind of global contexts do we want to create?

The embodiments of social work and social workers, in terms of their being, thoughts and actions,[2] have played their part in contributing to those contexts. We have to ask ourselves, what has been the role of social work in relation to the contexts of human rights and social justice, full employment and decent working conditions, gender and other forms of equality, and access to basic services such as nutritious food, health, education and housing, and the freedom and capacity for people to realise their full potential. To attain such a global context many significant actors and institutions are involved, with social work playing a not insignificant role. Much social work is engaged in patching-up work, remedying the adverse consequences of some other agents and institutions. Can social work afford to focus so much of its efforts on that patching-up work tradition? Some argue that it is important to break with that tradition and assume the role of addressing causes, not symptoms, and questioning those agents and institutions who are creating adverse consequences. Yet it is these adverse consequences that would seem to characterise the contemporary global context – global financial crises hurting especially the poor, irrespective of who was responsible for it, terrorist and war situations emerging and reemerging, environmental destruction and global warming, mass refugee and migrant movements, and all forms of human trafficking and exploitation. Often what is done is done in the name of liberalism and freedom, even though creating a more unequal world. Often it is done in the name of managerialism and corporatisation, freedom of the marketplace, or of greater economic growth and efficiency and other such ideologies. Yet sometimes what emerges is in effect a consequence of greed and narrow self-interests, with scant regard for the 'less important' members of societies.

In our current global context, with its negative impact on many communities, and in the hope of creating a better global context and better local communities[3] where human rights and social justice are upheld, this book is a timely and welcome addition to the literature. It seeks to redefine social work in our changing global context; for the question, 'what is social work?', continues to generate a lively and passionate debate in social work's quest to meet the demands and challenges of the dynamic global context and local realities we face today. Several chapters look at political and managerial factors affecting indigenous populations and human services. Part of the book clearly focuses on various vulnerable groups in different national contexts. Most importantly, the book is futuristic as the last section focuses on the next generation, drawing on developments in social work education in six countries. Synthesising contributors' views, the editors have developed sound arguments for adopting social development, international social work, and community engagement approaches in preference to the current over-emphasis on the remedial approach,[4] suggesting that professional organisations assume greater responsibilities 'to walk the talk'. I know some of the authors who have contributed chapters to this book and their work, and they are fine scholars.

Conceptualising an edited book, commissioning contributors and finding a publisher are not easy tasks. Having edited a few books myself, I am well aware of how much intellectual effort and hard work it calls for. The editors of this book, George Palattiyil, Dina Sidhva and Mono Chakrabarti, have brought together 28 authors from 10 countries, who have written 17 chapters, and they have organized their work in a most coherent and readable form. I congratulate them on editing this important and useful book, and I wholeheartedly recommend the book to social work students, educators, and practitioners. As there is a general dearth of social work literature, I hope that the book inspires others to work on and publish similar titles.

Manohar Pawar
Professor of Social Work
Charles Sturt University, Australia

Notes

1 The United Nations General Assembly proclaimed 20 February as World Day of Social Justice in 2007, inviting Member States to devote the day to promoting national activities in accordance with the objectives and goals of the World Summit for Social Development and the twenty-fourth session of the General Assembly. Observance of World Day of Social Justice should support efforts of the international community in poverty eradication, the promotion of full employment and decent work, gender equity and access to social well-being and justice for all. http:// undesadspd.org/InternationalDays/WorldDayofSocialJustice/2015.aspx
2 Pawar, M. and Anscombe, B. (2015). *Reflective Social Work Practice: Thinking, Doing and Being*. Melbourne: Cambridge University Press.
3 Pawar, M. (2014). *Social and Community Development Practice*. New Delhi: Sage.
4 Cox, D. and Pawar, M. (2013). *International Social Work: Issues, Strategies and Programs* (2nd edition). California: Sage; Midgley, J. (2014). *Social Development: Theory and Practice*. London: Sage; Lyons, K., Hokenstad, T., Pawar, M., Huegler, N. and Hall, N. (eds) (2012). *Sage Handbook of International Social Work*. London: Sage; Pawar, M. (2010). *Community Development in Asia and the Pacific*. New York: Routledge.

Foreword II

Like social work itself this book is both challenging and informative. It demonstrates clearly that the discipline of social work is both an art and a science. The diverse chapters take us from the raw emotional impact of poverty, ill-health, discrimination and abuse, where people share with practitioners the impact of these circumstances on their emotional and psychological well-being to the empirical evidence on the macro scale about how social work contributes to social justice and the building and sustaining of supportive communities. It illustrates how, in all its complexities, social work contributes to social development across national and international boundaries.

The book starts with the orthodoxy of social work rooted in the charities of the developed world. Later it talks about the social work in the communities that developed in response to natural disasters, pandemics and wars. Underlying all these roots are the principles and values of social workers across the world helping people find their sense of social justice that results in people feeling they belong and are full members of their local communities. This results in sustainable social development.

It is good to see developed in this book the return to the importance of anthropology, and in particular ethnography. An understanding of how people naturally form their communities and the importance of communication through expectation, providing care and protection to the vulnerable in indigenous and First Nation peoples is timely. It reminds us that these sustainable communities preceded social protection floors and were often wiped out by imported disease or another group of people exercising power and control in the search for valuable resources like precious metals and oil.

The book speaks to the reality that the wealth of any one nation does not guarantee that it can provide the best quality of life for its citizens. It takes us from the point in 2007 when UNICEF put the United States at the bottom of the list for child well-being in the world's economically advanced nations, through the spectrum to the development of caring societies in Botswana where people overcome the challenges of poverty and the trauma of the pandemic of HIV/AIDS using the cultural norms of how communities have traditionally communicated with each other and developed.

It provides contrasting discussions on social protection floors. Where there are good health care systems HIV/AIDS has evolved into a controlled chronic health condition. Where those health systems are absent, in India and Botswana, we are still dealing with a deadly pandemic where the victims are not just those with ill-health, but the children who are orphaned, the partners ostracised, and the consequences for the wider community are economically and socially devastating.

By contrast we also have an excellent chapter on Russia explaining how one form of social protection provided in the Soviet era has been dismantled and appears currently to be in that phase of instability that leads to change, with only the strongest elements surviving through the process. The example of growing old in Russia gives us a deeper understanding of some of the issues people who use social work services and social workers there face. It challenges us to rethink Western orthodoxy in social work intervention and rethink why we do certain things in our own systems. In this chapter we see the different approaches of the state, the NGO and the local municipalities as they struggle to find stable, sustainable social development. It was fascinating to read that in discussing new social work law the concern of the government was the place of the code of ethics. Herein, perhaps, lies the angst between politicians and social workers as they strive together to develop good social policies and then put them into practice.

The politics of social work and social development is discussed specifically in Chapter 6 but is an underlying theme through each chapter. The very privileged place that social workers have, listening to some of the most innermost thoughts and journeys people make through their lives, and our sense to search for social justice, mean social workers themselves have to navigate through often troubled political and structural waters regardless of where they live and work in the world.

As I read this chapter it was not long after the Scottish Referendum for independence where 98 per cent of those eligible registered to vote. On the day 84 per cent exercised this right. People who use social work services are usually from the most disenfranchised sectors of our societies. Bob Holman, a community social worker, was filmed on that day walking through Easterhouse in Glasgow, an estate of deprivation and low voter turnout, where he had lived and worked. A proud day for community engagement in politics and an illustration of how that sense of belonging is key to community well-being. This is an example of the importance of the political dimension in freeing silenced voices. There is an inherent challenge in this chapter to rethink our involvement with political process.

This theme of power and control links with 'who owns' social work. In the chapters on Iran and China there were clear demonstrations that community social work is alive and well! The questions that are raised by these chapters require us to re-examine the paternalism of charity-based NGO or state intervention to the power of community responsibility demonstrated in indigenous and First Nation societies. It underlines the ethics of empowerment in contrast to the impact of social control on people's lives. Power and control are fundamental issues in social work.

No book on global social work can ignore the movement of people across national boundaries and the chapter on post-9/11 was both moving and thought-provoking. People move either for enhancement of lifestyle, usually economic gain, or to escape from trauma, persecution and for safety and protection. Displaced people are already vulnerable from the impact of the journey and its underlying causes. To then experience a catastrophe not of their making, but the negative feelings of people caught up in their own grief in misplaced association with the offenders can be devastating. Envisaging the holistic picture of the total impact of such events on people requires multi-dimensional understanding. There continue to be war-torn parts of the world and refugees and asylum seekers in communities that may have little or no understanding of the journeys people have been forced to make. This chapter encourages thinking not just about working with the individual but the communities in which they live.

So the issues of how we measure the impact of the social work interventions on the development of societies is a complex multi-dimensional, multi-matrix task. Chapter 3 looks at the complexity of research across the diversity of cultural boundaries. It helps us focus on the importance, not just of work at the individual or community level, but also of evidence from our practice into the realm of policy-makers and planners. That evidence has to be robust, it has to be able to be integrated by people who may not understand our language. This chapter reminds us that we are also communicators and that one of our skills is helping others understand what is needed to make things better, to make that difference that every social worker aimed for when they first embarked into the profession.

This book, therefore, provides some really good material to provoke our thinking and development in this era of global social work. It acknowledges the contribution that the professions within social work, in all its diversity, can make to people's safety, well-being and sense of belonging to their communities. It takes us beyond charity, humanitarian aid and ad hoc responses to disasters to a proactive place where we can use our collective knowledge strategically in making the world a better place to live.

This is a book for people interested in the development of social capital to complement the other key pillars of society, like sound economic systems, in building sustainable and peaceful communities.

Ruth Stark
President
International Federation of Social Workers (IFSW)

Acknowledgements

Editing this book has been an enriching experience, albeit with a few challenges along the way. Engaging with social work academics from different corners of the world has been enlightening. Their experience has led to a wealth of diverse insights, some of which are reflected within this book.

We thank all our contributors for their valuable contributions. In particular, we appreciate the support from Amelia Derr, Bill Whyte, Edward Kruk, Eric Blyth, Kenneth Mclaughlin and Susan Hunter with peer reviewing chapters.

In addition, a big thank you to our colleagues and friends Cathy Macnaughton, Chris Jones, David Johnson, Deborah Menezes, Denise Smith, George Valiotis, Louisa Vahtrick (Routledge), Louise Morgan (Out of House Publishing), Manohar Pawar, Paul Rigby, Ruth Stark, Susan Wallace, Wendy Paterson for their helpful support at various stages with the book.

We gratefully acknowledge the many friends and family who supported us along the journey with their expertise, encouragement and stimulating suggestions: Almitra Billimoria, Anahita Kopet Sidhva, Anjali Kalgutkar, Beena Choksi, Danielle Piovano, Denise Schmutte, Freni Sidhva, Gemma and Peter Rebello, Jamie Billimoria, Janis Neil, Marcin Potepski, Marianne Mooljee, Ness Billimoria, Neville Billimoria, Pervez Sidhva, Shiraz Sidhva and Shubha Iyer.

Introduction

Social work: an emerging global profession

George Palattiyil, Dina Sidhva and Mono Chakrabarti

Social Work in a Global Context: Issues and Challenges endeavours to explore and depict the myriad shades of social work as conceptualised and practised in different parts of the world. With chapters from North America to New Zealand and several countries in between, the book makes a modest attempt at examining and critically analysing some of the current social work issues and policy drivers, and how these impact and inform local practice in a particular country context. It contemplates and reviews emerging trends, and issues that influence social work and the diverse challenges faced by social work practitioners, policy makers and academics in positioning social work as an internationally relevant profession fit for the twenty-first century.

Globalisation, while advancing the lives of many, has engendered a divide that starkly portrays the lives of the poor and marginalised. Social work across the world has been striving to advance the causes of the vulnerable and marginalised with the aim of promoting social justice, equality and human rights (IFSW, 2001). It is these issues that the book attempts to capture. In the UK, for example, some of the key issues that influence contemporary social work thinking are around the protection of vulnerable children and adults, greater integration of health and social care, involvement of service users and carers, personalisation of services, and the ever increasing managerialist approaches to practice, to name a few; while in the Asian and sub-Saharan African countries, issues of poverty and inequality, HIV and AIDS and other emerging epidemics, forced migration of people and human rights violations etc., have necessitated tremendous involvement and commitment from social work.

The idea for bringing out the book originated while talking to social work academics and practitioners from a number of countries, who felt the need for a publication that captures social work education and practice from different parts of the world. Linked to this, is the attempt by a number of higher education institutions from across the world to begin to offer degree programmes/courses in the emerging field of international social work; as such, a book that provides a glimpse of social work from around the world is seen as a welcome addition. *Social Work in a Global Context* thus is set in the international social work context and is an attempt to deepen the understanding of social work students, practitioners and academics, who have a passion for a transnational, comparative and cross-cultural analysis of social work.

Context of international social work

Social work originates variously from humanitarian, religious and democratic ideals and philosophies and has universal application to meet human needs and to develop human potential. Over the years, social work has been defined and re-defined to reflect its global reach and local impact, and several authors have written on the emerging field of international social work (see Lyons, 1999; Midgley, 2001; Healy, 2008; Dominelli, 2010; Gray and Webb, 2010; Cox and Pawar, 2013). While across the world, social work is concerned with eradicating the impact of poverty, inequality and promoting social justice, there is a diversity of ways in which the social work profession approaches these issues, which are context-dependent. Thus, there is no single way of defining what social workers do across the world, in a simple, single sentence. Nevertheless there is a shared understanding of social work's aspiration to promote social justice and human rights for all human beings. The global definition of the social work profession adopted by the International Federation of Social Workers and the International Association of Schools of Social Work (2014) states that:

> social work is a practice-based profession and an academic discipline that promotes social change and development, social cohesion, and the empowerment and liberation of people. Principles of social justice, human rights, collective responsibility and respect for diversities are central to social work. Underpinned by theories of social work, social sciences, humanities and indigenous knowledge, social work engages people and structures to address life challenges and enhance wellbeing.

It is evident that social work, while increasingly internationalised, is a context-dependent practice (Nikku and Pulla, 2014); on the other hand, social work education and training more generally draw on a wider, global theoretical literature base.

Globally the social work environment has greatly been impacted by issues of development, human rights and globalisation (Healy, 2008; Kendall, 2008; Dominelli, 2010). Social work has been responding to global social problems (Lalayants *et al.*, 2014) such as street children, human trafficking, disaster relief and humanitarian aid, food shortages, climate change, existing and emerging pandemics and forced migration and refugees, necessitating social workers to develop appropriate response strategies. As Kendall

(2008) notes, the social problems and conditions arising out of globalisation create significant areas of international responsibility and demands for expanded knowledge and understanding for the social work profession. The social work profession globally has increasingly been influenced by globalisation (Caragata and Sanchez, 2002; Dominelli, 2010) and its effects on social issues require social workers to be responsive and knowledgeable in addressing them (Lalayants *et al.*, 2014). Social work is a human rights-based profession and across the world it has been concerned with the impact of poverty and inequality on human development, and with promoting human rights and social justice. Professional social workers are on the frontline addressing some of today's most pressing international issues, and social work is becoming a more global profession rather than one dominated by its Western roots (see Lyons *et al.*, 2006, 2012; Weiss and Welbourne, 2007).

Globally, many social work schools have begun to internationalise their curricula (Lalayants *et al.*, 2014) and literature points to a growing interest in international exchange programmes for social work students. Such opportunities allow students to 'search for subjugated knowledge' by listening to the voices of the marginalised individuals, which prevents them from engaging in what Abram and Cruce (2007) call 'professional imperialism' (p. 14).

Given the increased emphasis on the internationalisation of the social work profession in recent years (Caragata and Sanchez, 2002; Johnson, 2004; Heron, 2005; Lalayants *et al.*, 2014) a number of authors have attempted to define what international social work entails. Over the years, these definitions have evolved from a narrow perspective to embrace more, broader aspects of international social work, such as working with asylum seekers and refugees to engaging in disaster relief efforts. For example, the US Council on Social Work Education in 1956 agreed that 'the term "international social work" should be confined to social work of international scope, such as those carried on by intergovernmental agencies, chiefly those of the U.N.; governmental or non-governmental agencies with international programmes' (Stein, 1957; cited in Healy, 2008). Others like Sanders and Pederson (1984) came up with a broader definition: 'international social work means those social work activities and concerns that transcend national and cultural boundaries' (p. xiv). However, there has been a greater emphasis on including social justice and human rights as a guiding principle for international social work. For example, Haug (2005) stated that 'international social work includes any social work activity anywhere in the world, directed toward global social justice and human rights, in which local practice is dialectically linked to the global context' (p. 133). In her book on international social work, Healy (2008) defined international social work as 'international professional action and the capacity for international action by the social work profession and its members. International action has four dimensions: internationally related domestic practice and advocacy, professional exchange, international practice, and international policy development and advocacy' (p. 10).

In what is perhaps the most recent definition, Cox and Pawar (2013) incorporate certain core themes and define international social work as:

> [the] promotion of social work education and practice globally and locally, with the purpose of building a truly integrated international profession that reflects social work's capacity to respond appropriately and effectively, in education and practice terms, to the various global challenges that are having a significant impact on the well-being of large sections of the world's population. This global and local promotion of social work education and practice is based on an integrated-perspectives approach that synthesises global, human rights, ecological, and social development perspectives of international situations and responses to them.
>
> (pp. 29–30)

In other words, international social work aims to advance the causes of the vulnerable and marginalised with the aim of promoting social justice, equality and human rights in a global context.

This broader definition helpfully encapsulates certain features that highlight the importance of local knowledge and practice over the ever-present danger of the West imposing on other countries its basic understanding of the nature and roles of social work (Cox and Pawar, 2013: 30). These include:

- action to address social work education and practice at global and local levels;
- links between education and international practice;
- integration of diverse practices rather than dominated by one country or culture;
- an integrated-perspectives approach to practice – that is, a synthesis of global, human right, ecological and social development perspectives;
- individual and collective well-being.

Thus, international social work entails social work intervention at many levels, from local to global, engaging to effect both social and structural changes with the aim of promoting human and social development, social justice and human rights. As Cox and Pawar (2006) emphasise, international social work should adopt an integrated perspective, drawing together issues of globalisation with human rights, ecological and social development perspectives. Such an approach will help extend the knowledge and skills required for operating at both local and global levels and promote effective services in the fields of international social development, social welfare and human services. In a globalised social environment, local social workers, wherever they are located, increasingly find that 'local practice is international' and international developments impact on local practice: 'international is local' (Jones, 2011, personal communication).

Social work as a significant global profession

Social workers are increasingly engaged in global social issues impacting human development and well-being, and trained social workers have occupied positions in many international development, humanitarian aid and human rights organisations. The significance of social work as a global profession has been gaining increased recognition from several global bodies including the United Nations (UN). The UN Under-Secretary General for Economic and Social Affairs, Mr Sha Zukang, in his keynote address to the World Conference on Social Work and Social Development 2010, emphasised the unique role of social workers in implementing global social policy at the grassroots, where social workers work with the poor, the voiceless and the disenfranchised, with the aim of eradicating poverty and inequality and promoting human rights (cited in Jones and Truell, 2012).

Helen Clark (Administrator of the United Nations Development Programme), while accepting the Global Agenda for Social Work and Social Development on behalf of the UN, reflected that:

> Across the United Nations, our organisations work to eradicate poverty, promote human rights, and advance sustainable development. The Global Agenda's vision mirrors many of the goals, rights, and agreements established by the United Nations – and the mandates of our agencies, funds, and programmes. We too are pledged to address the root causes of poverty, oppression, and inequality. We support the call in the Global Agenda 'to create a more socially-just and fair world which we will be proud to leave to future generations'.

She went on to highlight the significant role social workers play globally in promoting human rights and social justice:

> For more than a century, the social work profession has been at the forefront of promoting human rights and supporting people to realize their full potential. Various arms of the United Nations have worked with your organisations in global fora, and alongside social workers in-country to advance progress on the Millennium Development Goals, engage citizens in development, and strengthen social protection systems.
>
> (Clark, 2012)

Clark also anticipated enhanced partnerships between social workers and the United Nations in the years to come.

The importance of social work as a global profession gained much leverage with the establishment of World Social Work Day and the Social Work Day at the United Nations, which is now celebrated across the world as part of a global campaign to reposition the social work profession. In 2015, World Social Work Day highlighted the second theme of the Global Agenda for Social Work and Social Development – Promoting the Dignity and Worth of Peoples (IFSW, 2012). This growth and development of social work as a global profession owes much to the pioneering work of the three global bodies representing social work – the International Federation of Social Workers (IFSW), the International Association of Schools of Social Work (IASSW) and the International Council on Social Welfare (ICSW), whose vision, commitment and joint efforts culminated in developing the Global Agenda.

The Global Agenda for Social Work and Social Development

The Global Agenda for Social Work and Social Development (the Agenda) is a set of goals designed by the IFSW, IASSW and ICSW to strengthen the profile of social work and to enable social workers to make a stronger contribution to policy development (Jones and Truell, 2012: 454). It is the product of a three-year collaborative process by the above social work bodies working together with the United Nations to address the crucial problems perpetuating poverty, inequality and unsustainable human environments (Nikku and Pulla, 2014: 373).

The Agenda has been developed against the backdrop of globalisation (Dominelli, 2010) and new global challenges in human conditions that propel us into a search for new global responses (Jones and Truell, 2012). Jones and Truell (2012) argue that the worldwide recession, heightened inequality, extensive migratory movements, increased pandemics and natural catastrophes, and new forms of conflict, force us, as social work and social development professionals and educators, to be more aware of global realities and to act differently (p. 455). Widening social and economic inequality within most countries and across the world is now well-documented (UNDP, 2013) and there is an array of international reports and research studies all pointing in the same direction (e.g. Milanovic, 2005, 2011; Wilkinson and Pickett, 2009; Stiglitz, 2012). There is growing global consensus on the need to bridge the divide between the haves and the have-nots (Hongbo, 2013; UNDESA, 2013) and the Global Agenda has been developed as a shared commitment to address the worldwide dynamics that perpetuate poverty, inequality of opportunities and access to resources, and oppression, and to give greater prominence to the key contributions of social work and social development (IFSW *et al.*, 2014: 3). The Global Agenda is a major element in a decade-long commitment to focus worldwide attention on the four themes of:

- promoting social and economic equalities;
- promoting the dignity and worth of peoples;
- working towards environmental and community sustainability;
- strengthening recognition of the importance of human relationships.

The Global Agenda for Social Work and Social Development: Commitment to Action was formally released in March 2012 during the week of World Social Work Day (IFSW *et al.*, 2012). The three organisations have agreed an implementation strategy, including a commitment to promote a global network of regional centres to support implementation of the Agenda and to research the work environments which promote positive outcomes in social work and social development (Jones and Truell, 2012).

Despite this far-reaching policy aspiration, the challenge for achieving the Global Agenda outcomes depends on how a social work workforce can be developed, nurtured and equipped with the skills and expertise to implement these ambitious goals. This perhaps goes back to the question of how far we are prepared to include international social work in the social work curriculum. While international social work has begun to feature in some of the social work curricula globally, authors like Healy (1995) believe that schools of social work are not adequately exposing students to international content. Nagy and Falk (2000) further aver that the world's social work educational institutions do not appear to have moved steadily in the direction of incorporating a new vision of social work in the global context (p. 51); rather there is an overemphasis on the contextual aspects of social work (Nikku and Pulla, 2014) underpinned by local standards and regulations.

Nonetheless, the achievement of these shared global commitments depends on translating the four pillars of the Global Agenda, which needs the commitment of individual social work educators, schools of social work, global and regional organisations and policy makers (Nikku and Pulla, 2014: 383). A process of collective global engagement to make the Agenda a genuine, democratic and determined endeavour to provide a focus for social work; to reassert the specific contribution of social work knowledge and skills to a world in social crisis; and to encourage self-confidence among social work practitioners, educators and policy makers, is the need of the hour (Jones and Truell, 2012: 465).

Organisation of the book

Social Work in a Global Context: Issues and Challenges contains chapters from Australia, New Zealand, the United States of America, Canada, England, Botswana, India, Scotland, Russia, Hong Kong/China and Iran, in addition to the introduction and conclusion chapters by the editors. Together, these provide a lens through which an understanding can be gained of the colourful kaleidoscope of social work, continually evolving to become a global profession.

Given the range and breadth of chapters, the book has been divided into four parts:

Part I: Defining and redefining social work in a global context
Part II: Political, social and theoretical context of social work
Part III: Vulnerability and social work response in a global context
Part IV: Toward the next generation: developments in social work education.

Each part will be introduced with an overview that sets out the context of the section, followed by a brief summary of the chapters.

While attempts were made to secure contributions from many other countries of the world, particularly from the global South, it has not been possible to include some of these chapters due to editorial reasons. Therefore, we make no claim about the book representing a truly global perspective. Moreover, it would be undesirable and less effective to include social work contributions from several countries in a single volume, thus making the volume rather unwieldy. Thus, the book in its current version is a modest attempt at portraying social work as conceptualised and practised in different parts of the world; albeit the number of countries represented is limited.

The book is written for those who are interested in, or intend to work in, the field of international social work and social development with a view to providing a critical perspective on emerging issues informing the global social work agenda. We hope, in particular, that students doing comparative or international social work courses and those intending to undertake international social work exchange programmes find the collection of chapters interesting and insightful.

References

Abram, F.Y. and Cruce, A. (2007). A re-conceptualisation of 'Reverse Mission' for international social work education and practice. *Social Work Education*, 26(1), 3–19.

Caragata, L. and Sanchez, M. (2002). Globalization and global need: New imperatives for expanding international social work education in North America. *International Social Work*, 45(2), 217–38.

Clark, H. (2012). Opening remarks on the occasion of World Social Work Day at the United Nations, New York. Available at: www.undp.org/content/undp/en/home/presscenter/speeches/2012/03/26/helen-clark-opening-remarks-on-the-occasion-of-world-social-work-day.html.

Cox, D. and Pawar, M. (eds) (2006). *International Social Work: Issues, Strategies, and Programs*. Thousand Oaks: Sage.

Cox, D. and Pawar, M. (2013). *International Social Work: Issues, Strategies and Programmes*, 2nd edn. Thousand Oaks: Sage.

Dominelli, L (2010). *Social Work in a Globalizing World*. Cambridge: Polity Press.

Gray, M. and Webb, S.A. (2010). *International Social Work*. London: Sage.

Haug, E. (2005). Critical reflections on the emerging discourse of international social work. *International Social Work*, 48(2), 126–35.

Healy, L.M. (1995). Comparative and international overview. In T.D. Watts, D. Elliott and N. Mayadas (eds) *International Handbook on Social Work Education*, pp. 421–40. Westport: Greenwood Press.

Healy, L.M. (2008). *International Social Work: Professional Action in an Independent World*. New York: Oxford University Press.

Heron, B. (2005). Changes and challenges: Preparing social work students for practicums in today's sub-Saharan African context. *International Social Work*, 48, 782–93.

Hongbo, W. (2013). *Preface to Inequality Matters: Report on the World Social Situation 2013*. New York: United Nations.

International Association of Schools of Social Work, International Council on Social Welfare and International Federation of Social Workers (2014). Global agenda for social work and social development: First report. *International Social Work*, 57(S4), 3–16.

International Federation of Social Workers (IFSW) (2001). Global standards. Available at: http://ifsw.org/policies/global-standards/.

International Federation of Social Workers (IFSW) (2012). The global agenda for social work and social development – commitment to action. Available at: http://cdn.ifsw.org/assets/globalagenda2012.pdf.

International Federation of Social Workers and International Association of Schools of Social Work (2014). Global definition of social work. Available at: http://ifsw.org/get-involved/global-definition-of-social-work/.

International Federation of Social Workers, International Association of Schools of Social Work and International Council on Social Welfare (2012). *The Global Agenda for Social Work and Social Development: Commitment to Action*. Available at: www.globalsocialagenda.org/.

Johnson, A.K. (2004). Increasing internationalization in social work programs: Healy's continuum as a strategic planning guide. *International Social Work*, 47(1), 7–23.

Jones, D. (2011). Personal communication regarding international social work and social development. 19 May 2011.

Jones, D. and Truell, R. (2012). The global agenda for social work and social development: A place to link together and be effective in a globalised world. *International Social Work*, 55(4), 544–72.

Kendall, K. (2008). Foreword. In L.M. Healy, *International Social Work: Professional Action in an Independent World*. New York: Oxford University Press.

Lalayants, M., Doel, M. and Kachkachishvili, I. (2014). Pedagogy of international social work: a comparative study in the USA, UK, and Georgia. *European Journal of Social Work*, 17(4), 455–74.

Lyons, K. (1999). *International Social Work: Themes and Perspectives*. Aldershot: Ashgate Publishing.

Lyons, K., Manion, K. and Carlsen, M. (2006). *International Perspectives in Social Work: Global Conditions and Local Practice*. Basingstoke: Palgrave Macmillan.

Lyons, K., Hokenstad, T., Pawar, M., Huegler, N. and Hall, N. (2012). *The Sage Handbook of International Social Work*. London: Sage.

Midgley, J. (2001). Issues in international social work: Resolving critical debates in the profession. *Journal of Social Work*, 1(1), 21–35.

Milanovic, B. (2005). *Worlds Apart: Measuring International and Global Inequality*. Princeton: Princeton University Press.

Milanovic, B. (2011). *The Haves and the Have-Nots: A Brief and Idiosyncratic History of Global Inequality*. New York: Basic Books.

Nagy, G. and Falk, D.S. (2000). Dilemmas in international and cross-cultural social work education. *International Social Work*, 43(1), 49–60.

Nikku, B. and Pulla, V. (2014). Global agenda for social work and social development: Voices of the social work educators from Asia. *International Social Work*, 57(4), 373–85.

Sanders, D. and Pederson, P. (eds) (1984). *Education for International Social Welfare*. Manoa: University of Hawaii School of Social Work.

Stein, H. (1957, January). An international perspective in the social work curriculum. Paper presented at the annual meeting of the Council on Social Work Education, Los Angeles, CA. In L.M. Healy, *International Social Work: Professional Action in an Independent World*. New York: Oxford University Press.

Stiglitz, J.E. (2012). *The Price of Inequality: How Today's Divided Society Endangers Our Future*. New York: W.W. Norton & Company.

United Nations, Department for Economic and Social Affairs (UNDESA) (2013). *Inequality Matters: Report on the World Social Situation 2013*. New York: UNDESA, United Nations.

United Nations Development Programme (UNDP) (2013). *Humanity Divided: Confronting Inequality in Developing Countries*. New York: UNDP.

Weiss, I. and Welbourne, P. (2007). *Social Work as a Profession: A Comparative Cross-National Perspective*. Birmingham, AL: Venture.

Wilkinson, R. and Pickett, K. (2009). *The Spirit Level: Why Equality is Better for Everyone*. Harmondsworth: Penguin.

Part I

Defining and redefining social work in a global context

George Palattiyil, Dina Sidhva and Mono Chakrabarti

Social work is a people-centred profession, trying to help those in need to become independent and enable them to realise their full potential (IFSW, 2002). Social workers work with individuals, families and communities to help improve their lives. This may be to help protect children and adults from harm or abuse, or supporting people to live independently in the community or advocating for the rights of disadvantaged and marginalised people.

Social work originated in the West from a pre-modern charitable response of individuals or groups of people to address the problems of society, and over the years evolved to become the more modern profession of social work underlined by formal training in theory and practice (Palattiyil and Sidhva, 2012). Historically, the origins of social work are rooted in humanitarian and altruistic ideals that took the shape of voluntary work or charitable pursuits to help the poor and needy, for example the Victorian poor houses in Great Britain. While philanthropic and voluntary ideals continue to influence social work in some parts of the world, social work in most Western countries has undergone a radical transformation and has become more regulated, with statutory provisions underpinning social work education and practice.

Today, social work has become a major global profession; the Directory of Schools of Social Work compiled by the International Association of Schools of Social Work indicates that there are around 3,000 schools of social work and the website of the International Federation of Social Workers indicates that there are 1.5 million professional social workers practising in at least eighty-four countries (cited in Dominelli, 2010). Over the years, social work has been defined and redefined to reflect both the contextual and global imperatives affecting human lives. Several countries in the world with a national regulatory framework or a professional association for social workers have their own codes of practice (see British Association of Social Workers or the US Council on Social Work Education, for example). Social work is a contextually oriented profession, although several schools of social work are increasingly attempting to internationalise the social work curriculum (Nikku and Pulla, 2014). This contextual paradigm is very evident across the world in both social work education and practice. It is said, for example, that the individual paradigm is strongly represented in American social work (Cox and Pawar, 2013); that the mobilisation of the masses to address social problems is the focus of social work in China (Chow, 1997); that social work is underpinned by a strong emphasis on social justice and social action in Latin America (Kendall, 2000); and that social development is the focus of social work in Africa (Healy, 2008).

Social work across the world is committed to eradicating poverty and inequality and promoting social justice; nonetheless, the way in which social work approaches these challenges is contextually shaped. Thus, there is no single way of defining what social workers do across the world in a simple, single sentence. In what seems to be the latest definition, the International Federation of Social Workers and the International Association of Schools of Social Work (2014) adopted a broader vision which states that:

> social work is a practice-based profession and an academic discipline that promotes social change and development, social cohesion, and the empowerment and liberation of people. Principles of social justice, human rights, collective responsibility and respect for diversities are central to social work. Underpinned by theories of social work, social sciences, humanities and indigenous knowledge, social work engages people and structures to address life challenges and enhance wellbeing.

It is evident that issues of development, globalisation and human rights have impacted social work greatly (Healy, 2008; Kendall, 2008; Dominelli, 2010) and social work has been responding to global social problems (Lalayants *et al.*, 2014), trying to address the ever increasing inequality and poverty across the world. This global influence of social work was manifested in the joint work of the three global bodies representing social work when they agreed on the Global Agenda for Social Work and Social Development (Jones and Truell, 2012; IASSW *et al.*, 2014).

Part I of this book makes an attempt at exploring the conceptualisation of social work and examining some of the key issues and challenges facing social work in Australia, New Zealand and the United States.

Concern for social justice and human rights underpins social work practice on a global level. Chapter 1 illustrates the issues faced by social workers operating in the arena of mental health and disability, who have to continually manage the ongoing challenge of engaging productively with a variety of policy frameworks and practice scenarios.

Chapter 2 provides a brief review of social work in New Zealand, where issues of social justice for Maori people, along with the impact of poverty and marginalisation, create unique challenges. Social workers struggle with issues of professionalism and funding in a managerial environment, yet they continue to combat injustice in their everyday work as they advocate for the fair treatment of service users. On the other hand, Chapter 3 explores the concept of utilising evaluation in practice. This chapter discusses how evidence-based practice (EBP) has evolved globally, and in particular, how it has been utilized in practice with individuals, families and groups across the world and examines some of the inherent challenges in using EBP.

References

Chow, N. (1997). China. In N. Mayadas, T. Watts and D. Elliot (eds) *International Handbook on Social Work Theory and Practice*. Westport: Greenwood.

Cox, D. and Pawar, M. (2013). *International Social Work: Issues, Strategies and Programmes*, 2nd edn. Thousand Oaks: Sage.

Dominelli, L. (2010). *Social Work in a Globalizing World*. Cambridge: Polity Press.

Healy, L.M. (2008). *International Social Work: Professional Action in an Independent World*. New York: Oxford University Press.

International Association of Schools of Social Work, International Council on Social Welfare and International Federation of Social Workers (2014). Global agenda for social work and social development: First report. *International Social Work*, 57(S4), 3–16.

International Federation of Social Workers (IFSW) (2002). *Definition of Social Work*. Berne: Author.

International Federation of Social Workers and International Association of Schools of Social Work (2014). Global definition of social work. Available at: http://ifsw.org/get-involved/global-definition-of-social-work/.

Jones, D. and Truell, R. (2012). The global agenda for social work and social development: A place to link together and be effective in a globalised world. *International Social Work*, 55(4), 544–72.

Kendall, K. (2000). *Social Work Education: Its Origins in Europe*. Washington, DC: Council on Social Work Education.

Kendall, K. (2008). Foreword. In L.M. Healy, *International Social Work: Professional Action in an Independent World*. New York: Oxford University Press.

Lalayants, M., Doel, M. and Kachkachishvili, I. (2014). Pedagogy of international social work: A comparative study in the USA, UK, and Georgia. *European Journal of Social Work*, 17(4), 455–74.

Nikku, B. and Pulla, V. (2014). Global agenda for social work and social development: Voices of the social work educators from Asia. *International Social Work*, 57(4), 373–85.

Palattiyil, G. and Sidhva, D. (2012). Guest editorial – social work in India. *Practice: Social Work in Action*, 24(2), 75–8.

Chapter 1

Social work in Australia

Similarities as difference

Barbara Fawcett

Introduction

Social work in Australia is multifaceted and diverse. As a country, Australia encompasses six states – New South Wales, Victoria, Queensland, South Australia, Western Australia and Tasmania – and two territories – the Australian Capital Territory and the Northern Territory. The legislative context is informed by federal and state laws and although, for example, there is a federal Disability Discrimination Act dating from 1992, mental health legislation differs across and between states and territories. As a result, social workers have to take account of varying legislative and policy frameworks, they have to work with the tensions associated with the often conflicting federal and state priorities and funding schemes, and they also have to be fully cognizant of local contexts. There are also huge variations in terms of metropolitan and rural settings, with the latter often lacking the infrastructure and services taken for granted in the major urban conurbations of Sydney, Melbourne, Perth, Brisbane and Adelaide.[1]

In this chapter social work in Australia is critically examined to highlight prevailing issues, trends and challenges. There is recognition of the situation for Indigenous Australians as well as a particular focus on two fields of policy and practice – those of 'disability'[2] and mental health. An exploration of these arenas is used to appraise aspects of anti-oppressive practice, social inclusion and service user involvement. This discussion incorporates an appraisal of the tensions among federal, state and territory governments in the formulation, funding and rolling out of policy and practice initiatives. As part of this process, the way in which social work in Australia is both similar to, but also different from, social work in the United Kingdom is critically reviewed.

The Australian context

Australia's recent history is characterized by immigration and, as in many other countries, this has been to the severe detriment of the indigenous population. From the declaration of 'Terra Nullius' by the first European settlers, to the policies and practices that led to the Stolen Generation during the period from 1920 to 1969,[3] Aboriginal people have tended to be viewed by federal, as well as by state and territory, governments as a problem to be managed. As a result, marginalization, discrimination and social exclusion have continued to feature significantly. The decision by John Howard, the Federal Premier (representing the right-of-centre Liberal/National Coalition) to send in troops to address allegations of child sexual abuse within Aboriginal communities in the Northern Territory in 2007 can be seen as marking a recent regressive turn in the relationship between the federal government and Aboriginal people. It is also notable that this action was accompanied by the suspension of the Racial Discrimination Act of 1975 for Indigenous Australians living in the Northern Territory (Fawcett and Hanlon 2009b). A review of the Intervention by Peter Yu (2008), presented to the newly elected Labor administration of Kevin Rudd in 2008, tried to redress the balance. The report made it clear that whilst urgent action was needed to address the unacceptably high levels of disadvantage and social dislocation experienced by Aboriginal communities in the Northern Territory, this needed to be premised on genuine consultation, engagement and partnership.

The current situation remains complex, with injustice, structural inequality, ill-health and poverty fuelling intra- and inter-family and community dislocation. The way forward is an area beset by contestation, but as former Social Justice Commissioner, Tom Calma (2007) pointed out, in order to put in place the building blocks of long-term change, the recognition of human dignity, worth and social justice has to form the basis of all interaction. In a landmark statement on 12 February 2008, Kevin Rudd formally apologized for the abuse of the Stolen Generation. Nevertheless, Aboriginal people remain vastly overrepresented in all indices of social exclusion, including poverty levels, incarceration, child protection removals and lack of educational attainment, as well as in the arenas of 'disability' and mental health. There have been significant policy initiatives such as *Closing the Gap* (Committee on the Social Determinants of Health 2008), which have been supported by both the Rudd and Gillard Labor governments, but it is notable that even in relation to base line indicators such as life expectancy, there remains a significant disparity between Indigenous and non-Indigenous Australians (Australian Human Rights Commission 2007; Commonwealth of Australia 2010). Currently, addressing inequality is not a priority for the incumbent Liberal/National government. However, these are all areas that require ongoing commitment and support by social work, and social workers have a key role to play in promoting sustained interaction and building constructive partnerships.

The situation in relation to Indigenous communities in Australia draws attention to the struggle that social workers have across the globe to productively manage tensions between very different types of government intervention and the promotion of social justice and human rights. Often, these situations are not clear-cut but are beset by different agendas and conflicting interests. Accordingly, social work as a profession has to acknowledge complexity whilst managing the increasing pressure for 'quick fix' solutions. Social workers have to recognize the implications of marked power imbalances for particular groups and individuals and ensure that their practice addresses the effects of oppression and discrimination. The challenge is clearly considerable, and underpinning principles drawn from anti-oppressive and anti-discriminatory practice, as well as from critical reflection (both of which will be discussed later) have proved to be particularly important.

Mental health

When attention is turned towards areas such as mental health and 'disability', the overall canvas in Australia presents as being far more fragmented than is the case in the United Kingdom overall as well as in many European countries. With regard to mental health, the national policy context in Australia is based on an overarching mental health strategy. This was initially developed in the early 1990s following the 1991 United Nations Declaration, *Principles for the Protection of Persons with Mental Illness*. Australia was a signatory to this Declaration, and its publication drew attention to prevailing deficiencies leading to calls for a co-ordinated national approach. This was rolled out in 1992 and contained four major documents. The first was the *National Mental Health Policy* (Commonwealth of Australia 1992), which outlined the broad aims and the key underlying principles that were to provide the policy framework for service planning and development. The second was the *National Mental Health Plan* (Australian Government, Department of Health and Ageing 1992), which became the first five-year National Mental Health Plan for implementing the aims and principles of the National Mental Health Policy. The *National Standards for Mental Health Services* (Commonwealth of Australia 1996) were developed under this first plan as a means of assessing service quality and operating as a guide for continuous quality improvement. The remaining two documents were the *Mental Health Statement of Rights and Responsibilities* (Mental Health Consumer Outcomes Task Force 1991), which outlined the civil and human rights framework underpinning the strategy, and Medicare agreements, which revised funding agreements with general practitioners and psychiatrists.

As in many other countries, progress has not always kept pace with expectations, and when the first National Mental Health Plan was evaluated in 1997, although improvements in services were seen to have taken place, these were regarded as unevenly distributed across Australia with major problems remaining. Documented problems included an emphasis on serious mental illness, which excluded many who required support; primary care doctors continuing to view the mental health system as too insular; and slower than expected progress in implementing the National Standards for Mental Health Services, with consumers, 'carers'[4] and service providers giving negative feedback (Australian Government, Department of Health and Ageing 1997). The *Second National Mental Health Plan* (Australian Health Ministers 1998) ran from 1998 to 2003 and included the introduction of the *National Practice Standards for the Mental Health Workforce* (National Mental Health Education and Training Advisory Group 2002). These were seen as a means of building on and improving upon what was already in place and ensuring greater consistency in the practice of all those working in the field of mental health. The Second National Mental Health Plan was evaluated in March 2003, and a key finding was that there remained a substantial gap between principles, policy and practice in the implementation of the overall national mental health strategy (Steering Committee for the Evaluation of the Second National Mental Health Plan 2003). The *Third National Mental Health Plan* (Commonwealth of Australia, Department of Health and Ageing 2003) covered the period from 2003 to 2008. It aimed to build on the achievements of the First and Second National Mental Health Plans and address the areas highlighted in the two previous evaluations. However, the report *Not for Service*, published by the Mental Health Council of Australia (2005), was highly critical and drew attention to human rights issues and to consumers and carers either receiving insufficient support or not receiving the kind of support that they found helpful. The extent to which existing services were overstretched and underfunded was also highlighted (Mental Health Council of Australia 2005; Fawcett 2007; Fawcett *et al.*, 2012).

The *Fourth National Mental Health Plan* (Commonwealth of Australia, Department of Health and Ageing 2009), which covered the period from 2009 to 2014, was introduced by the Gillard-led Labor government in 2009. This plan prioritized five key areas: social inclusion and recovery; prevention and early intervention; service access, coordination and continuity of care; quality improvement and innovation; and accountability (measuring and reporting progress). The revised *National Standards for Mental Health Services* (Commonwealth of Australia, Department of Health and Ageing 2010) were also published in 2010, and the *National Practice Standards for the Mental Health Workforce* (National Mental Health Education and Training Advisory Group 2002) were also reviewed. Key changes related to the introduction of a new standard on supporting recovery and the inclusion of overarching principles for recovery-oriented practice. However, despite the continued rolling out of the National Mental Health Strategy, as in many other countries, problems remain. Reflecting the size of Australia and the federal system, these problems can be associated with the unevenness of improvements, the expansion of rural/urban divisions, continued tensions between national and state policies, lack of adequate funding overall and continued service fragmentation (Fawcett et al, 2012). There is also the need for continuing work with Indigenous Australians to develop services that are culturally appropriate, inclusive and adequately funded (Jorm *et al.* 2012). Social workers have a key role to play in this effort, providing mediation and advocacy and continuing to address pervasive power differentials.

It is also notable that in Australia there is a strong public/private divide, with support services either funded by health bodies or provided on a contractual basis, with non-government agencies (NGOs) competing for (often time-limited) state or federal funding (Hughes and Heycox 2010). Unlike the United Kingdom, which still has a National Health Service free at the point of delivery, Australia has a universal health insurance scheme. In this system, although some general practitioners have 'bulk billing' schemes that allow a patient to receive services without making an initial payment, for most, the system requires full payment at the time of consultation, with a proportion being reclaimable via the Medicare rebate scheme. Moves are also being made by the current Liberal/National administration to bring in co-payments across the board. However, in Australia, provided an individual has a Medicare card they can see a GP in any location in their state, unlike the UK which tends to have increasingly inflexible geographical boundaries. Another point of contrast is that in Australia there tends to be a greater reliance on private psychiatrists, consultants and counsellors, and many social workers, particularly in the field of mental health, now work in private practice. Provided there is a referral by a general practitioner (GP), a proportion of the costs are reclaimable by means of the Medicare scheme. The public system, meanwhile, has to concentrate on those who have few resources and face many challenges.

'Disability'

Before moving on to review the policy-to-practice interface with regard to social work in the arena of mental health, it is pertinent to provide an overview of national policy with regard to 'disability'. It is notable that Australia was one of the first countries to bring in federal anti-discrimination legislation regarding 'disability'. The Disability Discrimination Act (DDA) of 1992 pioneered the introduction of anti-discrimination legislation to fields such as recruitment, employment and the provision of goods and services. However, as in other countries, eligibility was determined on the basis of medical diagnostic criteria, with 'disability' also incorporating mental health 'disorders'.

From the outset, the DDA lacked widespread enforceability. One of the reasons for this was that the embedded complaints mechanism provided the only means of enforcing standards. With no independent monitoring and compliance arrangements in place, complaints had to be made by or on behalf of a 'person aggrieved' and not by any interested party. This effectively excluded disabled persons' organizations from influencing outcomes. There were also widespread exemptions to the Act. An example was that if an organization or business could claim that it would suffer 'unjustifiable hardship' by implementing the DDA, then the provisions of the Act could be waived. As a result, many public spaces that are privately owned have continued to be built or renovated without addressing accessibility issues.

The Australian Productivity Commission reviewed the DDA in 2004. The ensuing report maintained that the DDA recognized the implications of living in a disabling environment and stated that it had been reasonably effective in addressing disability discrimination. However, its overall impact was seen to be patchy, and the Commission acknowledged that there was still a long way to go. The Commission made two key recommendations. The first was to introduce an explicit duty for organizations to make reasonable adjustments to promote accessibility, and the second was to allow disability organizations to make representative complaints in their own right.

On 30 March 2008, Australia ratified the United Nations Convention on the Rights of Persons with Disabilities, and in 2009 amendments were made to the DDA based on the 2004 Australian Productivity Commission Report. However, although the amendments articulated a positive duty to make reasonable adjustments for a 'person with disability', the exclusionary clause was retained, absolving organizations of responsibility if they could claim unjustifiable hardship. The amendments also lacked any proactive obligations for service providers or government agencies to remove or alter existing structural features that could be regarded as disadvantageous. Perhaps most importantly, the recommendation to allow disability organisations to make representative complaints was not taken forward (Commonwealth of Australia Explanatory Memorandum 2008).

In terms of recent developments, the Rudd/Gillard-led Labor governments, as part of 'A Stronger, Fairer Australia' (Commonwealth of Australia 2009), promoted a social inclusion agenda and targeted mental health within the arena of 'disability'. This approach contrasted to the 'user pays' individualized and market-orientated policies of the previous Howard-led Liberal/National coalition. The underlying principles of social inclusion, linked to social investment, promoted by the Rudd/Gillard governments, were very similar to those taken forward under the Labour administrations of Blair and Brown in the UK (1997–2010). In Australia, this agenda resulted in the development of the National Disability Strategy with state and territory governments. This strategy was directed towards increasing social and economic participation, reducing discrimination, and improving support services for families and carers. As part of the overall initiative, mental health and disability employment strategies were linked, the Disability Employment Service put in place and an accompanying National Carers Strategy rolled out.

However, despite the presence of strong initiatives, particularly at the federal level during the Rudd/Gillard administrations in the arenas of mental health and 'disability', ongoing problems persited. These included disparities of access and outcomes across geographical areas, continued funding challenges, embedded tensions between federal and state governments, and service fragmentation. Addressing these has not been a priority of the succeeding Liberal/National administration. Additionally, although legislative and policy documents at national and state levels often use the language of the social model of disability, there are clear medicalized underpinnings, and both mental health and 'disability' services remain largely located within clinically orientated frameworks. This can be illustrated by the continued use of the term *person with disabilities* rather than *disabled person*. The former term clearly serves to acknowledge that the person takes precedence over the 'disability' but lacks the campaigning language and political message of the social model of disability. In 2011, the Australian Government Productivity Commission presented the National Disability Insurance Scheme (NDIS) as an alternative to the current system. The NDIS, which was given significant support by the Gillard-led Labor government, involved considerable federal funding and via a series of tiers, gave those assessed as eligible an entitlement to a variety of forms of support. This scheme was promoted as having the potential to provide far better coverage than that currently available and to redress geographical inequalities. The scheme, despite a change of federal government and some pairing back, continues to be rolled out across Australia and has had a considerable degree of state support. However, Fawcett and Plath (2012) argue that social workers have to play a crucial role in reframing the opportunities presented by this major policy change in order to ensure that the system operates in accordance with a rights-based social model and eschews a deficit-oriented approach. Fawcett and Plath maintain that social workers can significantly shape policy and practice in relation to three crucial areas highlighted within the scheme. These are: assessment processes, brokerage and local area coordination. As these areas have international relevance, they are discussed in greater detail below.

With regard to assessment, Fawcett and Plath (2012) draw attention to tensions relating to self-determination and autonomy being juxtaposed with professional definitions of need, functional criteria and eligibility. They maintain that starting from a human rights value base, a social work approach to assessment for the NDIS can assist in fairly assessing those who face multiple challenges by using a flexible but well-grounded framework, rather than an overly standardized assessment tool. They assert that social work assessments have to challenge functional 'tick box' approaches and to prioritize the social context in which individuals strive to achieve goals that have meaning for them, as well as to address the disabling social dimensions of structural barriers.

In relation to brokerage, Fawcett and Plath (2012) point to the tensions between 'brokers' who merely focus on cost, gate-keeping and functionally assessed 'need' and those who fully embrace social work ethics and practice principles in order to emphasize engagement, rights, self-determination and autonomy. They make it clear that promoting autonomy involves supporting individuals to define what is worthwhile and meaningful for them as well as incorporating an asset-orientated capacity-building approach.

The third area relates to local area coordination. Fawcett and Plath (2012) maintain that in relation to this aspect of the NDIS scheme, social work can ensure that the local area coordinator does not simply function as a mediator between government policy directives and communities, straightforwardly monitoring compliance and facilitating information exchange. Rather, they argue, this is where the goals of the social model of disability can be pursued, through ensuring that consumer groups have a voice in how services are accessed and in the diversity and quality of services; in advocating for more resources and flexible practices; and in community awareness-raising. With regard to the NDIS and elsewhere, there is potential for local area coordinators to engage with the politics of disability, rather than just with the mechanics of service coordination.

Translating policy into practice: the contribution of social work

In terms of the translation from policy to practice in the arenas of mental health and 'disability', a significant area that various agencies and organizations have struggled to address relates to consumer and carer involvement at all levels, ranging from that of the individual to levels associated with policy formulation and service development (Bland *et al.* 2009). Social workers often find themselves in situations where they have to struggle to represent social model orientations within clinical settings and to emphasize service user concerns over service or system responses. This is not a social work dilemma peculiar to Australia, but it is notable that social orientations and survivor movements have tended to have less impact in Australia than in the United Kingdom. In relation to mental health in Australia, the concept of consumer or service user involvement tends to be associated with a particular understanding of the term *social*. There is a tendency for this term to be linked to the social element of clinically orientated bio-psycho-social understandings rather than to campaigning, critically orientated, rights-based and user-focused perspectives. Munford and Bennie (2009), writing from an Australian and New Zealand perspective, have sought to clarify the situation by equating what they call a political model with a social model. Nevertheless, although survivor movements and more political social orientations are starting to influence policy and practice in

Australia, the foregrounding of the experiential knowledge and citizenship rights of service users has not developed as extensively as in the United Kingdom.[5] As a result, constructive challenges to clinical frameworks tend to remain underdeveloped.

This has led to social workers in Australia, as in many other countries, often finding themselves facing the challenge of promoting the rights and interests of service users whilst also being seen by members of clinical teams as both 'on board' and relevant. In these scenarios, the dangers of being sidelined are considerable.

In terms of the policy-to-practice interface, anti-oppressive and anti-discriminatory practice considerations (AOP/ADP) have formed a critical bridge between the demands of the system and the rights of the individual and between policy statements and practice developments. A range of perspectives have informed AOP/ADP, including critical theory, the various feminisms, structuralist critiques and social constructionist orientations. Although AOP/ADP has tended to acquire a prescriptive edge in some manifestations, more recently it has reflected a critical viewpoint drawn from social constructionist perspectives, with the result that AOP/ADP continues to be re-forged. Accordingly power imbalances, particularly those between service users and professionals, have been subject to more intense critical scrutiny, human rights issues have been brought to the fore and the importance of context has been emphasised. As a result, AOP/ADP in the UK context has supported the incorporation of social model and survivor perspectives into practice developments.

In Australia, although AOP/ADP has been influential, it has developed more as an approach[6] rather than a set of underpinning principles for analysis and action. In its stead, critical reflection has proved to be a constructive means of developing social work practice. It incorporates many of the deconstructive elements associated with the underpinning principles of AOP/ADP and, in a similar manner, is influenced by a range of perspectives. Fook (2002, 2009), for example, emphasizes that critical reflection requires examining fundamental assumptions, reintegrating experiences, reformulating meaning and using these as a guide for action. Pockett *et al.* (2011) draw attention to the importance of social workers utilizing critical thinking at all levels in all contexts. They particularly highlight the need to work collaboratively with all those involved in any situation.

The utilization by social workers of both AOP/ADP and critical reflection can effectively serve to counter social exclusion and promote social inclusion. However, in Australia, as well as in the United Kingdom during the Blair/Brown administrations (1997–2010), the view that paid employment leads to greater inclusion and equality has predominated. This view has served to send very mixed messages to service users and has presented challenges for social workers. Fawcett *et al.* (2012) point out that the attention paid to employment and productivity, somewhat paradoxically, can be seen to further reinforce, rather than reduce, the focus on compliance. An example is that the requirement to become a job seeker can be linked to compliance with regard to medication. Both can then be associated with the responsibilities and the rights of citizenship, with the latter being premised on the former. Bellamy and Cowling (2008) argue that, in the context of welfare-to-work policies, using work as the basis of social inclusion fails to systemically address those pervasive inequalities associated with low income, the casualization of the workplace, poor educational opportunities and unequal access to health services. They maintain that countering marginalization and exclusion has to have a much wider agenda, with the experiential knowledge of those excluded by overt and covert processes playing a significant part. Clearly at all levels social work has an important role to play in this process, with its knowledge base, as well as the tools provided by AOP/ADP and critical reflection, featuring significantly.

Concluding remarks

Concern for social justice and human rights underpins social work practice on a global level. Social workers operating in the arena of mental health and 'disability' have to continually manage the ongoing challenge of engaging productively with a variety of policy frameworks and practice scenarios. As Fawcett and Hanlon (2009b) point out, policy spaces, such as those opened up by new initiatives, can enable social workers to draw from AOP/ADP and critical reflection to enhance inclusivity and service user participation and to influence policy and practice development and service delivery. There will always be significant challenges, but social workers in Australia and worldwide are well placed to make a difference.

Notes

1 At the outset, it is useful to note that the situation regarding accreditation for social workers and for social work courses is very different from that in many other countries. In Australia, social workers are accredited by a non-government professional body, the Australian Association of Social Workers (AASW), and eligibility for membership is obtained by successfully completing a four-year AASW-accredited undergraduate degree in social work or, for those with experience in social welfare and a relevant undergraduate degree, by means of a two-year qualifying Master of Social Work degree. Currently, Australia, unlike New Zealand, does not have a National Registration Board for social workers.
2 Throughout this chapter, 'disability' is placed in inverted commas to acknowledge the ongoing tension between medicalized and social models of disability. This tension can be seen as particularly apparent in Australia.
3 During this period, in order to take forward what has now become the very controversial policy of assimilation, children, largely of mixed Aboriginal and white parentage, were forcibly removed from their families and placed in state and religious institutions and with white families. This resulted in a loss of identity, and many children found themselves in abusive situations.

4 'Carers' have been placed in inverted commas at this point to highlight the continuing debates manifested in the disability literature in particular about the
multifaceted nature of caring and how 'care' can be presented in a unidimensional
manner and be associated with loss of self-determination and control. Although
'care' and 'carers' will not continue to be placed in inverted commas, the controversial nature of these terms is recognized throughout this chapter.

5 It is accepted that there is variation in both nations.

6 An approach is akin to a method of practice, such as crisis intervention for
example.

References

Australian Government, Department of Health and Ageing (1992) *National Mental
Health Plan*, Canberra: Commonwealth of Australia.

Australian Government, Department of Health and Ageing (1997) *Evaluation of
the First National Mental Health Plan 1993 – 1998*, Canberra: Commonwealth
of Australia.

Australian Government Productivity Commission (2004) *Productivity Commission's
Inquiry into the Disability Discrimination Act 1992*, Melbourne: The Productivity
Commission.

Australian Health Ministers (1998) *Second National Mental Health Plan*,
Canberra: Department of Health and Family Services.

Australian Human Rights Commission (2007) *Achieving Aboriginal and Torres
Strait Islander Health Equality within a Generation – A Human Rights Approach*,
Canberra: AHRC.

Bellamy, J. and Cowling, S. (2008) 'The Lived Experience of Welfare Reform: Stories
from the Field', paper presented to ARACY AR/NHMRC Research Network supported Workshop on the Impact of Welfare-to-Work and Workplace Reforms on
Young People and Children at Risk, University of Sydney, Sydney, February 2008.

Bland, R., Renouf, N. and Tullgren, A. (2009) *Social Work Practice in Mental Health*,
Crows Nest: Allen & Unwin.

Calma, T. (2007) 'Comment', *Sydney Morning Herald*, 10 July 2007: 1.

Committee on the Social Determinants of Health (CSDH) (2008) *Closing the Gap
in A Generation: Health Equity through Action on the Social Determinants
of Health*, Final Report of the Commission on Social Determinants of Health,
Geneva: World Health Organization.

Commonwealth of Australia (1992) *National Mental Health Policy*, Canberra:
Australian Government Publishing Service.

Commonwealth of Australia (1996) *National Standards for Mental Health Services*,
Canberra: Australian Government Publishing Service.

Commonwealth of Australia (2009) *A Stronger Fairer Australia: National Statement
on Social Inclusion*, Canberra: Department of Prime Minister and Cabinet Office.

Commonwealth of Australia (2010) *Closing the Gap – Prime Minister's Report
2010*, Canberra: Commonwealth of Australia.

Commonwealth of Australia, Department of Health and Ageing (2003) *Third
National Mental Health Plan*, Canberra: Commonwealth of Australia.

Commonwealth of Australia, Department of Health and Ageing (2009) *Fourth
National Mental Health Plan*, Canberra: Commonwealth of Australia.

Commonwealth of Australia, Department of Health and Ageing (2010) *National Standards
for Mental Health Services (Revised)*, Canberra: Commonwealth of Australia.

Commonwealth of Australia Explanatory Memorandum (2008) *Disability Discrimination and Other Human Rights Legislation Amendment Bill 2009*, Canberra: Commonwealth of Australia.

Fawcett, B. (2007) 'Consistencies and Inconsistencies: Mental Health, Compulsory Treatment and Community Capacity Building in England, Wales and Australia', *British Journal of Social Work*, 37(6): 1027–42.

Fawcett, B. and Hanlon, M. (2009a) 'Child Sexual Abuse and Indigenous Communities in Australia: A Case Study of Non-Inclusive Government Intervention, European Journal of Social Work, Vol 12, Issue 1, ISSN 13691457: 87–100, Routledge.

Fawcett, B. and Hanlon, M. (2009b) 'The "Return To Community": Challenges for Human Service Professionals', *Journal of Sociology*, 45(4): 433–44.

Fawcett, B. and Plath, D. (2012) 'A National Disability Insurance Scheme: What Social Work Has to Offer', *British Journal of Social Work*, Online. doi: 10.1093/bjsw/bcs141.

Fawcett, B., Weber, Z. and Wilson, S. (2012) *International Perspectives on Mental Health*, Basingstoke: Palgrave Macmillan.

Fook, J. (2002) *Social Work: Critical Theory and Practice*, Thousand Oaks: Sage.

Fook, J. (2009) *Critical Reflection: Overview and Latest Ideas*, AASSWE Workshop, Melbourne: Monash University.

Hughes, B. and Heycox, K. (2010) *Older People, Ageing and Social Work: Knowledge for Practice*, Crows Nest: Allen & Unwin.

Jorm, A.F., Bourchier, S.J., Cvetkovski, S. and Stewart, G. (2012) 'Mental Health of Indigenous Australians: A Review of Findings from Community Surveys', *Medical Journal of Australia*, 196(2): 118–21.

Mental Health Consumer Outcomes Task Force (1991) *Mental Health Statement of Rights and Responsibilities*, Canberra: Australian Government Publishing Service.

Mental Health Council of Australia (2005) *Not for Service*, report prepared in association with the Brain and Mind Research Institute and Human Rights and Equal Opportunities Commission, Canberra: MHCA.

Munford, R. and Bennie, G. (2009) 'Social Work and Disability', in M. Connolly and L. Harms (eds) *Social Work: Contexts and Practice*, South Melbourne: Oxford University Press.

National Mental Health Education and Training Advisory Group (2002) *National Practice Standards for the Mental Health Workforce*, Canberra: Commonwealth of Australia.

Pockett, R., Napier, L. and Giles, R. (2011) 'Critical Reflection for Practice', in R. Pockett and A. O'Hara (eds) *Skills for Human Service Practice*, South Melbourne: Oxford University Press.

Steering Committee for the Evaluation of the Second National Mental Health Plan (2003) *Evaluation of the Second National Mental Health Plan 1998–2003*, Canberra: Commonwealth of Australia.

United Nations (1991) *Principles for the Protection of Persons with Mental Illness and the Improvement of Mental Health Care in Human Rights: A Compilation of International Instruments*, vol. 1, New York and Geneva: United Nations, adopted by The General Assembly, Resolution 49/119, 13 December 1991.

Yu, P. (2008) *The Northern Territory Emergency Response Review Board*, Canberra: Commonwealth of Australia.

Chapter 2

Social work in Aotearoa New Zealand

Social policy, risk and professionalization

Liz Beddoe and Phil Harington

Introduction

New Zealand social work shares with other countries many of the challenges to identity and autonomy in a mixed welfare system. Social workers work in statutory child welfare services, public health services, youth justice and corrections and in a very broad range of services delivered by non-government organizations, many in partnership with state ministries. New Zealand is a former British colony and is in the Commonwealth. It has a Westminster-style government and has had coalition governments under a mixed-member proportional voting system since 1993. New Zealand is a small country experiencing growing ethnic diversity, especially in the North Island and the region of Auckland.

Staniforth, Fouché and O'Brien noted, 'One of the defining features of social work is that it sits within the social context in which it is practised' (Staniforth *et al.* 2011: 196). Thus, while subject to many global influences, social work in New Zealand has its own unique history and character, having developed from colonial models of welfare, but with the increasing impact of indigenous traditions (Nash 2009; Ruwhiu 2009). Social work is a relatively young profession in New Zealand. The first university-based educational preparation began in 1949, and the professional association, the Aotearoa New Zealand Association of Social Workers (ANZASW), was formed in 1964 (Nash 2009). In 2011, less than half of an estimated 6,000 social workers were registered in New Zealand under a limited system of voluntary registration, based on legislation enacted in 2003 (Beddoe and Duke 2009). The precise size of the social work qualified workforce is difficult to obtain, as there is a limited system of regulation without 'protection of title' and thus people who would not be eligible for registration can describe themselves as social workers.

In a complex local context, moves to strengthen expertise in an increasingly risk-averse climate and a continuing commitment to bicultural practice (incorporating Maori and Western models) have engaged New Zealand social work in a challenging professional project, the preoccupation of the profession with its education, social standing and regulation of its territory. For an increasingly global profession, international issues of risk, contested claims to professional expertise, globalization and indigenization have their local resonances in social work. The profession in New Zealand has been slow to move towards registration, in large part because professionalism was frequently associated with elitism (Beddoe 2007; Beddoe and Randal 1994). In a prolonged debate during the 1980s and 1990s, calls for regulation and educational benchmarks were perceived as acts of occupational closure and seen as antithetical to local aspirations that more Maori, Pacific Islander and working class people would enter the profession. Decisions about levels of education for social work were caught up in debates that seemed to remain unresolved (Nash and Munford 2001), although with every passing decade the professionalization project gained momentum.

By the turn of the twenty-first century, the call for regulation strengthened; over the period 2001–2003 the profession gained the support of government, and regulation was introduced in 2003 (Beddoe and Duke 2009). In large part, the relative ease with which regulation was established was a consequence of a government mindful of increasing public concern over high levels of child abuse, family and community violence and social dislocation. Continuing public demand for action on child abuse created new challenges for policy makers and social workers. At a time when social work was building its case for greater professional status, the demand for practitioners to gain those credentials that signify expertise and scholarship became more acute (Nash and Munford 2001). Starting from these observations, this chapter will endeavour to explore how local and global forces have shaped the professionalization of New Zealand social work.

Social work and professionalization

In the last three decades, scholars have renewed long-standing debates about the nature of professions. Earlier trait models, in which the characteristics of professions are defined and enumerated (for example, Flexner 1915; Greenwood 1957) have been replaced by concern with process and power relations (for example, Johnson 1972). Much literature focuses on the major themes such as the impact of 'neo-liberal politics and welfare state reforms' drawing professional services into organizational settings (Noordegraaf 2011: 1350); the impact of public failures in producing risk-averse environments where trust is lessened (Giddens 1999; O'Neill 2002); and significantly, the challenges to professional autonomy via the management of professionals (Noordegraaf and Schinkel 2011).

While other professions were regulated much earlier, social work has struggled with both the internal and external conditions that would facilitate complete occupational closure, although many countries have developed systems of licensing and regulation over recent decades. Based on different theorizations of professions, several possible explanations for social work's position can be offered: (1) gender and power constraints on social workers' ability to influence lawmakers; (2) social workers' qualms about the politics of professionalizing; (3) the lack of a clearly articulated and particular body of knowledge; and lastly, (4) the associated low levels of autonomy within highly managerial public service environments. This state of affairs might have lasted for many more decades but for the changes in the public sector brought about through the 'audit culture' (Power 1997), in which governments faced a crisis of trust in the professions. In spite of the marginalized nature of social work, by the turn of the century the importance to governments of at least being seen to be 'doing something' about ensuring high standards for public services outweighed any concerns about adding to the number of occupations able to professionalize. In the 'risk society' (Beck 1992; Giddens 1999) social work needed to be subject to regulatory scrutiny. For social workers (political patronage aside) the professional project was inextricably enmeshed with aspirations to greater power and control. This unhappy prospect of diminished government and public confidence is often intensified when applied to social work, despite practice traditionally being located in highly managed organizational contexts since the very beginnings of the welfare state. Social work (perhaps alongside teaching) suffers more than other professions from the fate of being at the mercy of fickle government policy. Social work is particularly influenced by policy forged within the risk society (Kemshall 2002; Webb 2005) as uncertainty and anxiety nibble at its confidence. It is vulnerable to diminished autonomy (Powell and Gilbert 2007) and increasingly controlled via technologies of practice (Garrett 2005). Governments are perhaps less inclined to let the social work profession manage its own education and standards. Education for social work was and remains an area of contestation (Nash and Munford 2001), and in New Zealand as elsewhere concerns about child protection failures drove government action on the regulation of social work to reduce risk (Beddoe 2007).

The focus on risk is fairly central to the ideology of welfare. Management practices shaped by government expectations have seen social work influenced by the discourses of the risk society. In New Zealand as elsewhere, there was a shift to surveillance and targeting schemes that screen vulnerable categories of people in order to pinpoint application of service. Stanley (2007) describes three distinct periods wherein 'risk' in social work is characterized in different ways. Stanley suggests that in the 1970s, risk 'entered the official discourse of child protection, and social workers were increasingly expected to diagnose and identify risks for particular children and families' (2007: 165). During the last two decades of the twentieth century, technological solutions were sought and 'increasingly proceduralized models of practice were introduced to help social workers manage the uncertainty and ambiguity associated with assessment work', and thus risk assessment was employed to organize and determine services provided (Stanley 2007: 165). In the current era, there is a shift away from the third risk discourse, which Stanley argued legitimized an approach where there was less emphasis on relationship in the assessment process (2007: 166). The critique of such defensive practice is summed up clearly by Dominelli, who argues that 'risk management involves regulation not only of the client, but also of the worker' (Dominelli 2004: 118). Perhaps a fourth discourse acknowledges our anxiety about risk but recognizes that losing sight of the importance of relationship hinders effective responses to vulnerable people (Ruch 2012). What then has been the New Zealand social work experience within this challenging international climate for social work?

Social policy and social work in New Zealand

The journey of social work cannot be separated from political history in any national context. Decades of political change in New Zealand saw social welfare segue to a social development approach committed to fostering greater social participation. Changes in government in New Zealand (and the shift to a mixed-member proportional electoral system (Elections New Zealand 2015)) and policy efforts to foster 'social participation' in response to high levels of abuse, violence and social dislocation have created challenges for and demands on social service practitioners over the last two decades. At the turn of the century a Labour-led government won office, running on a platform of a small increase in taxes for the wealthy, the re-nationalization of a core government agency, a return of rights to unions to operate in the labour market, and a commitment to engage with social services and communities of need on the basis of contractual partnerships. These measures have readily been characterized as 'Third Way' strategies between full state provision of welfare and a neo-liberal market model of provision (Craig 2006). The focus on community partnerships can be read as first steps in an effort to reconstruct a progressive, centre-left tradition to social policy, while eschewing a return to big government and universalism. To form a stable government, Labour embraced the policy preferences of smaller parties to form a coalition able to look to 'confidence and supply'.

The emergent social policy became known as the 'Social Development' approach and forms the background against which this discussion of professionalism within New Zealand social work takes place. The new government set off with a series of initiatives aimed at cultivating a new contract with the community while maintaining the confidence of markets with stable monetary and fiscal policy. The new public management approach gained considerable momentum and Treasury policy favoured 'organisational efficiency and effectiveness' (Boston *et al.* 1991: ix) with diminished public provision of services. This was tempered by the very real and long-standing claims by Maori, women, and those whose economic hardship was caused by the blunt impact of deregulation and privatization. Social workers were challenged to stay close to calls for social justice in a changing professional environment (O'Brien 2005). While there were political twists and turns over the next decade, Labour held office in coalition with various combinations of partners, always with a broad social development consensus. Labour lost office in 2008 to a conservative coalition led by the National Party, which began its second term in 2012.

The demand for greater confidence in the performance of social services, invariably at less cost, has continued. Simultaneously, communities have been encouraged to have greater input in determining the services that will apply to their circumstances. There is tension between strengthening the dependability of professional practice and at the same time cultivating the impression that community capacity can be activated via lay and local input. A further unique feature of New Zealand is social policy designed to liberate indigenous practices, in response to the claims and rights of Maori (Walker 2004). New Zealand was one of the last outposts of an empire built on colonizing the indigenous people and the appropriation of land sought for agriculture. That history, symbolized in the Treaty of Waitangi signed in 1840 between Maori and the governor acting as an agent of the Crown, had given expression to the view of partnership soon to be denied in the realpolitik that followed. A renaissance of Maori autonomy, stemming from a 1987 High Court declaration, which clarified state obligations under the Treaty of Waitangi (Baragwanath 2007), required the state to honour the long-neglected commitment to protect the rights of Maori. Significant support for Maori initiatives led to devolution of services to Maori tribal bodies and other communities (Walker 2004). The intention was to restore traditional community bonds and build safer lives for children and young people, and the rhetoric was grounded in issues of identity and cultural recognition.

New Zealand social services policy in the first decade of the new century could thus be viewed as a trade-off between two distinct discourses: partnerships at the community level and professionalization of social workers. The partnerships discourse seeks to reduce the distance between state agencies and communities willing to take responsibility for their own challenges. For such partnerships to be effective, governance must be cognizant of issues of trust and control (Walker 2007). In this effort, social work and social policy were aligned by supporting the embedding of practice in the traditions of the communities where services are applied. These policies conveyed the notion that practice can be inappropriate if constructed as merely the imposition of the will of the state, without the engagement of those communities deemed vulnerable. It thus demonstrates less than full confidence in a professional model. The partnership rhetoric in practice, however, was not without significant tensions. Walker notes that in the approaches developed during the early part of the 2000s, 'power imbalances between the players that lead to domination under the contract model might well still be present' (2004: 166). State agencies retained significant powers external to the partnerships 'to define who the target groups were ... [and] what services were relevant' and to determine the qualifications and experience required of those working in Maori welfare organizations (Walker 2004: 166).

The second discourse is that of professionalization. While the partnerships narrative suggests many elements that can be recognized as part of the de-professionalization thesis (Healy and Meagher 2004), in the midst of the effort to reconstruct the relationship between the state and community, the government introduced legislation to define social work as a registered profession (Beddoe 2007). In a period when there was stringent oversight of social service costs, the government committed resources into framing the professionalism of social work, especially in the non-government sector, where funds were made available to expand participation in social work education. The Social Workers Registration Act of 2003 introduced a system of voluntary registration, motivated in part by the political imperative to answer mounting criticism of state sector social work and its failure to prevent child abuse deaths. The Act requires the social work registration board (SWRB) to establish a schedule of recognized New Zealand social work qualifications for purposes of registration. The SWRB decided that from 2006, a bachelor's level degree in social work would be required (Social Workers Registration Board [SWRB] 2012).

When looking back from some distance, it seems entirely plausible that improving the services to communities would also lead to moves to strengthen the workforce. The first point to note here is that the pervading socio-political climate was making this relationship take a particular form. In the new political construction of the 'Third Way', the drive was to disaggregate generic and universalistic notions of service so that new approaches could be created which valued diversity, rapport and targeting (Walker 2007). The New Zealand government responded to the global trend to reform the state in a neo-liberal vein and also appreciated the shift to greater regulation of social work in other jurisdictions (Orme and Rennie 2006). Social work in the New Zealand setting had itself been engaged in its own professionalization project, and despite considerable resistance to professional status (Beddoe and Randal 1994), there had been a willingness to form a unique stance on what might constitute professionalism in the New Zealand context (Nash 2009).

The social work profession in post-colonial societies faces compelling arguments to indigenize practice and teaching (Briskman 2007; Coates et al. 2006). Tensions occur between a traditional professional model characterized by the drive for 'scientific' practice and the call from indigenous people to make space for culturally and spiritually derived practices (Coates et al. 2006; Passells 2006). Webb has argued that for all the rhetoric about global social work, the promotion of relationships at the level of 'local cultural practice' (2005: 202) is a social work strength. In New Zealand social work has experienced strains between the push for practice and education to become more indigenous in order to better serve local service users, and the pull to prepare graduates for the growing global labour market (Beddoe 2007). Ruwhiu (2009) argues that bicultural practice in New Zealand must understand and implement three significant recognition points in order to fully support the aspirations of Maori people, who are generally most adversely affected by health disparities and social inequalities (Ruwhiu 2009: 107). The first recognition point is the significance of the history of colonization in New Zealand and the impact on Maori rights, well-being and socioeconomic status. The second recognition point is the strength of narratives, stories and cultural practices of indigenous people considered alongside the colonial narratives of 'displacement, discontinuity and cultural oppression' (Ruwhiu 2009: 113). The third recognition point asks for bicultural social work to understand and incorporate Maori concepts of well-being, which are multifaceted and include spiritual, physical, psychological, philosophical, relational and political aspects of worldview and the cultural practices and customs that support these aspects of humanity.

In New Zealand, these dimensions of identity and recognition have led to significant change in practice. They require a reconciliation of Western individualist perspectives and the more collectivist worldviews of indigenous people. The ANZASW Code of Ethics, for example, while inclusive of international principles, addresses the tensions between these paradigms by having two sections. The first is the International Federation of Social Workers (IFSW) Code of Ethics, and the second is a Code of Bicultural Practice, unique to New Zealand (ANZASW 2008). In two significant respects, the Bicultural Code of Practice extends the codification of indigenous rights further than most codes. The first is an explicit requirement to acknowledge and engage with extended family as the primary source of care and nurturing of individuals. The second extension of an indigenous rights perspective into professional ethics is the assertion of the rights of Maori service users to have access to Maori social workers. Thus, the code has taken an explicit stance in relation to indigenous rights and rejected the generalization of individual self-determination that is frequently central to the Western perspective.

Professionalization and social justice

Social work in New Zealand continues in its journey to professionalizing. The results of a consultation in 2012 suggested that mandatory registration of all social workers, with 'protection of title', had considerable support (SWRB 2012). Of the 422 submissions received, 95 per cent were in support of moving to mandatory registration, with only 5 per cent of submissions supporting the continuation of the current system, under which most government-employed social workers are registered, but registration remains voluntary in the non-governmental sector. The most commonly cited benefits of registration are: compulsory minimum standards, account-ability and qualification levels for all social workers; improved social work practice as practitioners meet, maintain and develop standards; and greater protection for vulnerable people by minimizing the risk of poor social work practice (SWRB 2012). In spite of this strong support the New Zealand government decided not to pursue comprehensive mandatory registration and protection of title, with a major report citing concerns about 'possible negative consequences of mandatory registration include the financial costs involved, the reduction in the social work workforce, and the possibility that people will change job titles to avoid registration' (Ministry of Social Development 2012: 148).

The debates about registration continue, despite this support. In New Zealand there has been concern that preoccupation with professionaliza-tion has had an adverse effect on the mission of social work to work for social justice. Professional associations, being located in civil society and driven by their membership, are often thought to enable greater social activ-ism. O'Brien (2005) in New Zealand and Gillingham (2007) in Australia both noted that in the first decade of the twenty-first century, professional associations' activities reflected preoccupation with structure and govern-ance. Membership activity has been more focused on improving the public position of the profession and 'achieving professional legitimacy' (O'Brien 2005: 17). Both commentators also suggest that professionalization does not automatically mean diminished public advocacy; rather they suggest that greater legitimacy can be applied to a strong public voice in partner-ship with groups disadvantaged by structural inequality, poverty and mar-ginalization. The moral imperative remains in the codified tenets of the profession.

Traditionally, social work in former colonies has derived many of its values and principles, theories and practices from the United Kingdom and the United States. Until the 1990s, New Zealand social work was taught largely from overseas texts. New Zealand social work, as a member of the IFSW, adheres to the international definition, although this is currently under review (IFSW 2000). Staniforth et al. note that there is pressure to move away from attempts to have one global definition but to develop 'strengths based non-exclusively on Western perspectives that recognize the importance of local and indigenous cultures' (Staniforth et al. 2011: 196). More recently, a growing literature and increasing links with Australian social work, along with the writings of indigenous and Pacific scholars, has led to the growth of more local perspectives, echoing the call to keep 'glo-bal' social work in perspective and not accept uncritically the claims for a global profession (Webb 2003). These trends to develop the local will expand; however, the fundamental commitment to human rights and social justice continues to underpin social work in countries like Australia and New Zealand.

The struggle of indigenous people in Australasia has kept some degree of social work focus on structural inequalities, in spite of an avalanche of risk-focused individualising discourses. As elsewhere, most social workers often struggle to articulate 'doing' social justice work, given their location in managerially dominated contexts. This prompts the question: are social workers doing what they say they do in the public statements of their mission? Staniforth *et al.* (2011) report on the analysis of more than 300 responses from social workers in New Zealand to the question 'what is your definition of social work?' In this study, 53 per cent of respondents indicated that 'the aspect of helping individuals, groups or families to change' formed part of their definition, while 27 per cent of respondents reported 'social change' as part of their definition (Staniforth *et al.* 2011: 202). Staniforth *et al.* suggest that results may also be 'at odds with the current IFSW definition that places social change at the forefront of social work's core business' (Staniforth *et al.* 2011: 202). In order to explore social justice in the everyday work of social workers, two recent studies in Australasia have explored the way social workers constructed and defined their practice with a view to understanding where social justice ideals fit.

In the first example, O'Brien (2009) asked New Zealand social workers about their definition of social justice, the factors which had shaped their thinking about and approach to social justice and the current social justice priorities affecting practice (2009: 4). The practitioners in O'Brien's study gave examples of social justice underpinning practice actions, though he notes that this was almost entirely about 'individual actions aimed at more socially just outcomes and experiences for users' (2009: 9). Only occasionally did the data provide examples of actions aimed at 'broad structural levels around issues of redistribution and recognition and respect' (O'Brien 2009: 9). It was notable from this research that social workers who participated in the study retained a clear expression of a social justice orientation, while their actions focused on the individual worlds of service users, rather than at the structural level. Thus O'Brien notes that reports of the 'death of social justice in social work' are premature; 'social justice is in fact alive in the work of these practitioners' though not at the level of structured social action (O'Brien 2011: 177).

In a second study carried out in Australia, Zufferey interviewed 39 social workers from diverse settings who were known to work with homeless people and asked them about the 'unique contributions' that social workers could make in the homelessness field and what were the 'tensions and dilemmas' faced in their practice in this field (2011: 9). Zufferey was interested in how social workers constructed their professional identities in this context. The main themes emerging from her study were that social workers struggled to define the 'contribution of social work as a profession independent of organizational contexts' and struggled with the profound influence of 'tensions created by managerialist organizational processes' (Zufferey 2012: 518). Zufferey found that a critical social work knowledge base enabled resistance to 'dominant managerial and individualist practices'. She also found individual examples of workers resisting managerialist domination and use of 'merged individualist and collective approaches' in their advocacy for homeless people (Zufferey 2012: 525).

Conclusions

In a very brief review of social work in New Zealand, there are mixed conclusions. On the one hand, there are strong signals of a commitment to social justice in respect to the rights and aspirations of Maori people: bicultural practice is embedded in professional and educational requirements. On the other hand, patterns of employment and the perpetuation of a persistent managerial environment in social services seem to engage social workers in a never-ending struggle to rise above a preoccupation with delivering the services that governments are prepared to fund. Such services increasingly focus on targeted 'at risk' populations, with little attention paid to the impact of poverty and marginalization. Social workers' voices seem muted in the public realm. And yet in everyday practice, the analysis of injustice and the stubborn determination of social workers to get fair treatment for users of services remains a powerful motivating force in New Zealand social work.

References

Aotearoa New Zealand Association of Social Workers (ANZASW) (2008) *Code of Ethics and Bicultural Code of Practice* (reprinted, first edn 1997), Christchurch: ANZASW.

Baragwanath, D. (2007) 'New Zealand Maori Council V Attorney-General [1987] 1 NZLR 687: A perspective of counsel'. Paper presented at the 'In Good Faith' Symposium, University of Otago, 29 June 2007. Available at: www.otago.ac.nz/law/conferences/otago037106.html (accessed 29 July 2013).

Beck, U. (1992) *Risk Society: Towards a New Modernity*, London: Sage.

Beddoe, L. (2007) 'Change, complexity and challenge in social work education in Aotearoa New Zealand', *Australian Social Work*, 60(1): 46–55.

Beddoe, L. and Duke, J. (2009) 'Registration in New Zealand social work: The challenge of change', *International Social Work*, 52(6): 785–97.

Beddoe, L. and Randal, H. (1994) 'NZASW and the professional response to a decade of challenge', in R. Munford and M. Nash (eds) *Social Work in Action*, Palmerston North: Dunmore Press.

Boston, J., Martin, J., Pallott, J. and Walsh, P. (eds) (1991) *Reshaping the State: New Zealand's Bureaucratic Revolution*, Auckland: Oxford University Press.

Briskman, L. (2007) *Social Work with Indigenous Communities*, Sydney: Federation Press.

Coates, J., Gray, M. and Hetherington, T. (2006) 'An "ecospiritual" perspective: Finally a place for indigenous approaches', *British Journal of Social Work*, 36(3): 381–99.

Craig, D. (2006) 'Community wellbeing strategy and the legacies of new institutionalism and new public management in third way New Zealand', in L. Bauld, K. Clarke and T. Maltby (eds) *Social Policy Review 18*, Bristol: Policy Press.

Dominelli, L. (2004) *Social Work: Theory and Practice for a Changing Profession*, Cambridge: Polity Press.

Elections New Zealand (2015) New Zealand Voting System. New Zealand Government. Available at: www.elections.org.nz/voting-system (accessed 30 April 2015).

Flexner, A. (1915, reprint 2001) 'Is social work a profession?', *Research on Social Work Practice*, 11(2): 152–65.

Garrett, P.M. (2005) 'Social work's "electronic turn": Notes on the deployment of information and communication technologies in social work with children and families', *Critical Social Policy*, 25(4): 529–53.

Giddens, A. (1999) 'Risk and responsibility', *Modern Law Review*, 62(1): 1–10.

Gillingham, P. (2007) 'The Australian Association of Social Workers and the social policy debates: A strategy for the future?', *Australian Social Work*, 60(2): 166–80.

Greenwood, E. (1957) 'Attributes of a profession', *Social Work*, 2(3): 45–55.

Healy, K. and Meagher, G. (2004) 'The reprofessionalization of social work: Collaborative approaches for achieving professional recognition', *British Journal of Social Work*, 34(2): 243–60.

International Federation of Social Workers (IFSW) (2000) 'Definition of social work'. Available at: http://ifsw.org/resources/definition-of-social-work/ (accessed 8 April 2012).

Johnson, T. (1972) *Professions and Power*, Basingstoke: Macmillan.

Kemshall, H. (2002) *Risk, Social Policy and Welfare*, Buckingham: Open University Press.

Ministry of Social Development (2012) *White Paper on Vulnerable Children Volume 2*, Wellington: Ministry of Social Development.

Nash, M. (2009) 'Histories of the social work profession', in M. Connolly and L. Harms (eds) *Social Work: Contexts and Practice*, 2nd edn, Melbourne: Oxford.

Nash, M. and Munford, R. (2001) 'Unresolved struggles: Educating social workers in Aotearoa New Zealand', *Social Work Education*, 20(1): 21–34.

Noordegraaf, M. (2011) 'Risky business: How professionals and professional fields (must) deal with organizational issues', *Organization Studies*, 32(10): 1349–71.

Noordegraaf, M. and Schinkel, W. (2011) 'Professional capital contested: A Bourdieusian analysis of conflicts between professionals and managers', *Comparative Sociology*, 10(1): 97–125.

O'Brien, M. (2005) 'A just profession or just a profession', *Social Work Review*, 17(1): 13–22.

O'Brien, M. (2009) 'Social work and the practice of social justice: An initial overview', *Aotearoa New Zealand Social Work*, 21(1&2): 3–10.

O'Brien, M. (2011) 'Social justice: Alive and well (partly) in social work practice?', *International Social Work*, 54(2): 174–90.

O'Neill, O. (2002) *A Question of Trust*, Cambridge: Cambridge University Press.

Orme, J. and Rennie, G. (2006) 'The role of registration in ensuring ethical practice', *International Social Work*, 49(3): 333–44.

Passells, V. (2006) 'Pasifika location and privilege: Conceptual frameworks from first year Pasifika social work students', *Aotearoa Social Work Review (Tu Mau II)*, 18(1): 14–21.

Powell, J.L. and Gilbert, T. (2007) 'Performativity and helping professions: Social theory, power and practice', *International Journal of Social Welfare*, 16(3): 193–201.

Power, M. (1997) *The Audit Society: Rituals of Verification*, Oxford: Clarendon Press.

Ruch, G. (2012) 'Where have all the feelings gone? Developing reflective and relationship-based management in child-care social work', *British Journal of Social Work*, 42(7): 1315–32.

Ruwhiu, L. (2009) 'Indigenous issues in Aotearoa New Zealand', in M. Connolly and L. Harms (eds) *Social Work: Contexts and Practice*, 2nd edn, Melbourne: Oxford.

Social Workers Registration Board (SWRB) (2012) Mandatory social worker registration: A discussion paper. Available at: www.swrb.govt.nz/news-and-publications/publications (accessed 31 August 2013).

Staniforth, B., Fouché, C. and O'Brien, M. (2011) 'Still doing what we do: Defining social work in the 21st century', *Journal of Social Work*, 11(2): 191–208.

Stanley, T. (2007) 'Risky work: child protection practice', *Social Policy Journal of New Zealand*, 30: 163–77.

Walker, P. (2004) 'Partnership models within a Maori social-service provider', *International Journal of Social Welfare*, 13(2): 158–69.

Walker, P. (2007) 'Trust, risk and control within an indigenous–non-indigenous social service partnership', *International Journal of Social Welfare*, 16(3): 281–90.

Webb, S. (2003) 'Local orders and global chaos in social work', *European Journal of Social Work*, 6(2): 191–204.

Webb, S. (2005) *Social Work in a Risk Society: Social and Political Perspectives*, New York: Palgrave Macmillan.

Zufferey, C. (2012) '"Jack of all trades, master of none?" Social work identity and homelessness in Australian cities', *Journal of Social Work*, 12(5): 510–27.

Chapter 3

Evidence-based social work practice

Challenges and opportunities in the global context

Mark J. Macgowan and Sheila P. Vakharia

Introduction

At the forefront of the international definition of social work is that the profession 'promotes social change, problem-solving in human relationships, and the empowerment and liberation of people to enhance wellbeing' (Hare 2004: 409). However, it is a challenge to determine whether social work practitioners are successful in achieving these aims. To do this in their work with individuals, families and groups, social workers often employ practice evaluation in order to 'provide feedback about client change and enhance the client's outcome' (Corcoran *et al.* 2001: 67). The concept of utilizing evaluation in practice, specifically in the form of evidence-based practice (EBP), has gained momentum throughout the world, but is not without challenges. This chapter discusses how EBP has evolved globally, and in particular, how it has been utilized in practice with individuals, families and groups across the world. We begin by defining EBP and its relevance for social work across cultures. We then review how EBP has been used by practitioners in various global contexts, explore the barriers to its implementation and discuss ways in which it can be advanced globally.

Defining EBP

EBP is essentially an effort to integrate the best research into practice. It is rooted in medicine's effort to provide the best medical care to patients, requiring the 'conscientious, explicit and judicious use of current best evidence in making decisions about the care of individuals' (Sackett *et al.* 1996: 71). EBP has made substantial inroads in social work, especially in the United States. There is a growing body of literature on EBP in social work in general and in specific areas such as family work (Corcoran 2003), group work (Macgowan 2008; Pollio and Macgowan 2011) and the field practicum (Edmond *et al.* 2006; Thomlison and Corcoran 2007). Yet, there have also been strong critiques of EBP in the global literature, which have raised questions about the nature of knowledge and science and what is appropriate for social work practice (Nevo and Slonim-Nevo 2011; Petr and Walter 2009; Taylor and White 2005; Webb 2001). Some of the criticisms are based on particular conceptualizations of EBP and about what can be considered 'evidence'. For the purpose of this chapter, there are two conceptualizations of EBP.

First, there are empirically supported interventions (ESIs), which are also known as empirically supported treatments, empirically validated treatments or research-supported treatments. These are interventions (including prevention approaches) shown to be efficacious for specific problems (or risk factors) through randomized clinical trials (RCTs), meta-analyses and/ or through the consensus of experts based on critical reviews of research evidence. These treatments often get designated as 'evidence-based' or 'evidence supported' (e.g. Chambless and Ollendick 2001; Weisz and Kazdin 2010). 'Evidence' here is exclusively based on the rigour of the quantitative research and strength of the findings showing improved outcomes. The use of ESIs may be considered a 'top-down' approach to implementing EBP, because they are recommended or required for practice, and these decisions are non-participatory. ESIs are often products, such as manuals or treatment guidelines.

There are concerns when this model of EBP is mandated, particularly for the local practitioner. Whereas ESIs may meet a high standard of research rigour (i.e. limit rival explanations for improved client outcomes), they might not be suitable for the local practice situation. Most ESIs require that practitioners receive training or ongoing supervision in order to maintain fidelity to the model, which may not be available in many international settings. Implementing an ESI without training and supervision could render the intervention ineffective.

In addition, there are important cultural issues that should be considered before utilizing an ESI. Practitioners may not find ESIs developed within their own country, and this could impact client outcomes if the interventions are implemented without consideration. This is also a challenge within culturally and ethnically diverse nations such as the United States. For example, both authors are located in Miami, Florida, where the largest population group comes from Latin America. Practitioners in Miami often deal with the question of the relevance of research that has been undertaken with other non-immigrant, non-Latin American groups. To cite a specific example from the literature:

> If social workers encounter a Central American woman suffering from *susto* (a cultural syndrome akin to 'fright' that emerges after experiencing or witnessing a frightening event), should the practitioner promote the treatment commonly prescribed in her culture (i.e., calming teas and rituals that restore the soul's balance)? Or should the therapist go with what she has been trained in such as a psychodynamic model that

focuses on transferential phenomenon and unexpressed libidinal desires or with a cognitive based intervention that reconditions her thinking?

(Zayas *et al.* 2011: 404)

Utilizing an ESI may not be acceptable in that context because of the immediate relevance to the client of her own indigenous understanding of the problem (i.e. a spiritual imbalance) and her culture's prescribed treatment for it (i.e. consuming teas, partaking in certain rituals). Studies about attending to client characteristics and client preferences for treatment challenge the notion that all interventions will work equally well with all ethnic and racial groups (Benish *et al.* 2011; Swift *et al.* 2011; Zayas *et al.* 2011). An ESI that 'lacks relevance to the needs and preferences of a sub-cultural group, even if the intervention could be administered with complete fidelity, would exhibit low levels of effectiveness' (Castro *et al.* 2010: 218). Thus, practice judgment (practice wisdom) that attends to cultural issues is required before an ESI is implemented.

The second conceptualization of EBP, the one the authors support, is a *process* model, which may incorporate ESIs, but only after critical review. In social work, this model has been defined as:

> The mindful and systematic identification, analysis, evaluation, and synthesis of evidence of practice effectiveness as a primary part of an integrative and collaborative process concerning the selection and application of service to members of target client groups. The evidence-based decision-making process includes consideration of professional ethics and experience as well as the personal and cultural values and judgments of consumers.
>
> (Cournoyer 2004: 4)

This is a 'bottom-up' model, as it is embedded in the practice context rather than imposed upon the practitioner. The practitioner utilizes evidence that is determined to be not only rigorous and impactful, but also applicable and appropriate to the practitioner's abilities, clients and setting. This model is often operationalized through a series of steps that practitioners can follow; namely, to (1) develop a practice question that is answerable and searchable; (2) search for evidence that answers the practice question; (3) critically appraise the evidence in the three areas of research rigour, impact (significant effects) and applicability (relevant and appropriate for practice context); (4) apply the evidence in consideration of client values, preferences, strengths and circumstances; and (5) evaluate effectiveness and efficiency and seek ways to improve (Cournoyer 2004; Gibbs 2003; Mullen *et al.* 2007a). In this model, the 'best available' evidence is the most rigorous, has the greatest impact, and is applicable (Cournoyer 2004; Gibbs 2003; Haynes *et al.* 1996; Macgowan 2008). Evidence can be research-based (based on formal qualitative or quantitative study) or authority-based (e.g. opinions of others, anecdotal experience), and there are guides that help practitioners evaluate the rigour, impact and applicability of a variety of authority- and research-based evidence (Gibbs 2003; Lee *et al.* 2010; Macgowan 2008; Rubin 2008).

This process model of EBP requires practice expertise (i.e. clinical expertise, practice wisdom) that includes consideration of authority- or research-based evidence, practice circumstances and client preferences and actions, which include client culture and preferences (Chen *et al.* 2008; Haynes *et al.* 2002; Morales and Norcross 2010). Practice expertise is essential as practitioners review the applicability of research evidence from other countries, and how to adopt or adapt it for the host culture (Barrera *et al.* 2013; Bass *et al.* 2007). Practice expertise also draws on the most rigorous evidence or knowledge derived from the local culture (indigenous knowledge), which has the potential for the development of more effective interventions.

These two models of EBP are distinct but related. They are distinct in that one is a product and the other is a process. They are related in that ESIs may be used as part of the process model for efficacious practice. For example, a social work practitioner may determine that an ESI is rigorous, impactful and applicable, and will use it in his or her practice. Yet, the two conceptualizations of EBP are often confused by practitioners and academics (Rubin and Parrish 2007; Stewart *et al.* 2012). For example, almost equal proportions of academics in a national survey in the United States reported that EBP was either 'a way to designate certain interventions as empirically supported under certain circumstances' or 'a process that includes locating and appraising evidence as a part of practice decisions' (Rubin and Parrish 2007: 116). Almost half in the survey reported that it was both. It is important to know the differences. The process model avoids the potential ethical issues involved in mandating particular interventions without considering applicability and cultural issues.

Global perspectives in implementing evidence-based practice

The definition of social work provided by the International Federation of Social Workers (IFSW) states that 'Social work bases its methodology on a systematic body of evidence based knowledge derived from research and practice evaluation, including local and indigenous knowledge specific to its context' (Hare 2004: 419). The concept of 'evidence-based' knowledge is presented alongside 'indigenous' knowledge, thereby validating the significance of both in clinical decision making in countries around the world. The inclusion of 'indigenous knowledge' means that social workers can and should engage in a critical examination of how the research evidence fits within local cultural wisdom, realities and needs (Hare 2004). As noted above, this is not just relevant in determining whether a piece of Australian research evidence might be relevant for practice in Singapore, but also whether knowledge generated in urban Malaysia is relevant for rural Malaysia.

The remainder of this chapter deals with factors that have promoted or hindered the use of EBP globally, based on a review of recent social work literature on EBP and practice evaluation. Commonly reported factors include socio-political-economic climate, professional factors affecting social work practice and education, research access and utilization of social work knowledge, and diverse organizational contexts.

Socio-political-economic climate

Governments in Australia, Hong Kong, Italy, Norway and the United Kingdom have placed pressure upon social service organizations to provide interventions with demonstrated efficacy, to ensure the survival of the most effective programmes (Fook *et al.* 2011; McNamara and Neve 2009; Morago 2010). Nationalized social care allows governments to establish unilateral requirements about making particular information accessible, when they are supportive of EBP (Gambrill 2004). Despite vigorous debates in the literature about EBP, the government of the United Kingdom has placed top value on EBP to replace 'individual discretion based on professional experience and personal preference' (Payne 2008: 78). South Korea has experienced tremendous economic growth in the past decade, creating an awareness of its diverse social problems. This has resulted in an increase in government expenditure on social programming, and social workers have been involved in the provision of these services, although little efficacy data exists about the approaches used (Choi *et al.* 2009). In contrast, political factors are one of the three major obstacles to EBP dissemination in Canada, where the authorities' desire for re-election has determined that funding priorities lie elsewhere (Holosko 2004).

Major political changes can also affect priorities related to EBP. Large political changes have created nations within a single generation (e.g. Israel, South Africa and the former Soviet Republics). Much of the focus of social work in those countries has been on establishing and building their social welfare systems (Ronen 2004; van Zyl 2004). In Northern Ireland, the work has been focused on responding to major political changes (e.g. decommissioning, the restructuring of the police force), with little attention to practice evaluation and EBP (Dillenburger 2004). However, political progress has given the opportunity for discussion about what is evidence, and the charge for developing EBP is putting pressure on academics to produce research for practice (Dillenburger 2004).

The socio-political systems of different countries may support some research philosophies over others, which may affect the full development of EBP. For example, leadership within South Africa has tended to support postmodern perspectives on knowledge, making qualitative methods the preferred, if not required, approach to research (van Zyl 2004). Yet, for EBP to fully develop, both qualitative and quantitative research designs are needed, as each has different purposes (Fraser *et al.* 2009). Indeed, mixed-methods designs combining both qualitative and quantitative approaches can yield richer information about intervention processes and outcomes than either can alone. However, this requires recognition of the value and place of quantitative designs in intervention design and development.

Similarly, support for EBP depends on the specific social characteristics of the countries. In South Africa, there is an emphasis on developmental social work at the community level (van Zyl 2004). As a result, there has been relatively little outcome research on practice with individuals, families and small groups. Although some socio-political systems may be perceived as challenges to traditional conceptions of EBP, they also provide an opportunity to creatively expand methods of EBP so that they are more culturally sensitive and expansive.

Professional

Social work practice

The presence of professional accrediting bodies for social work practice and education affect the dissemination and implementation of EBP. However, many countries do not have accrediting bodies, and those that do lack strong mandates for EBP. Social workers from countries such as the United States, Canada and the United Kingdom, where social work has a long history, are more likely to be accountable to national accrediting bodies. Social workers in these countries tend to have developed their own body of empirical knowledge, which is disseminated through numerous professional publications, conferences and continuing education opportunities. These social workers receive specific training on various skills and in research and evaluation. For example, in the United States the National Association of Social Workers (NASW) includes in the Code of Ethics as part of social work's ethical responsibility to the profession (5.02), that:

> Social workers should monitor and evaluate policies, the implementation of programs, and practice interventions ... Social workers should critically examine and keep current with emerging knowledge relevant to social work and fully use evaluation and research evidence in their professional practice.
>
> (NASW 2008)

Although there are many member organizations of the IFSW,[1] few have accessible websites, which limits the promulgation of standards that may support practice evaluation and EBP. Except for NASW, few organizations have websites and many do not explicitly promote or require practice evaluation and EBP. The Canadian Association of Social Workers (CASW 2005) mentions competence in professional practice and encourages effective strategies, but it does not specifically mention a requirement to evaluate practice or integrate the best available research into practice. Schisms in the profession between researchers and practitioners have been a barrier to adoption of EBP in Canada (Holosko 2004). The British Association of Social Workers website[2] clearly notes that one of the duties of social workers is to 'facilitate and contribute to evaluation and research'. The Australian Association of Social Workers[3] website notes the importance of including communities and clients in programme evaluation, but there is no statement that social workers should monitor and improve direct practice. Social work is still a relatively young profession in many countries, such as China, Israel and Japan (Akiyama and Buchanan 2007; Leung 2007; Ronen 2004). Initiatives that promote evaluation and EBP in these countries tend to be localized, often associated with the interests of particular universities, so practitioners in those communities may be better prepared than those in other geographical locations (Ronen 2004).

Social work education

An important foundation for the use of EBP is for students to be trained in it (Mullen *et al.* 2008; Stewart *et al.* 2012). There are specialized methods that must be learned to effectively seek, find, critically appraise and apply evidence in practice. Social work education is not standardized internationally; thus, social workers graduate with different levels of proficiency with practice evaluation and EBP. In the United States, the Council on Social Work Education (CSWE) has required curriculum content on practice evaluation since 1984 (Baker *et al.* 2010; CSWE 2008). The most recent credentialing document from CSWE requires programmes to educate students to 'engage in research-informed practice and practice-informed research. Social workers use evidence-based interventions, evaluate their own practice' (Educational Policy 2.1.6, CSWE-ACFTS 2008). In a survey of faculty in master's programmes in the United States, a large majority (73 per cent) had a favourable view of EBP, but saw differences in how EBP was defined (Rubin and Parrish 2007). Many schools in the United States include EBP in their curricula, and at least one school has adopted EBP as the primary learning model in its curriculum (Edmond *et al.* 2006; Howard *et al.* 2003).

The specific requirement for EBP is not consistent across North America. Canada does not require accredited programmes to teach EBP, but there is a general requirement for students to have research competence (with no mention of which research competencies) and to engage in practice evaluation as part of field education (SM 6.02, CASWE-ACFTS 2008). As a result, EBP has not been adequately integrated into coursework: 'in general, Canadian social work educational settings have not successfully promoted, taught, or trained their professionals to understand or use evidence-based practice to any great extent' (Holosko 2004: 154). There have been notable exceptions, such as in the University of Toronto, which has established an institute for evidence-based social work (Regehr *et al.* 2007).

The few advances in EBP in North America have not been shared globally. In much of the United Kingdom, preparation for EBP has not been part of mainstream academic coursework and has been relegated to post-qualifying courses (Petch 2004; Sheldon *et al.* 2005). Although evaluation and the use of research in practice is a qualifying requirement for social work professionals in the United Kingdom, how much has appeared in practice is uncertain (Morago 2010). In England, surveys of university-educated social workers have reported that relatively few were familiar with current research publications or had critical appraisal skills for quantitative research (e.g. concept of statistical significance, difference between experimental or quasi-experimental designs (Sheldon *et al.* 2005)). In Northern Ireland, where social work training began a century ago, programmes offer a range of research courses, but mostly at post-qualifying levels (Dillenburger 2004). A survey of MSW students in Northern Ireland noted that students were well-prepared in research and most found it to be a valuable component of their professional training, but the type of research training was not suited for implementing EBP (McCrystal and Wilson 2009).

Sweden has had an accrediting body for social work since the beginning of the twentieth century, although the training has been mostly vocational (Sundell *et al.* 2010). There have been advancements since the 1970s, but academics there have not promoted EBP (Sundell *et al.* 2010). Some of the lack of adoption may be due to intellectual academic traditions that do not promote outcome evaluation (related to socio-political systems, noted above). Some countries, rather than teaching about philosophies of science conducive to outcome evaluation, support phenomenological approaches, which has created, at least in Germany, a reticence to adopt helping approaches (such as EBP) that may focus on specific problems and their outcomes (Kindler 2008; Otto *et al.* 2008). In Germany, this has been framed as the issue between interpretative (*verstehen*) understanding and causal explanation (*erklären*), so that EBP has not taken root there (Otto *et al.* 2008). This has led to few native outcome studies that practitioners could draw on (Kindler 2008).

In Finland, there has been no national organization for social work education. Thus, curriculum content has been left to the university departments (Rostila and Piirainen 2004). Social work faculty has tended to teach qualitative research methods, with quantitative research methods taught by faculty from other disciplines (Rostila and Piirainen 2004). Evaluation research has not been an essential part of social work practice (Rostila and Piirainen 2004). This has resulted in relatively few graduates knowing how to rigorously evaluate process and outcomes in social work practice.

In Holland, social work education has not emphasized research methods. To overcome this deficiency, it has been recommended that work groups be formed in which academics and practitioners work together to generate the best evidence (Garretsen *et al.* 2005). In Hong Kong, EBP is not a core orientation and there has been only a nominal effort to teach the critical review of interventions (Shek *et al.* 2004). In Israel, there is no uniform requirement for students to enrol in research courses; many social work faculty do not utilize research and evaluation themselves, and field supervisors do not promote the use of evaluation in practice (Ronen 2004). There is a similar situation in Japan, where social workers are not typically trained to be research-minded, which has affected their receptiveness to EBP (Akiyama and Buchanan 2007).

Research knowledge and its accessibility

Additional factors that affect the utilization of EBP around the world include the accessibility of research knowledge, the availability of research by and for social work, and the availability of culturally relevant research. Access to the latest evidence begins with a required infrastructure. Even in North America, where there are many resources, EBP requires access to journal databases and the technology to readily access them, which are often fee-based. Accessibility of libraries has been a concern in developing countries and in rural areas of most countries. Lack of access to online and physical resources is a real barrier to the implementation of EBP.

In the countries in which social workers are not well trained in quantitative research methods, there are relatively few outcome studies by social work researchers. Although the United Kingdom has been producing good quality empirical research, the quality of outcome research in its leading social work journal has not been rigorous. Surveys of the quantitative research in the *British Journal of Social Work* reported improvements over the years, but there were still relatively weak quantitative designs and poor-quality mixed methods studies (McCambridge *et al.* 2007). A review of Japan's academic journal, *Studies on Social Work of Japan*, revealed that most of the published papers were predominantly exploratory or descriptive, rather than aiming to 'demonstrate the efficacy and effectiveness of practice and intervention' (Akiyama and Buchanan 2007: 260). Evidence yielded by qualitative research methods is important, particularly in the process of intervention design and development (Fraser *et al.* 2009), but rigorous effectiveness and efficacy studies also require quantitative methods, which require adequate training.

Access to materials that are culturally relevant is important (Baker *et al.* 2010; Choi *et al.* 2009; McNamara and Neve 2009). In Hong Kong, there is a lack of literature on psychosocial interventions from within that country (Shek *et al.* 2004). There is also the problem of a lack of assessment instruments in native languages, such as in Finland (Rostila and Piirainen 2004) and Israel (Ronen 2004). In numerous countries there are many dialect groups. South Africa has over ten official languages and different dialects within each language group (van Zyl 2004), thus requiring different versions of instruments. Kee (2004: 339) wrote about the difficulty with 'linguistic and cultural equivalence' in translating Western, English-based measures in Malaysia, where certain concepts do not exist or are differently interpreted. Literacy rates affect the suitability and types of assessment instruments as well. In countries with high numbers of people with low literacy, such as South Africa, text-based measures cannot be self-administered or should be replaced by visual measures (van Zyl 2004). Others have also written about the desire to acknowledge client strengths, individuality, diversity and uniqueness without homogenizing them through the use of standardized measures (McNamara and Neve 2009).

Organizational factors

While many practitioners have acknowledged the value of practice evaluation and EBP (Edmond *et al.* 2006; Moncoske and Pui-Fong 1990; Morago 2010; Sheldon *et al.* 2005), they also note significant barriers related to the work environments. Factors in social service organizations are important in the adoption and advancement of EBP globally (Sheldon and Chilvers 2004). Many practitioners report that they do not feel adequately equipped or supported to do EBP (Morago 2010; Steyaert *et al.* 2011). Studies of agency administrators in the United States have reported correlations between favourable adoption of EBP and organizational culture, climate and leadership (Aarons 2006; Aarons and Sawitzky 2006; Proctor *et al.* 2007). Organizational culture and climate can influence whether individual practitioners decide to engage in evaluation, whether they feel as though they may be judged or criticized due to outcomes, and whether they have access to the resources needed to engage in evaluation (Aarons and Sawitzky 2006). Supervisor support is important, as engaging in evaluative processes can utilize practitioner time that perhaps would have been allocated to other tasks (Baker *et al.* 2010). Social workers are more likely to evaluate their practice if it is normalized and also done by colleagues (Moncoske and Pui-Fong 1990). In addition, time to engage in EBP has been a major barrier in many countries, such as Australia, Israel, Italy, the United Kingdom and the United States (Edmond *et al.* 2006; McNamara and Neve 2009; Morago 2010; Ronen 2004; Sheldon *et al.* 2005).

Surveys of social workers in England found that most respondents thought they had little encouragement from their departments to keep abreast of the research literature (Sheldon *et al.* 2005). According to the surveys, organizations provided little or no access to library facilities, and almost half had no access to computer databases. To increase the practical use of research, the suggestion of over one third of survey respondents was 'increased availability of technical research facilities (36%), with protected study time (20%) and opportunities to attend research meetings (21%)' (Sheldon *et al.* 2005: 32).

Summary, recommendations and conclusions

This descriptive review has explored and summarized how EBP has been adopted globally, noting the barriers and facilitators to its implementation. In general, the adoption of EBP has been slow and uneven. There are, however, promising practices that may advance EBP. Lessons can be learned from the experiences of countries with relative success in the implementation of EBP, and strategies can be developed to enhance the use of EBP in countries where it is limited or non-existent. Recommendations may be made in the three areas noted above. However, it should be noted that these domains are interrelated. For example, the intellectual traditions in Germany are not unrelated to the few rigorous outcome studies in that country. The socio-political climate clearly affects the viability of professional accrediting bodies and social welfare organizations to deliver services that are outside political mandates and economic priorities. Thus, changes in broader systems are likely to have the biggest impact.

Perhaps the most important area where social workers can start to raise awareness about the importance of EBP is at the macro level, addressing social, economic and political barriers which can trickle down and affect mezzo- and micro-level changes. This can be done by engaging in political advocacy to stress the importance of providing effective social services, thereby appealing to political and economic stakeholder interests. For EBP to be more fully disseminated and implemented in developing countries, a comprehensive approach is also needed in which research, education and organizations work together (Manuel *et al.* 2009; Mullen *et al.* 2008; Proctor 2004).

Additionally, social workers can organize themselves within their own countries to establish credentialing for social work professionals, standards of practice, and accreditation for social work education. The presence of a national professional organization which includes a mandate for evaluating practice is instrumental for EBP to be legitimized within social work in those countries. This includes professional accrediting bodies for practice and for education, nationally or regionally.

Social work education will require coursework in EBP, which should be part of mainstream social work education and not relegated to post-qualifying courses. The training to develop practitioners in the EBP process model requires a different approach than what is usually taught in research methods courses. Students need skills in critical appraisal for evaluating assessment tools and interventions, appropriate intervention designs, and when and how to adapt ESIs for particular practice situations. Educational programmes should provide opportunities to learn critical skills in finding, critiquing, implementing and evaluating evidence in practice. Social work education also needs to have a comprehensive approach in teaching the principles of EBP, including well-established and coordinated linkages with field settings for EBP education to be fully realized in social work education (Howard *et al.* 2007; Mullen *et al.* 2007b; Proctor 2007). Where academia is not teaching the elements of practice evaluation and EBP, continuing education programmes can take over. Training in the important elements of EBP can be done successfully, as attested in empirical studies of workshops in the United States (Parrish and Rubin 2011) and in Britain (CEBSS; Sheldon *et al.* 2005).

There is a need for more within-country outcome research and the development of culturally appropriate, reliable and valid measures. To develop practice-useful research, institutes and centres can be formed. Institutes and centres for EBP have helped generate research and practice in various countries, such as Australia (Barber and Dunston 2004), Canada (Regehr *et al.* 2007), Holland (Garretsen *et al.* 2005), South Korea (Choi *et al.* 2009) and Sweden (Sundell *et al.* 2010). In the United States, there are many sites that offer research-based evidence, but one focused on the process model of EBP is at Columbia University's Wilma and Albert Musher Program.[4] In the United Kingdom, there is the Institute for Research and Innovation in Social Services,[5] the Social Care Institute of Excellence,[6] and Oxford's Centre for Evidence-Based Intervention[7].

In countries where EBP is well established, more research is needed that is compatible with the values and practices of countries where EBP is not regularly practised. For example, research is needed (1) on beneficial processes that can improve direct practice outcomes (e.g. common factors such as the therapeutic alliance); (2) where the target of intervention is not only the individual (who becomes potentially labelled and victimized), but larger systems that may have affected them; and (3) on models that are community-based and incorporate both quantitative and qualitative approaches (e.g. community based participatory research).

A culture of evaluation can be developed within social service organizations, 'wherein evaluation is an integral part of practice and encouraging dialogues on barriers and benefits, creating a positive climate for evaluation as one component of implementing EBP' (Baker *et al.* 2010: 972). This has also been referred to as the 'organizational excellence model', in which there is a research-minded culture among leadership, management and structure (Walter *et al.* 2004). To get there, large-scale agency adoption of EBP is needed: 'multi-level implementation strategies, leveraging not only key organizational resources but the agency directors' authority, interpersonal influence, and leadership' (Proctor *et al.* 2007: 487). Support will require protected time for practitioners to engage in EBP, or at least a structure and process within the organization for someone to seek, acquire and critically evaluate evidence. In addition, agency–academic partnerships are needed to offset some of the barriers to EBP that exist within organizations (Regehr *et al.* 2007). A knowledge-sharing team within the organization ('link officers'; Austin *et al.* 2012: 191) could have the function of serving as the liaison to a university and can also help direct practitioners to find, evaluate and apply best evidence into practice.

A limitation of this review has been its reliance on English-language publications. This has resulted in a partial glimpse of the actual literature that exists on EBP. Another limitation is its emphasis on EBP with individuals, families and small groups. This has excluded a discussion about the relevance of EBP to other levels of practice (e.g. communities, policy) which, in some countries, may be the desired focus of change. Although the scope of this review was limited, EBP in its various forms has been used and discussed across the world. The global discussions around EBP have stirred up discussion and debate about how to best serve our clients and how to best evaluate the quality of our services.

Notes

1 www.ifsw.org.
2 www.basw.co.uk/.
3 www.aasw.asn.au/.
4 www.columbia.edu/cu/musher/EBP%20Resources.htm.
5 www.iriss.org.uk/.
6 www.scie.org.uk/.
7 www.spi.ox.ac.uk/research/centre-for-evidence-based-intervention.html.

References

Aarons, G.A. (2006) 'Transformational and transactional leadership: Association with attitudes toward evidence-based practice' [Research Support, N.I.H., Extramural], *Psychiatric Services*, 57(8): 1162–9.

Aarons, G.A. and Sawitzky, A.C. (2006) 'Organizational culture and climate and mental health provider attitudes toward evidence-based practices', *Psychological Services*, 3(1): 61–72.

Akiyama, K. and Buchanan, A. (2007) 'A comparison between Japanese and British research papers in key academic journals', *International Social Work*, 50: 255–64.

Austin, M.J., Dal Santo, T.S. and Lee, C. (2012) 'Building organizational supports for research-minded practitioners', *Journal of Evidence-Based Social Work*, 9(1–2): 174–211.

Baker, L.R., Stephens, F. and Hitchcock, L. (2010) 'Social work practitioners and practice evaluation: How are we doing?' *Journal of Human Behavior in the Social Environment*, 20(8): 963–73.

Barber, J.G. and Dunston, R. (2004) 'Evidence-based practice in Australia', in B.A. Thyer and M.A.F. Kazi (eds) *International Perspectives on Evidence-Based Practice in Social Work*, Birmingham: Venture.

Barrera, M., Castro, F.G., Strycker, L.A. and Toobert, D.J. (2013) 'Cultural adaptations of behavioral health interventions: A progress report', *Journal of Consulting and Clinical Psychology*, 81(2): 196–205.

Bass, J.K., Bolton, P.A. and Murray, L.K. (2007) 'Do not forget culture when studying mental health', *The Lancet*, 370(9591): 918–19.

Benish, S.G., Quintana, S. and Wampold, B.E. (2011) 'Culturally adapted psychotherapy and the legitimacy of myth: A direct-comparison meta-analysis', *Journal of Counseling Psychology*, 58(3): 279–89.

Castro, F.G., Barrera, M. and Steiker, L.K.H. (2010) 'Issues and challenges in the design of culturally adapted evidence-based interventions', *Annual Review of Clinical Psychology*, 6(1): 213–39.

CASW (2005) *Canadian Association of Social Workers (CASW) Code of Ethics*. Available at: http://casw-acts.ca/sites/default/files/attachements/CASW_Code%20 of%20Ethics.pdf (accessed 2 August 2013).

CASWE-ACFTS (2008) *Canadian Schools for Social Work Education/Association Canadienne pour la Formation en Travail Social, Standards for Accreditation*. Available at: http://caswe-acfts.ca/wp-content/uploads/2013/03/COAStandardsMay2012.pdf (accessed 2 August 2013).

Chambless, D.L. and Ollendick, T.H. (2001) 'Empirically supported psychological interventions: Controversies and evidence', *Annual Review of Psychology*, 52: 685–716.

Chen, E.C., Kakkad, D. and Balzano, J. (2008) 'Multicultural competence and evidence-based practice in group therapy', *Journal of Clinical Psychology*, 64(11): 1261–78.

Choi, J.S., Choi, S. and Kim, Y. (2009) 'Improving scientific inquiry for social work in South Korea: The Center for Social Welfare Research at Yonsei University', *Research on Social Work Practice*, 19(4): 464–71.

Corcoran, J. (2003) *Clinical Applications of Evidence-Based Family Interventions*, New York: Oxford University Press.

Corcoran, K., Gingerich, W.J. and Briggs, H.E. (2001) 'Practice evaluation: Setting goals and monitoring change', in H.E. Briggs and K. Corcoran (eds) *Social Work Practice: Treating Common Client Problems*, 2nd edn, Chicago: Lyceum Books.

Cournoyer, B.R. (2004) *The Evidence-Based Social Work (EBSW) Skills Book*, Boston: Allyn & Bacon.

CSWE (2008) *Educational Policy and Accreditation Standards (EPAS)*, Alexandria: Council on Social Work Education.

Dillenburger, K. (2004) 'Evidence-based practice in Northern Ireland', in B.A. Thyer and M.A.F. Kazi (eds) *International Perspectives on Evidence-Based Practice in Social Work*, Birmingham: Venture.

Edmond, T., Megivern, D., Williams, C., Rochman, E. and Howard, M. (2006) 'Integrating evidence-based practice and social work field education', *Journal of Social Work Education*, 42(2): 377–96.

Fook, J., Johannessen, A. and Psoinos, M. (2011) 'Partnership in practice research: A Norwegian experience', *Social Work*, 9(1): 29–43.

Fraser, M.W., Richman, J.M., Galinsky, M.J. and Day, S.H. (2009) *Intervention Research: Developing Social Programs*, New York: Oxford University Press.

Gambrill, E.D. (2004) 'The future of evidence-based social work practice', in B.A. Thyer and M.A.F. Kazi (eds) *International Perspectives on Evidence-Based Practice in Social Work*, Birmingham: Venture.

Garretsen, H., Bongers, I. and Rodenburg, G. (2005) 'Evidence-based work in the Dutch welfare sector', *British Journal of Social Work*, 35(5): 655–65.

Gibbs, L. (2003) *Evidence-Based Practice for the Helping Professions*, Pacific Grove: Brooks/Cole-Thomson Learning.

Hare, I. (2004) 'Defining social work for the 21st century', *International Social Work*, 47(3): 407–24.

Haynes, R.B., Devereaux, P.J. and Guyatt, G.H. (2002) 'Physicians' and patients' choices in evidence based practice', *British Medical Journal*, 324(7350): 1350.

Haynes, R.B., Sackett, D.L., Gray, J.M., Cook, D.J. and Guyatt, G.H. (1996) 'Transferring evidence from research into practice: 1. The role of clinical care research evidence in clinical decisions', *American College of Physicians Journal Club*, 125(3): A14–16.

Holosko, M.J. (2004) 'Evidence-based practice in Canada', in B.A. Thyer and M.A.F. Kazi (eds) *International Perspectives on Evidence-Based Practice in Social Work*, Birmingham: Venture.

Howard, M.O., Allen-Meares, P. and Ruffolo, M.C. (2007) 'Teaching evidence-based practice: Strategic and pedagogical recommendations for schools of social work'. *Research on Social Work Practice*, 17(5): 561–8.

Howard, M.O., McMillan, C.J. and Pollio, D.E. (2003) 'Teaching evidence-based practice: Toward a new paradigm for social work education', *Research on Social Work Practice*, 13(2): 234–59.

Kee, L.H. (2004) 'The search from within: Research issues in relation to developing culturally appropriate social work practice', *International Social Work*, 47(3): 336–45.

Kindler, H. (2008) 'Developing evidence-based child protection practice: A view from Germany', *Research on Social Work Practice*, 18(4): 319–24.

Lee, E., Mishna, F. and Brennenstuhl, S. (2010) 'How to critically evaluate case studies in social work', *Research on Social Work Practice*, 20(6): 682–9.

Leung, J.C.B. (2007) 'An international definition of social work for China', *International Journal of Social Welfare*, 16(4): 391–7.

McCambridge, J., Waissbein, C., Forrester, D. and Strang, J. (2007) 'What is the extent and nature of quantitative research in British social work?' *International Social Work*, 50(2): 265–71.

McCrystal, P. and Wilson, G. (2009) 'Research training and professional social work education: Developing research-minded practice', *Social Work Education*, 28(8): 856–72.

Macgowan, M.J. (2008) *A Guide to Evidence-Based Group Work*, New York: Oxford University Press.

McNamara, P. and Neve, E. (2009) 'Engaging Italian and Australian social workers in evaluation', *International Social Work*, 52(1): 22–35.

Manuel, J.I., Mullen, E.J., Lin Fang, Bellamy, J.L. and Bledsoe, S.E. (2009) 'Preparing social work practitioners to use evidence-based practice', *Research on Social Work Practice*, 19(5): 613–27.

Moncoske, R.J. and Pui-Fong, Y.L. (1990) 'Practice evaluation attitudes: Hong Kong social workers', *International Social Work*, 33(4): 311–24.

Morago, P. (2010) 'Dissemination and implementation of evidence-based practice in the social services: A UK survey', *Journal of Evidence-Based Social Work*, 7(5): 452–65.

Morales, E. and Norcross, J.C. (2010) 'Evidence-based practices with ethnic minorities: Strange bedfellows no more', *Journal of Clinical Psychology*, 66(8): 821–9.

Mullen, E.J., Bellamy, J.L. and Bledsoe, S.E. (2007a) 'Evidence-based social work practice', in R.M. Grinnell and Y.A. Unrau (eds) *Social Work Research and Evaluation: Quantitative and Qualitative Approaches*, New York: Oxford University Press.

Mullen, E.J., Bledsoe, S.E. and Bellamy, J.L. (2008) 'Implementing evidence-based social work practice', *Research on Social Work Practice*, 18(4): 325–38.

Mullen, E.J., Bellamy, J.L., Bledsoe, S.E. and Francois, J.J. (2007b) 'Teaching evidence-based practice', *Research on Social Work Practice*, 17(5): 574–82.

NASW (2008) *Code of Ethics of the National Association of Social Workers*. Available at: http://naswdc.org/pubs/code/code.asp (accessed 10 November 2012).

Nevo, I. and Slonim-Nevo, V. (2011) 'The myth of evidence-based practice: Towards evidence-informed practice', *British Journal of Social Work*, 41(6): 1176–97.

Otto, H.-U., Polutta, A. and Ziegler, H. (2008) 'Struggling through to find what works: Evidence-based practice as a challenge for social work', in H.-U. Otto, A. Polutta and H. Ziegler (eds) *Evidence-Based Practice: Modernising the Knowledge Base of Social Work?* Farmington Hills: Barbara Budrich.

Parrish, D.E. and Rubin, A. (2011) 'An effective model for continuing education training in evidence-based practice', *Research on Social Work Practice*, 21(1): 77–87.

Payne, M. (2008) 'Knowledge, evidence and the wise person of practice: The example of social work and social care in palliative care', in H.-U. Otto, A. Polutta and H. Ziegler (eds) *Evidence-Based Practice: Modernising the Knowledge Base of Social Work?* Farmington Hills: Barbara Budrich.

Petch, A. (2004) 'Evidence-based practice in Scotland', in B.A. Thyer and M.A.F. Kazi (eds) *International Perspectives on Evidence-Based Practice in Social Work*, Birmingham: Venture.

Petr, C.G. and Walter, U.M. (2009) 'Evidence-based practice: A critical reflection', *European Journal of Social Work*, 12(2): 221–32.

Pollio, D.E. and Macgowan, M.J. (eds) (2011) *Evidence-Based Group Work in Community Settings*, New York: Routledge.

Proctor, E.K. (2004) 'Leverage points for the implementation of evidence-based practice', *Brief Treatment and Crisis Intervention*, 4(3): 227–42.

Proctor, E.K. (2007) 'Implementing evidence-based practice in social work education: Principles, strategies, and partnerships', *Research on Social Work Practice*, 17(5): 583–91.

Proctor, E.K., Knudsen, K., Fedoravicius, N., Hovmand, P., Rosen, A. and Perron, B. (2007) 'Implementation of evidence-based practice in community behavioral health: Agency director perspectives', *Administration and Policy in Mental Health and Mental Health Services Research*, 34(5): 479–88.

Regehr, C., Stern, S. and Shlonsky, A. (2007) 'Operationalizing evidence-based practice: The development of an institute for evidence-based social work', *Research on Social Work Practice*, 17(3): 408–16.

Ronen, T. (2004) 'Evidence-based practice in Israel', in B.A. Thyer and M.A.F. Kazi (eds) *International Perspectives on Evidence-Based Practice in Social Work*, Birmingham: Venture.

Rostila, I. and Piirainen, K. (2004) 'Evidence-based practice in Finland', in B.A. Thyer and M.A.F. Kazi (eds) *International Perspectives on Evidence-Based Practice in Social Work*, Birmingham: Venture.

Rubin, A. (2008) *Practitioner's Guide to Using Research for Evidence-Based Practice*, Hoboken: John Wiley and Sons.

Rubin, A. and Parrish, D. (2007) 'Views of evidence-based practice among faculty in master of social work programs: A national survey', *Research on Social Work Practice*, 17(1): 110–22.

Sackett, D.L., Rosenberg, W.M., Gray, J.A., Haynes, R.B. and Richardson, W.S. (1996) 'Evidence based medicine: What it is and what it isn't', *British Medical Journal*, 312(7023): 71–2.

Shek, D.T.L., Lam, M.C. and Tsoi, K.W. (2004) 'Evidence-based practice in Hong Kong', in B.A. Thyer and M.A.F. Kazi (eds) *International Perspectives on Evidence-Based Practice in Social Work*, Birmingham: Venture.

Sheldon, B. and Chilvers, R. (2004) 'Evidence-based practice in England', in B.A. Thyer and M.A.F. Kazi (eds) *International Perspectives on Evidence-Based Practice in Social Work*, Birmingham: Venture.

Sheldon, B., Chilvers, R., Ellis, A., Moseley, A. and Tierney, S. (2005) 'A pre-post empirical study of obstacles to, and opportunities for, evidence-based practice in social care', in A. Bilson (ed.) *Evidence-Based Practice and Social Work: International Research and Policy Perspectives*, London: Whiting and Birch.

Stewart, R.E., Chambless, D.L. and Baron, J. (2012) 'Theoretical and practical barriers to practitioners' willingness to seek training in empirically supported treatments', *Journal of Clinical Psychology*, 68(1): 8–23.

Steyaert, J., Spierings, F. and Dorier, C.A. (2011) 'Promoting a practice-minded culture in research organizations', *European Journal of Social Work*, 14(1): 123–39.

Sundell, K., Soydan, H., Tengvald, K. and Anttila, S. (2010) 'From opinion-based to evidence-based social work: The Swedish case', *Research on Social Work Practice*, 20(6): 714–22.

Swift, J.K., Callahan, J.L. and Vollmer, B.M. (2011) 'Preferences', *Journal of Clinical Psychology*, 67(2): 155–65.

Taylor, C. and White, S. (2005) 'What works and about what works? Fashion, fad and EBP', in A. Bilson (ed.) *Evidence-Based Practice in Social Work*, London: Whiting and Birch.

Thomlison, B. and Corcoran, K. (2007) *The Evidence-Based Internship: A Field Manual for Social Work and Criminal Justice*, New York: Oxford University Press.

van Zyl, M.A. (2004) 'Evidence-based practice in South Africa', in B.A. Thyer and M.A.F. Kazi (eds) *International Perspectives on Evidence-Based Practice in Social Work*, Birmingham: Venture.

Walter, I., Nutley, S., Percy-Smith, J., McNeish, D. and Frost, S. (2004) *Improving the Use of Research in Social Care Practice*, London: Social Care Institute for Excellence. Available at: www.scie.org.uk/publications/knowledgereviews/kr07.asp (accessed 8 August 2013).

Webb, S. (2001) 'Some considerations on the validity of evidence-based practice in social work', *British Journal of Social Work*, 31(1): 57–79.

Weisz, J.R. and Kazdin, A.E. (2010) *Evidence-Based Psychotherapies for Children and Adolescents*, 2nd edn, New York: Guilford Press.

Zayas, L., Drake, B. and Jonson-Reid, M. (2011) 'Overrating or dismissing the value of evidence-based practice: Consequences for clinical practice', *Clinical Social Work Journal*, 39(4): 400–5.

Part II

Political, social and theoretical context of social work

George Palattiyil, Dina Sidhva and Mono Chakrabarti

Although it is difficult to fix a date to mark the origins of social work, it is clear that social work originated in the philanthropic and charitable ideals of individuals and communities to respond to the social ills of the time (Healy, 2008). Through generations, social work developed and evolved to become a professional discipline, particularly as the Western economies became industrialised and the welfare of citizens became part of the post-war state provision. In contrast, social work continued to be a charitable and humanitarian act in many developing countries until it was 'introduced into countries in Asia and Africa by the American and European experts to address the problems of underdevelopment' (Healy, 2008: 136).

Today, social work is taught and practised in several countries of the world that share a commitment to tackle poverty and inequality and to promote social justice and human rights (Jones and Truell, 2012; IFSW and IASSW, 2014). The teaching and practice of social work has also undergone massive transformation in response to changing needs and other social and political forces impacting social work. For example, many countries in the West have formalised social work education and practice with regulatory frameworks and codes of practice, with a view to raising standards. This has necessitated that social work practitioners be registered with the country's regulatory authority in order to be able to work as a social worker. Similarly, social work has assumed a managerialist role – as in the UK, for example, with outcomes and performance indicators as barometers of social work involvement. On the other hand, social work teaching and practice in most of the developing countries continue to be linked to social action movements and radical approaches with a view to effecting structural changes to the deep-rooted issues of poverty, inequality, caste and class divisions (Palattiyil and Sidhva, 2012).

The recent past has also witnessed an emerging interest in and emphasis on the importance of indigenous knowledge in social work education and practice; much as a reaction characterised by a rejection of Western models and a search for an indigenous form of social work (Healy, 2008: 153). This approach strives to appreciate the local needs and the cultural, political and economic realities of the local context in social work education in preference for what is otherwise seen as a colonial model of understanding social issues. Moreover, there has also been an increasing interest in First Nations and aboriginal social work in response to the need for social work that is sociologically relevant to aboriginal people. Such education incorporates aboriginal history and is premised upon traditional sacred epistemology in order to train both aboriginal and non-aboriginal social workers who can understand and meet the needs of aboriginal people (Sinclair, 2004).

Part II provides a bird's-eye view of the changing landscape of social work theory and practice, underpinned by the political forces and trends impacting social work endeavours.

Chapter 4 traces the historical context and the contemporary challenges to social work practice of the legacy of the oppression and colonisation of the First Nations peoples, and highlights responses by the social work profession to address these challenges, with particular attention to the efforts of the Indigenous communities in Canada. Chapter 5 examines the issues and challenges facing Canadian child and family social workers in the context of neo-liberalist social and economic policies and discusses a policy framework and practice approach that directly supports parents in the fulfilment of their parenting responsibilities. Chapter 6 explores the increasing role of the state in controlling individual behaviour. Intervention into the minutiae of people's lives is a key aspect of social work, whether in the guise of community, charity or social worker. Increasingly, however, the state, in various guises, is encroaching ever further onto this terrain. This chapter examines the debate over the extent to which social work is, or should be, political. It outlines the fundamental problem: the extent to which, in contemporary society, politics has become social work.

References

Healy, L.M. (2008). *International Social Work: Professional Action in an Independent World*. New York: Oxford University Press.

International Federation of Social Workers and International Association of Schools of Social Work (2014). Global Definition of Social Work. Available at: http://ifsw.org/get-involved/global-definition-of-social-work/.

Jones, D. and Truell, R. (2012). The Global Agenda for Social Work and Social Development: A Place to Link Together and be Effective in a Globalised World. *International Social Work*, 55(4), 544–72.

Palattiyil, G. and Sidhva, D. (2012). Guest Editorial – Social Work in India. *Practice: Social Work in Action*, 24(2), 75–8.

Sinclair, R. (2004). Aboriginal Social Work Education in Canada: Decolonizing Pedagogy for the Seventh Generation. *First Peoples Child & Family Review*, 1(1), 49–61.

Chapter 4

Canadian social work and First Nations people

Michael A. Hart and Denis C. Bracken

Social work practice in Canada increasingly reflects the diversity of the country. But this diversity is not based only on the successive waves of immigrants who have arrived continuously since the first European contact with the indigenous populations in the seventeenth century. Contemporary Canadian social work practice also is a reflection of the issues surrounding the colonization of those Indigenous populations from the time of first European contact to the present day. Although this has been long neglected in discussions of policy and practice, the last three decades have seen an increasing awareness of the impact of two centuries or more of colonization policy, and in the twentieth century, of social work's role in that colonization process. Further, the ongoing transmission to successive generations of the damage done by the residential schools, which operated from the 1860s until the 1990s, continues to play a significant role in shaping policy and practice. This chapter will trace both the historical context and the contemporary challenges to social work practice of the legacy of oppression and colonization of the First Nations peoples[1] and highlight responses by the social work profession to address these challenges, with attention given to the efforts of the Indigenous communities in Canada.

The chapter begins with an overview of the historical context of First Nations peoples in the parts of North America that were to become Canada after 1867. Beginning with the Royal Proclamation of 1763, it will trace the relationships between First Nations peoples and governments up to the development of the post-Second World War welfare state. It will then focus on the role of the emerging profession of social work in the post-war period and beyond. Social work's role included considerable involvement in the imposition of Euro-Canadian values on First Nations peoples with respect to child welfare, and acceptance of these peoples' economic and social marginalization from Canadian society. The chapter will also consider the gradual recognition by the profession, and other sectors of Canadian society, of the destructive impact of colonialism on First Nations peoples and the initial steps to overcome this impact.

At the time of contact between First Nations peoples and European settlers, there were over 50 languages covering all of the territory of what is now referred to as Canada. The linguistic diversity between some of the languages was a great as that between English and Mandarin. This diversity is also reflected in ways the various First Nations peoples developed and expressed their own cultural, economic, social and political structures. What unites First Nations peoples is their experiences with the European settlers. This experience has not been positive. As outlined by Paul (2006), the Eastern First Nations faced such subjugation that many of the smaller First Nations were left on the verge of extinction or past it. While the means of subjugation has changed over time and has been enforced to varying degrees, the oppression of First Nations peoples throughout Canada has nevertheless remained as a central pillar in the relationship between First Nations and the European settlers (Miller 2000).

Frideres (2011) noted that by the early seventeenth century, the French and English had established themselves in lands that would be called Canada. These conflicts changed significantly when the war between the British and French ended with a peace treaty signed in 1763. At this time several First Nations who were allied with the French were angered by this development and were active in developing an inter-nation Indigenous force to wipe out all British as they encroached upon their territories. Partially in an effort to address this confrontation by the First Nations, King George III issued the Royal Proclamation of 1763, which, among other things, recognized First Nations rights to the land, set the Crown as the only legitimate force to enter treaty negotiation with the First Nations for land, and unilaterally placed First Nations peoples and lands under the dominion and protection of the British Crown. The mentality evident in the wording of the Proclamation reflected the perspectives of the British and emerging colonial governments, in which they recognized First Nations peoples, but deemed them to be inferior to the British.

This positioning of First Nations peoples as inferior was also reflected in changes in the economic relationship between First Nations and European settlers (Frideres 2011; Miller 2000). During the late seventeenth and eighteenth centuries, many First Nations were drawn into the European economy, particularly the fur trade, to the degree that First Nations economies moved from their more traditional structures to becoming significantly dependent upon the fur trade. When the two main trading companies in British North America, the Northwest Company and the Hudson Bay Company, amalgamated, they removed the competition for furs, thus reducing First Nations' beneficial economic position between the two rival companies. These events reflected the shift in the balance of power in the relationship between First Nations and European peoples.

When the British government changed its relationship with First Nations and moved responsibilities for dealing with First Nations from military to civil authorities in 1830, the colonial attitudes based upon paternalistic oppression fully emerged. Propaganda campaigns emerged that focused on the need to develop and civilize First Nations people (Tobias 1991). These campaigns were the basis for experimenting with ways to civilize and 'protect' First Nations peoples. Among these ways were the establishment of the reserve system, where First Nations peoples could be taught to farm and receive religious and educational instruction. In the middle of the nineteenth century, two acts were passed by the colonial legislature that directly reflected this paternalism, specifically 'An act for the better protection of the lands and property of Indians in Lower Canada' and 'An act for the protections of Indians in Upper Canada from imposition, and the property occupied or enjoyed by them from trespassing and injury'. This action was profoundly significant in that for the first time, a body outside the control of First Nations peoples arrogated the authority to define who was an 'Indian' (Miller 2000). This concept was directly reflected in the passing of the British North America Act of 1867, which established federal jurisdiction over 'Indians and lands reserved for Indians'. Non-Status and Metis peoples were excluded from this clause and were seen as falling under the jurisdiction of the provincial governments. Inuit peoples were also not included in this clause, but fell under the jurisdiction of the federal government when northern territories were ceded by Britain to the Dominion of Canada in 1880.

In order to access and exploit the land in the manner they deemed worthy, the Government of Canada had to address the Royal Proclamation of 1763, which recognized First Nations rights to the land. The necessity to access the land was heightened as the United States was growing in the western part of North America, and there was concern that they would appropriate the lands of what is now Western Canada. Between 1870 and 1921, treaties were signed with the First Nations in what is now the Canadian prairies so as to annex their lands. The initial western 'numbered' treaties followed the format of the Robinson Superior and Robinson Huron treaties of 1850 and covered the southern part of Western Canada. While the treaties remained as recognized agreements between the First Nations and the Crown and were held in a sacred manner by First Nations peoples, it is suggested that the Crown representative participated in bad faith and imposed rather than negotiated the agreements (Frideres 2011). Even with the limited commitments that included the provision of education, medicine and agricultural supplies, annuities in perpetuity, and the access to, and a say in the use of, Crown lands, First Nations quickly found themselves threatened or redefined as non-First Nations and the treaties ignored or forgotten (Frideres 2011).

This period of establishing treaties coincided with the Government's efforts to further its control over First Nations, for example the passage of the 1876 'Act to Amend and Consolidate the Laws Respecting Indians', commonly referred to as the Indian Act. It was through this Act that 'Indians would lose control of every aspect of their corporate existence' (Milloy 1991: 152). The laws and policies reflected Canada's paternalism towards First Nations, Metis and Inuit peoples. These include the 'Indian Advancement Act' that incorporated a clause that appointed the Indian Agent in each band, or First Nation, as the chairman of the band's council. First Nations' cultural structures were also suppressed. Those activities found to be central to First Nations, such as the potlatch held by many First Nations of the west coast and the give-away ceremonies conducted by First Nations in prairies, were outlawed (Miller 2000).

Even when First Nations adapted the imposed systems, such as farming, efforts were taken by the Canadian Government on behalf of petitioning persons to limit the success of First Nations peoples. Specifically, First Nations who were producing high yielding crops and selling them at lower rates than the settlers were forced by law to stop selling their produce for profit and farm for subsistence only (Carter 1993). Policies were also developed to suppress First Nations peoples' social systems. While completely ignoring First Nations' social structures, the Government of Canada, along with several Christian denominations, established a system that would seek to assimilate Indian children to produce 'a generation of English speaking Indians, accustomed to the way of civilized life' (quoted in Frideres 2011: 59).

The residential school system made attendance compulsory by 1920, forbade the speaking of any Indigenous languages, and suppressed cultural practices while providing some time for learning and often more than half of the day at labour (Milloy 2000). The intent of the school was well captured by Duncan Campbell Scott, the head of the Department of Indian Affairs from 1913 to 1932. He stated, 'Our objective is to continue until there is not a single Indian in Canada that has not been absorbed into the body politic and there is no Indian question, and no Indian Department, that is the whole objective of this Bill' (Titley 1986: 50). Coupled with the industrial schools that were the forerunners to the residential schools, the entire system was in effect for a time frame spanning more than 100 years, ending in 1996. Many students of these former schools have recounted harrowing experiences of sexual, physical, emotional and mental abuses (Deiter 1999; Fontaine 2010; Fournier and Crey 1997; Milloy 2000) and the negative intergenerational impact remains today (Deiter 1999; Fournier and Crey 1997; Truth and Reconciliation Commission of Canada 2012).

Despite this political, economic, cultural and social oppression and the extreme poverty that resulted, many First Nations people followed through with their commitment to the treaties that included their loyalty to the Crown. It was noted that the enlistment during the First World War by individuals from First Nations communities was approximately one in three able-bodied First Nations men, an amount equal to or greater than that of individuals in other communities (CBC News Online 2006; Dempsey 1999).

Thousands more were enlisted in Canada's armed forces during the Second World War (Scheffield 2001). While veterans almost universally claimed that they were treated as equals during their time in service, when they returned to civilian life they were either ignored or confronted with the 'old society prejudices, stifling government policies and overbearing administration they had know before they enlisted' (Dempsey 1999; Scheffield 2001: iii). As explained by the War Amps, approximately 1,800 First Nations persons were offered the sum of $39 million on 21 June 2002 as compensation for how they were treated after the war. While not an admission of liability, the compensation was clearly based upon the failure of the Government of Canada to provide the same provisions to First Nations veterans that had been offered to other veterans under the Veteran Land Act (War Amps n.d.).

The growth of the welfare state in the immediate aftermath of the Second World War included the rare occasion that Canadians looked at the way they treated First Nations peoples. In light of the exceptionally large number of First Nations individuals who enlisted in the armed forces during World War II, and with the significant push by First Nations leaders for the just recognition of their rights, Canadians began to look at the way they treated First Nations peoples. In 1946, the Canadian Parliament established a joint committee of the Senate and House of Commons with the purpose of reviewing the Indian Act. While they were consistently hindered from participating in this process, this was the first time that First Nations people were permitted to present on their own behalf. The Committee heard from various organizations and people over two years and this resulted in recommendations of revisions to the Indian Act in 1951. However, to the ongoing detriment of First Nations peoples, their contributions were ignored and the revisions were unattached to First Nations' aspiration. Instead, the revisions resulted in the Act returning to the philosophy and content of the original Indian Act, which encouraged assimilation, enfranchisement and integration (Miller 2000).

The social work profession

Social work as a profession in Canada grew from the experiences of both urbanization and industrialization. Rapid population growth due to immigration in the late nineteenth and early twentieth centuries, and increase in industrialization and resulting urban population in Ontario and Quebec, and economic downturns, especially after the First World War, all contributed to the growth of social work, especially in urban Canada. There was also the influence of the Charity movement (as exemplified in Charity Organizations Societies) and the settlement house movement in contributing to the idea of a profession dedicated to helping the 'needy'. The Depression of the immediate pre-Second World War years, combined with the expansion of the welfare state after the war, facilitated a rapid expansion of the profession of social work. A 1941 census reported 1,767 social workers in Canada, a number which grew continuously into the 1990s. Yet during much of this expansion, First Nations people were largely invisible. The attention of the social work profession in the first half of the twentieth century was largely focused on the industrial urban poor and the immigrant populations. The reserve system kept those defined under the Indian Act and its predecessors generally on reserve, and legislation made movement off reserve subject to a loss of legal status. The Metis and Non-Status groups were effectively invisible as distinct and separate cultural and linguistic groups. The forced removal of First Nations children from their families into residential schools that were largely based outside urban centres, while devastating to the children and their families, meant that they were ignored by urban-based social work professionals. It was a combination of the increase in an urban First Nations population, especially in Western Canada, and policy developments with respect to the post-Second World War welfare state that meant that the profession began to pay closer attention to First Nations peoples.

The development of the welfare state and the related increase in members of the social work profession was paralleled by the recognition of the rights of First Nations people as citizens who had a claim to the same level of welfare services as non-First Nations Canadians. However, the structure of the Canadian federation placed at cross purposes the responsibilities of the Federal Government for First Nations peoples, in particular those defined under the Indian Act, and the responsibility for the provision of social welfare services, which rested squarely on the provinces. First Nations people live in all ten provinces and the three territories. Ongoing disputes over which level of government, therefore, had responsibility for First Nations people (and whether those responsibilities extended to those not living on reserves) have continued to the present day. The expansion and provision of social welfare services to First Nations people during this period can be seen as a two-edged sword. Shewell (2004) describes the dilemma that First Nations people faced as social services were expanded to include them:

> On the one hand, they welcomed the new spirit of optimism, and they recognized an opportunity to address historical grievances and to take advantage of new state benefits and programs ... On the other hand, First Nations did not unconditionally accept the new benefits and increased rights; they continued to resist federal attempts to integrate them into the mainstream.
>
> (Shewell 2004: 172)

In particular, talk of assimilation into the mainstream of Canadian society, in large measure through the efforts of provincially administered social welfare programmes, suggested that the historical rights of the First Nations peoples, ignored though they frequently were, would be lost if the Federal Government abandoned them to the provinces. However, the movement toward extension of provincial social welfare policy and its application to First Nations people as the welfare state expanded was apparently unstoppable. A joint brief by the Canadian Welfare Council and the Canadian Association of Social Workers (CASW), submitted in 1947 to a committee of the Canadian Parliament examining the Indian Act, strongly recommended the extension of provincial social services, including child welfare, to First Nations people on reserves (Johnson 1983: 3). Jennissen and Lundy point out that the brief was in favour of 'full assimilation of Canada's First Nations population' (Jennissen and Lundy 2011: 97) as an end goal. Further recommendations from CASW in 1950 similarly promoted the extension of all education and social rights of Canadians to First Nations peoples, as part of a movement for full assimilation into Canadian life, a position that seems naive with the benefit of hindsight. First Nations people then and now see 'full assimilation' as an attack on their culture and way of life. Amendments to the Indian Act in the 1950s gave legal authority to the provinces under section 87, which stated, 'Indians are subject to the provisions of child welfare legislation on the same basis as other residents of a province' (Indian and Northern Affairs Canada 1967: 326).

A study undertaken for the Department of Indian Affairs by H.B. Hawthorn considered the difficult position that social workers found themselves in when attempting to impose provincial child welfare policies on First Nations people:

> In general, social workers have found that it requires much skill and time to establish a therapeutic relationship with members of Indian communities. The weak nuclear family unit but sometimes strong extended kinship bonds of Indians frequently produces behaviour on the part of Indian parents that the Childrens Aid workers find difficult to accept.
> (Indian and Northern Affairs Canada 1967: 329)

It is interesting to read in this quote the position attributed by the author to social workers that they in general rejected the notions of kinship and tribe common to First Nations peoples. These were and are important factors in child rearing in First Nations communities, and yet appear to have been completed rejected by social workers in the 1950s and afterwards. Further, these cultural traditions and values as expressed by parents were 'difficult to accept' for social workers who were seeking to develop 'theraputic relationships' as a foundation for practice. Shewell makes this point in terms of the establishment of hegemony by the dominant group over the subordinate one. Assimilation required First Nations people to become individual wage-dependent persons, and when this did not happen, the 'problems' of First Nations people, including child welfare-related problems, had to be addressed through the culture of the dominant group. Hawthorne thought that the passage of time would help to alleviate some of the tension between social workers and First Nations peoples, and even went so far as to suggest that the 'appointment of Indians to Boards of Directors of the Societies, and consultation with the chief and council would undoubtedly contribute to improved relations between the Societies and Indian communities' (Indian and Northern Affairs Canada 1967: 329).

This expansion of child welfare services brought the social work profession directly into contact with Aborginal people like never before. The story of what has become known as the '60s Scoop' is told in detail elsewhere (Alston-O'Connor 2010; Johnson 1983; McKenzie and Hudson 1985). Briefly, a combination of the impact of residential schools on the parenting skills of a generation or more of First Nations peoples, combined with the overt policy of assimilation (best exemplified by the residential school system) and an assumption by social workers that First Nations culture essentially had no place in a modern Canada, led to a major increase in the number of children apprehended and placed in care by provincial child welfare authorities. Johnson points out that in British Columbia alone the percentage of First Nations children in care increased from less than 1 per cent in 1955 to 34 per cent in 1964. What some have labelled 'cultural genocide' (Alston-O'Connor 2010) is said to have occurred[2] in particular through the practice of arranging adoptions of First Nations peoples to non-First Nations families, and in some cases adoptions to families outside of Canada.

This shift was given greater emphasis by First Nations organizations, which began in the 1970s to (re)assert their rights under the treaties and other commitments made in the nineteenth century and to express strong criticism of the way they had been treated by successive governments. For example, the Manitoba Indian Brotherhood, an organization of First Nations peoples in Manitoba, stated in 1971: 'The pattern of educational development was predicated upon the *false* belief that to educate the Indian child you must *separate* him from the parents and environment in which he lived' (Manitoba Indian Brotherhood 1971: 8, emphasis added). Through the late 1970s, different First Nations bands in Manitoba negotiated with the Federal and provincial governments to establish their own child welfare organizations on reserve (Manitoba 2001). None of these organizations initially had the legal power to apprehend children and place them in alternative care arrangements. If the band agency were to recommend an apprehension, an outside (i.e. provincial government-sanctioned) agency like the Children's Aid Society would be called in. By 1977, there was sufficient pressure on the Province of Manitoba and the Federal Government to establish a 'tripartite' committee, which included representatives of the political leadership of First Nations people, to consider ways of meeting the demand for a more culturally relevant approach to child welfare services. This was for many simply the next step.

The movement toward the delivery of child welfare services to Indian people by Indian people graphically illustrates and establishes the principle *that Indian people must be involved at all levels and in all aspects of child welfare services.* The challenge is therefore clear: Indian people, working through their bands, their councils, their communities, the Manitoba Indian Brotherhood and the senior levels of government must, together, deliver child welfare services to Registered Indians in Manitoba.

(Tripartite Committee 1980: i)

Public policy also began to shift. By 1981, the Dakota-Ojibway Child and Family Services had been given a mandate from the province, and thus became the first First Nations organization to be fully recognized by the provincial and Federal governments as capable of delivering child welfare services to the Council's six reserves.

In 1982 sufficient pressure regarding out-of-province adoptions (another legacy of the '60s Scoop') led the Manitoba Government to establish a judicial enquiry into the practice (Kimmelman 1985). Patrick Johnson's work for the Canadian Council on Social Development (Johnson 1983) also provided a systematic examination of the over-representation of First Nations children in provincial child welfare systems.

The 1970s brought the beginning of a shift in perspective on the part of the social work profession, and especially social work higher education programmes. There was also an expansion of social work training programmes in the same period, with over 34 university-based social work education programmes extant by 2000. In 1976, the Federation of Saskatchewan Indians established the Saskatchewan Indian Federated College (now the First Nations University of Canada) that included a Bachelor of Social Work (BSW) programme. By 1979, the University of Manitoba School (now Faculty) of Social Work had a 'special consideration' category of admissions, which gave priority to First Nations people applying for the BSW programme. While it would be incorrect to see these changes as a reflection of changes in social welfare policy (out-of-country adoptions and residential schools continued into the 1980s), it would appear that the social work training programmes were beginning to acknowledge that social work education, at least, had to become more culturally sensitive. Courses on First Nations traditions, history and culture are common in social work education programmes in Canada. The notion of 'cultural competency' (Lundy 2011) is now more or less an accepted standard for social work practice. What is not always clear is whether First Nations peoples ought to be seen as somehow fitting into a diversity approach to social work practice in the twenty-first century. The historic context of their relations with Canadian governance structures and their social and economic marginalization suggests recognition of and approaches to practice that differ from cultural competency in a multicultural framework.

From culturally 'sensitive' to culturally based practices

As social work continued developing its practice orientation, it has centred itself in the dominant perspectives of helping. It has a history of and connection to psychoanalysis, cognitive-behavioural theory, problem-solving methods, and systems and ecological perspectives. Much of these were challenged for their privileging of male universalist perspectives by feminist scholars and practitioners. Later, often with the support of post-modern critiques, these centring positions were challenged for their emphasis on Western notions of universality and individualism (Pease and Fook 1999). As part of the response, the social work profession began to include the idea of culturally sensitive practice. This emerging caveat for practice with people from cultures other than those previously centred tended to focus on tinkering with the centred approaches so that they are appeasing to marginalized groups. Even today, this focus remains as evident in Roysircar's (2009) explanation of culturally sensitive treatment, which may include specific interventions developed for a particular culture, or may involve the adaptation of an established European American method to a particular culture, such as the therapeutic alliance, group therapy and family therapy.

Culturally sensitive practice has been questioned for its continued reliance on a universal focus, thus potentially creating a chasm between the practitioner and the recipients of services (Hart 2003). As stated by Martinez-Brawley, 'in our commitment to liberal traditions, for example, we have left little room to value and appreciate the traditions of those groups that may differ' (Martinez-Brawley 2000: 2004). In recognition of this gap, aspects of the social work profession in Canada further developed to meet the challenge of ideas of cross-cultural practice and acknowledged that they are working from a cultural space that included their practice. Through greater awareness to culture, including their own cultural background, social workers would be more open to differences and restrain their own cultural influences (Yan 2005).

It soon evolved that practitioners could develop a set of skills, or competencies, from which to practice cross-culturally. However, it was later recognized that cultural competent social work practice missed a significant matter of concern for social work, namely how power fits into the equation. In light of the experiences of First Nations peoples in Canada with the oppressive use of power by professions, including social work, this omission was problematic. This concern extended to many groups facing oppression, and social work responded with greater attention to how power is used in practice. Critical theory, with expressions in social justice, anti-oppressive practice and anti-racist practice, centred matters of power in society. Such a centring has been directly relevant to Indigenous peoples, as their experiences with oppression continue at the present time in Canada.

However, it has been recognized that while these approaches are beneficial, they still ignore a key factor for Indigenous peoples. Indigenous understandings, perspectives and practices still remain on the periphery of the theoretical world in social work. So instead of tinkering with non-Indigenous practice methods, often based within European worldviews, efforts emerged to centre Indigenous practices within social work.

Morrissette *et al.* (1993) were among the first to identify a framework for working with Indigenous peoples. Their model was based upon four key principles. First, they emphasized the recognition of distinct First Nations worldviews and traditions. Second was the 'development of First Nations consciousness about the process and effects of colonialism' (Morrissette *et al.* 1993: 93). The third principle was the importance of 'cultural knowledge and traditions as active components of retaining First Nations identity and collective consciousness' (Morrissette *et al.* 1993: 92). Fourth was the emphasis on participation and empowerment through developing critical consciousness, overcoming self-blame, and using group processes as a means of collective power.

Other models emerged as well. From his 1997 master's thesis, Hart published an approach to working with First Nations peoples (Hart 1999). This approached was based upon the understanding of First Nations practitioners utilizing a culturally based method of helping. It had several key concepts, namely wholeness, balance, relationships, harmony, growth, healing and *mino-pimatisiwin*, or the good life. This approach identified that much of First Nations philosophy emphasized certain values, of which respect and sharing were centred for this approach. Hart outlined several presuppositions of the approach relating to perception of people, the characteristics of the helpers and relevant techniques. This approach was further developed by Hart in 2002, 2008 and 2009. In these later developments, it was identified that the approach had a central pillar, namely the recognition of the central role of spirituality for First Nations people. The approach was also deemed to be framed within First Nations worldviews, particularly the philosophical orientation of respectful individualism and communalism.

Recently, a text has been published identifying aspects of First Nations social work in Canada (Sinclair *et al.* 2009). This text includes the expansion of the *mino-pimatisiwin* approach initially developed by Hart. Baikie's (2009) framework of Indigenous-centred social work includes several practice models for working in relation to different Indigenous peoples and issues. Indeed, there have been efforts by individuals not only to centre First Nations people as a whole, but to recognize that particular Indigenous nations have their own helping philosophies and practices. Such a stance reflects the work of Hart (2007), who has developed a Cree model of practice.

At the same time, Indigenous authors have moved to centre Indigenous perspectives and practices while incorporating those non-Indigenous theories and practices deemed to be supportive of Indigenous peoples. Baskin (2011) is one of these authors and has published a text that significantly includes post-modernism, anti-oppressive and structural social work theories along with Indigenous knowledge.

Future directions

These developments in the past 50 years in the field of social work in relation to First Nations peoples have been a movement from one of facilitating oppression, with the end goal of assimilation, to one of creating room for the development of Aboriginal-centred critiques and practices. The profession has moved from advocating for the assimilation of Aboriginal people and facilitating this assimilation through the removal of Aboriginal children from their communities, to recognition of the importance of Aboriginal peoples' cultures in relation to their well-being, as demonstrated in the CASW submission to the Royal Commission on Aboriginal Peoples (CASW 1994). This recognition is evident in the increase of Aboriginal content in social work curricula. There are Aboriginal-centred programmes that are likely to support an increase in Aboriginal people reaching doctoral-level studies and academic positions. With such an increase in the numbers of Aboriginal academics, the breadth and depth of Aboriginal theories and practices are certain to increase. Indeed, much of the recent theoretical developments have been led by Aboriginal academics, particularly those who have been maintaining close ties to Aboriginal nations and communities. Such development will not be without challenges.

There will be a need for increased research on Aboriginal social work practices. Such research will require continued attention to the development of Indigenous research paradigms and methods that have emerged (Absolon 2011; Hart 2009; Kovach 2009) for consistency and relevance. There will also be a need for the non-Aboriginal social work profession and society to further recognize Aboriginal peoples, perspectives and challenges, particularly the colonial challenges that remain. This recognition should take into consideration the recent adoption of the United Nations Declaration of the Rights of Indigenous Peoples and similar supports for Indigenous peoples and perspectives. There is a need for the wider profession to understand its history in relation to Aboriginal peoples, its role in the oppression and how, more often than not in the past 30 years, it has been silent on the challenges faced by Aboriginal people. As Aboriginal people continue to contribute to the development of the profession, the wider professional body, as well as the Canadian population generally, must recognize that they are in a long-standing relationship with Aboriginal peoples and that for the most positive changes to occur, the profession and society must not only make room for Aboriginal peoples' contributions, they must participate in, and contribute to, the changes themselves.

Notes

1 The Constitution Act of 1982 Section 35 defines Aboriginal persons as follows: 'In this Act, "Aboriginal Peoples of Canada" includes the Indian, Inuit and Métis peoples of Canada'. This chapter addresses the First Nations peoples, a name used by those First Nations peoples themselves that refers to what the Constitution refers to as 'Indians'. This chapter does not address issues specific to the Inuit or Metis peoples.
2 Although for a different perspective, see Swidrovich (2004).

References

Absolon, K. (2011) *How We Come to Know*, Halifax: Fernwood.

Alston-O'Connor, E. (2010) 'The sixties scoop: Implications for social workers and social work education', *Critical Social Work* 11(1): 53–61.

Baikie, G. (2009) 'Indigenous-centered social work: Theorizing a social work way of being', in G. Bruyere, M.A. Hart and R. Sinclair (eds), *Wichitowin: Aboriginal Social Work in Canada*, Halifax: Fernwood.

Baskin, C. (2011) *Strong Helpers' Teachings: The Value of Indigenous Knowledges in the Helping Professions*, Toronto: Canadian Scholars Press.

Canadian Association of Social Workers (CASW) (1994) 'The social work profession and the Aboriginal peoples: CASW presentation to the Royal Commission on Aboriginal Peoples', *The Social Worker/Le Travailleur social* 62(4): 158.

Carter, S. (1993). *Lost Harvest: Prairie Indian Farmers and Government Policy*, Montreal, Kingston: McGill-Queen's University Press.

CBC News Online (2006) 'Aboriginals and the Canadian military', *CBS News Online*, 21 June 2006. Online. Available at: www.cbc.ca/news2/background/aboriginals/aboriginals-military.html (accessed 13 January 2015).

Deiter, C. (1999) *From Our Mothers' Arms: The Intergenerational Impact of Residential Schools in Saskatchewan*, Toronto: United Church Publishing House.

Dempsey, L.J. (1999) *Warriors of the King: Prairie Indians in World War I*, Regina: Canadian Plains Research Center.

Fontaine, T. (2010) *Broken Circle: The Dark Legacy of Indian Residential Schools*, Calgary: Heritage House Publishing.

Fournier, S. and Crey, E. (1997) *Stolen from Our Embrace: The Abduction of First Nations Children and the Restoration of First Nations Communities*, Vancouver: Douglas & McIntyre.

Frideres, J.S. (2011) *First Nations in the Twenty-First Century*, Toronto: Oxford University Press.

Hart, M.A. (1999) 'Seeking minopimatisowin: An Aboriginal approach to social work practice', *Native Social Work Journal* 2(1): 91–112.

Hart, M.A. (2002) *Seeking Mino-Pimatisiwin: An Aboriginal Approach to Helping*, Halifax: Fernwood.

Hart, M.A. (2003) 'Am I a modern day missionary? Reflections of a Cree social worker', *Native Social Work Journal* 5(November): 299–313.

Hart, M.A. (2007) *Cree Ways of Helping: An Indigenist Research Project*, unpublished doctoral thesis, University of Manitoba.

Hart, M.A. (2008) 'Critical reflection on an Aboriginal approach to helping', in J. Coates, M. Grey and M. Yellowbird (eds), *Indigenous Social Work around the World: Towards Culturally Relevant Education and Practice*, Aldershot: Ashgate.

Hart, M.A. (2009) 'For Indigenous peoples, by Indigenous peoples, with Indigenous peoples: Towards an Indigenist research paradigm', in R. Sinclair, M.A. Hart and G. Bruyere (eds), *Wicihitowin: Aboriginal Social Work in Canada*, Winnipeg: Fernwood.

Indian and Northern Affairs Canada (1967) *A Survey of the Contemporary Indians of Canada Economic, Political, Educational Needs and Policies Part 1* (The Hawthorn Report). Online. Available at: www.aadnc-aandc.gc.ca/eng/1291832488245/1291832647702 (accessed 21 October 2013).

Jennissen, T. and Lundy, C. (2011) *One Hundred Years of Social Work: A History of the Profession in English Canada 1900–2000*, Waterloo: Wilfred Laurier University Press.

Johnson, P. (1983) *Native Children and the Child Welfare System*, Toronto: Canadian Council on Social Development and James Lorimer and Company.

Kimmelman, E.C. (1985) *No Quiet Place: Final Report of the Review Committee on Indian and Metis Adoptions and Placements*, Winnipeg: Manitoba Community Services.

Kovach, M. (2009) *Indigenous Methodologies – Characteristics, Conversations, and Contexts*, Toronto: University of Toronto Press.

Lundy, C. (2011) *Social Work, Social Justice and Human Rights: A Structural Approach to Practice* (2nd edn), Toronto: University of Toronto Press.

McKenzie, B. and Hudson, P. (1985) 'Native children, child welfare, and the colonization of native people', in K. Levitt (ed.) *The Challenge of Child Welfare*, Vancouver: UBC Press.

Martinez-Brawley, E.E. (2000) 'Social work, transculturality, and etiquette in the academy: Implications for practices', *Families in Society* 81(3): 197–210.

Manitoba (2001) *Aboriginal Justice Implementation Commission – Final Report*. Online. Available at: www.ajic.mb.ca (accessed 21 October 2013).

Manitoba Indian Brotherhood (1971) *Wabung: Our Tomorrows*. Online. Available at: www.trcm.ca/wp-content/uploads/Wabung-Our-Tomorrows-1971.pdf (accessed 14 January 2015).

Miller, J.R. (2000) *Skyscrapers Hide the Heavens: A History of Indian-White Relations in Canada* (3rd edn), Toronto: University of Toronto Press.

Milloy, J.S. (1991) 'The early Indian Acts: Development strategy and constitutional change', in J.R. Miller (ed.) *Sweet Promises: A Reader on Indian-White Relations in Canada*, Toronto: University of Toronto Press.

Milloy, J. (2000) *A National Crime: The Canadian Government and the Residential School System, 1879–1986*, Winnipeg: University of Manitoba Press.

Morrissette, V., McKenzie, B. and Morrissette, L. (1993) 'Towards an Aboriginal model of social work practice', *Canadian Social Work Review* 10(1): 91–108.

Paul, D. (2006) *We Were Not the Savages: Collison between European and Native American Civilizations* (3rd edn), Halifax: Fernwood.

Pease, B., and Fook, J. (1999) *Transforming Social Work Practice: Post-Modern Critical Pespectives*, London: Routledge.

Roysircar, G. (2009) 'Evidence-based practice and its implications for culturally sensitive treatment', *Journal of Multicultural Counseling and Development* 37: 66–82.

Scheffield, R.S. (2001) *A Search for Equity: A Study of the Treatment Accorded to First Nations Veterans and Dependents of the Second World War and the Korean Conflict*, a report prepared for the National Round Table on First Nations Veterans' Issues.

Shewell, H. (2004) *'Enough to Keep Them Alive': Indian Welfare in Canada, 1873–1965*, Toronto: University of Toronto Press.

Sinclair, R., Hart, M.A, and Bruyere, G. (eds) (2009) *Wicihitowin: Aboriginal Social Work in Canada*. Halifax, NS: Fernwood Publishing.

Swidrovich, C.M. (2004) *Positive Experiences of First Nations Children in Non-First Nations Foster or Adoptive Care: De-Constructing the 'Sixties Scoop'*, Master of Arts thesis, University of Saskatchewan, Saskatoon.

Titley, L.B. (1986) *A Narrow Vision: Duncan Campbell Scott and the Administration of Indian Affairs in Canada*, Vancouver: UBC Press.

Tobias, J.L. (1991) 'Protection, civilization, assimilation: An outline history of Canada's Indian policy', in J.R. Miller (ed.) *Sweet Promises: A Reader on Indian-White Relations in Canada*, Toronto: University of Toronto Press.

Tripartite Committee (1980) *Report of the Indian Child Welfare Subcommittee Manitoba*, Winnipeg: Author.

Truth and Reconciliation Commission of Canada (2012) *They Came for the Children*, Winnipeg: Author.

War Amps (n.d.) *Aboriginal Veterans Essential Facts and Time Line*. Online. Available at: www.waramps.ca/newsroom/archives/abvet/back.html (accessed 21 October 2013).

Yan, M.C. (2005) 'How culture awareness works: An empirical examination of the interaction between social workers and their clients', *Canadian Social Work Review* 22(1): 5–29.

Chapter 5

Child and family social work in Canada

Issues and challenges within a neo-liberal political context

Edward Kruk

Introduction

Over the past two decades in Canada, within the social and economic context of neo-liberalism, a programme of legislative and policy change has been undertaken, designed to reduce social spending and to dismantle programmes aimed to support children and families. This policy change has had a profound effect on the well-being of children. This chapter examines the impact of changing child and family policies in Canada in three major areas of concern to child and family social work: child protection, child custody and child care. I will argue, first, that the retrenchment of national welfare structures in each of these domains has contributed to a precipitous decline in direct parental involvement in children's lives in Canada; second, that declining parental involvement levels are a significant contributing factor to compromised child well-being; and third, that new directions for social policy and direct practice are desperately needed to recognize state agencies' duty of care and responsibility to support parents in the fulfilment of their parenting roles. The chapter concludes with a discussion of new directions for child welfare policy that place a primary emphasis on actively supporting responsible parental involvement in children's lives. These include increased family support, preservation and reunification programmes for children at risk in the child protection arena, promotion of shared parental responsibility for children after divorce in the child custody realm and reestablishment of universal family allowance payments and other incentives to encourage parental involvement in the child care domain.

Current levels of parental involvement in children's lives in Canada fall far short of what parents actually desire, as parents want to spend more time with their children but encounter a multitude of constraints (Bibby 2003). Canadians report that their family responsibilities are more important to them than their political convictions, religious beliefs, jobs and wages. For most Canadians, family life is about relationships in which they are taken care of and take care of others, and parents' responsibility to their children's needs remains paramount (Bibby 2003).

Yet with rising levels of parental role strain, role overload and role conflict, and the lack of adequate state support for addressing these problems, children are bearing the brunt of decreased parental involvement. In the 2007 UNICEF report on the well-being of children in the economically advanced nations, despite the fact that Canada ranks relatively high in regard to children's material and educational well-being, it ranks extremely low, eighteenth out of 21 countries, in regard to family relationships, particularly with respect to parental involvement. As a result, Canadian children score high on problematic behavioural and risk measures such as substance abuse, violence and risk-taking (Statistics Canada 2007). In regard to subjective well-being, Canadian children rank very low; the rate of youth suicide in Canada and depression in children is of particular concern. Depression is most acute among Aboriginal youth, with an incidence seven times higher than the national average, and 11 times higher among Inuit youth. Although 'child poverty' continues to be defined primarily in financial terms by Canadian child advocacy groups such as Campaign 2000, 'poverty of parental involvement' is increasingly being recognized as central to the compromising of children's emotional well-being (UNICEF 2007).

Child protection policy

Canadian child protection policy and practice is the first arena in which parental involvement in children's lives is devalued. This is evident in dramatically increased rates of placement of children in government care, at a time when other jurisdictions are focusing on a family preservation approach to child protection. A large increase in children apprehended and taken into government care has occurred since the mid-1990s in Canada, to the degree that relative to other economically advanced nations, Canada has an extremely high proportion of children in state care and in the justice system (Trocme *et al.* 2005). In Ontario alone, a 56 per cent increase occurred in a five-year period, with 11,609 children in care in 1998, rising to 18,126 in 2003 (Swift and Parada 2004). The number of children in care across Canada increased from 40,000 in the early 1990s to 76,000 in 2000 (Farris-Manning and Zandstra 2003); whereas in New York, which implemented a family preservation policy, the number dropped from 49,365 in 1992 to less than 19,000 in 2002 (Office of the Public Advocate of New York 2002), and the overall number of child abuse complaints declined by 52 per cent. Trocme *et al.* (2005) noted a 125 per cent increase in substantiated child abuse in Canada from 1998 to 2003.

It seems clear that taking a family preservation and support approach to child protection is associated with decreases in child abuse rates, whereas rising rates of child removal, originally intended as a last resort, are not. Physical abuse is not the primary reason that children are removed from parental care in Canada; according to Trocme *et al.* (2005), physical harm to children occurred in only 10 per cent of cases of substantiated maltreatment, with only 3 per cent of cases requiring medical intervention. Apprehensions are generally the result of parents' struggles with poverty, addiction and mental health problems (Eamon and Kopels 2004), with Aboriginal children being nearly ten times more likely to be in government care than non-Aboriginal children (Pivot Legal Society 2008). Trocme *et al.* (2005) found that First Nations children were vastly overrepresented in the child protection system at every point of intervention, despite the fact that they were not any more likely than other children to have been victims of physical, emotional and sexual abuse, or exposure to family violence. The high rates of placement of Aboriginal children in care are not due to higher rates of abuse, but because of the less clear-cut category of neglect, fuelled by poverty, poor housing and parental substance abuse. Children from single-parent families and families in poverty constitute the vast majority of children removed from parental care by child protection authorities in Canada (Swift and Callahan 2009).

In tandem with legislation expanding the definition of a 'child in need of protection' (such as adding 'is likely to be in need of protection' to the definition), most Canadian child protection authorities have embraced the use of standardized risk assessment tools, heralded as providing an objective, standardized method to assess risk of abuse and neglect. There is no research, however, that has demonstrated the effectiveness of such risk technologies as predictors of future harm to children, and numerous concerns have been expressed about relying on such deficit-based approaches to assessment (Swift and Callahan 2009). Focusing on the past rather than the present, on parental weaknesses rather than strengths, and on individual faults rather than structural factors contributing to parents' struggles have been cited as fundamental flaws of the risk assessment approach (Pivot Legal Society 2008). The inquisitorial and coercive nature of risk assessment, which stands in contrast with the helping responsibilities of social workers, reinforces oppressive relationships, reduces social work to the issue of standardized recommendations, and demands an inordinate amount of time on paperwork at the expense of face-to-face time with clients (Swift and Callahan 2009). Parents are held accountable for factors external to themselves, such as poverty and lack of adequate housing, deflecting attention away from the responsibilities of social institutions to redistribute resources to ensure that parents have adequate resources to raise their children. Clearly, new assessment tools are needed that take into account family strengths and the systemic barriers to parents being able to effectively address their children's needs.

Once children are in state care, little emphasis is placed on reunification planning, as social workers have too many cases and too few resources to address underlying social and economic problems. The prescribing of psychotropic medication for children in government care is a widespread practice, parental visits with children are not being prioritized by social workers, and supervised visits (one component of the larger web of surveillance to which parents of children in government care are subject) are a strong barrier for many parents of children in care (Pivot Legal Society 2008). The outcomes for children in the foster care system have been described as 'devastating'; in British Columbia, 73 per cent of youth offenders are involved in the child protection system, and only 21 per cent graduate high school, compared with 78 per cent of the general population (Pivot Legal Society 2008).

Parents have not found redress within the court system in regard to flawed child protection policies. The Supreme Court of Canada ruled in 2007 that the child protection system can take and keep children in government care without a finding of abuse or unfitness, saying that there is no general basis in Canadian law under which a family can claim that a 'duty of care' is owed to them by child welfare agencies or their employees (*Syl Apps Secure Treatment Centre* v. *B.D.*, 2007 SCC 38).

Family support, preservation and reunification programmes for children at risk

Clearly, Canadian child protection policy and practice has strayed far from the goals of family preservation, support and reunification as central to the child protection mandate, particularly in cases where physical or sexual abuse are not primary concerns. Parents are being removed from children's lives due to social problems such as poverty, addiction and mental health struggles, and family preservation programmes, respite care and shared parenting, all of which motivate parents to take voluntary action towards reducing the risk of harm to their children, are not being utilized to the same degree as in other jurisdictions. The lack of funding parity between foster caregivers and family caregivers is also a major problem, as the financial resources made available to family members caring for children are minimal. Foster care rates are set at $800–$900 per child per month, with additional supplements for special needs; the rates are $250–$450 for children placed in the home of a relative (Pivot Legal Society 2008).

Research has demonstrated that child protection agencies with explicit formal goals of building more cooperative helping relationships with families will be more successful in doing so (Cameron *et al.* 2007). There are several collaborative alternatives that promote responsible parental involvement in children's lives via a family preservation approach to child protection: family group conferencing, child protection mediation, culturally specific healing circles, and family development responses. When parents require respite care for their children, 'shared parenting' foster care models between birth parents and foster parents provide an alternative to child removal. These focus on respite care support and emphasize co-parenting alliances between foster carers and birth parents, who are sometimes given the option of continuing to reside with the child, with a respite carer or 'mentor family' available when needed. The key to such programmes is encouraging parents to be actively involved in their children's care, while building supportive and trusting relationships with child protection social workers. Parents retain primary responsibility for their children, but are able to approach parenting as a team with a foster family.

When children are in state care and parents demonstrate a commitment to making changes to address child protection concerns, it is imperative that their commitment be recognized and supported by means of facilitating a family reunification process as quickly as possible, with required supports made available. The current impasse of inadequate resources to support parents must be addressed. Part of this involves addressing the emotional consequences of child apprehension on parents, which, when unaddressed, present a significant barrier to successful family reunification.

Challenges for social work

Numerous challenges present themselves to social work practitioners within a residual child protection system located in an increasingly mean-spirited social and economic context. Child protection workers find themselves as agents in a highly litigious and adversarial system, in which ever-increasing numbers of children are being removed from parental care and brought into already burdened alternative care arrangements, in the context of an increasingly lowered threshold for child protection intervention. The previous requirement that actual harm to children has occurred (to warrant child protection intervention) was replaced with the requirement of substantial risk of harm, which has now been replaced with simply risk of harm.

It is thus no surprise that recruitment and retention of staff has become a serious problem in the child protection field in Canada. Caseload numbers have been climbing steeply. Worker discretion and professional judgment have been largely replaced by standardized risk assessment models and standardized recommendations such as parent education programmes, anger management groups and short-term drug and alcohol programmes, none of which have been empirically demonstrated to achieve their objectives. Time spent on paperwork outstrips by far time spent in direct service to children and families, as 70–80 per cent of the workday is spent at computers. When things go wrong, social workers are blamed, while systemic problems are glossed over. And the adversarial nature of child protection has resulted in situations where parents who need support minimize their struggles and avoid getting the help they need.

There are, however, beginning attempts to adopt community approaches to child protection, such as locating child protection workers in community settings where they can practice in a less threatening, more supportive and collaborative fashion. Programmes and services that build community capacity to provide support to parents who are struggling are on the increase, with parent education, child protection mediation, material support and other resources made available. An important development is the transfer of authority for child protective services to community systems; First Nations organizations have been pioneering this approach. Within Aboriginal child protection agencies in particular, family group conferencing (based largely on the New Zealand model) and other family strengths-based approaches have taken hold, and the use of extended family and kin-based care, along with placement in the child's home community as the first choice in alternate care arrangements, has been established. These and other innovations are signalling a paradigm shift in the delivery of child protection services, from a residual model favouring child removal in high risk situations to a community-based preventive approach emphasizing family preservation and reunification and culturally specific practice.

Child custody policy

Child custody is another arena in which routine parental care of children is discouraged by current policy. Divorcing parents who cannot agree on the post-separation living arrangements for their children are forced into a 'winner-takes-all' adversarial battle as courts award primary child care responsibility to one parent only. This practice results in significantly less overall parental involvement for children, as the non-custodial parent is relegated to the status of a visitor in his or her child's life. Regardless of whether parents shared child care responsibility while living together, judges routinely remove one of the parents as a custodial parent.

The sole custody model prevalent in Canadian courts flies in the face of recent research on child and family outcomes in divorce, which indicates that the most salient factor in children's adjustment to the consequences of their parents' divorce is the protection and continuation of parental involvement in children's lives, along with shielding children from parental conflict. The notion that children's interests will best be served by sole custody is not in accord with child development theory; children form primary attachment bonds with each of their parents, and their well-being primarily depends on maintaining these relationships (Kelly 2000).

In recent years a consensus has emerged among divorce researchers on the issue of child custody (Fabricius et al. 2010). A legal presumption of shared parental responsibility, rebuttable in cases of family violence and child abuse, is an evidence-based, child-focused alternative to the sole custody model. Shared parenting preserves children's relationships with both parents, and children in shared custody fare significantly better than children in sole-custody arrangements on every measure of adjustment, both general and divorce-specific (Bauserman 2002). They also spend more time in parental as opposed to substitute care (Melli and Brown 2008). Shared parenting also decreases parental conflict and prevents post-separation family violence. Conflict between parents in shared custody arrangements lessens over time, and increases in sole-custody arrangements, as parents threatened by the loss of their children and their parental identity continue to battle years after their actual physical separation. According to several studies (Ellis and Wight-Peasley 1986; Hotton 2003; Statistics Canada 2014), fifty per cent of first-time family violence occurs after separation within the current adversarial 'winner-takes-all' forum. Further, shared parenting reflects children's preferences and views about their needs and best interests; a recent large-scale study of young adult children who have lived through parental divorce (Fabricius 2003) concluded that most children want to spend roughly equal amounts of time with each of their parents after separation, and consider shared parenting to be in their best interests. In addition, shared parenting reflects parents' preferences and views about their children's needs and best interests, as Canadian public opinion polls indicate 80 per cent support for a legal presumption of shared parental responsibility (Nanos Research 2009). Shared parenting reflects child caregiving arrangements before divorce; with the gender convergence of child care roles, shared parental responsibility has emerged as the norm in two-parent families (Bianchi *et al.* 2006; Higgins and Duxbury 2002; Marshall 2006). Shared parenting decreases parental focus on 'mathematizing' time, 'one shoe fits all' outcomes, and litigation (Bonach 2005). This arrangement provides an incentive for inter-parental negotiation, mediation and the development of individualized parenting plans (Kaspiew *et al.* 2009). It provides a clear and consistent guideline for judicial decision-making; reduces the risk and incidence of parental alienation; enables the enforcement of parenting orders; and addresses social justice imperatives regarding protection of children's rights, as well as social justice imperatives regarding parental authority, autonomy, equality, rights and responsibilities (Kruk 2011, 2012).

Canada lags behind several US states, Australia, France, Belgium, the Netherlands, Sweden and other countries in reforming child custody law and practice in a manner that positions children's needs for the active involvement of both parents in their lives at the forefront of child custody legislation. In Canada, children and other family members remain at risk within the dominant sole-custody 'primary residence' framework.

Shared parental responsibility for children in contested child custody

A rebuttable legal presumption of shared parental responsibility is defined as children spending equal amounts of time in each parent's household, in contested child custody cases. The presumption incorporates a four-stage process of child custody determination, as follows (Kruk 2011). The first stage is a legal expectation that parents develop a parenting plan before a family court hearing is held. The role of the court would be to legally sanction the parenting agreement, whether sole, shared or equal parenting. Parents would retain the options of developing the plan jointly though negotiation, legal negotiation or family mediation; family mediation and family support services would be focused on assisting parents in the development of the plan. Parental autonomy and self-determination in regard to post-divorce parenting arrangements would thus be the cornerstone of family law. The second stage is a legal expectation that in cases where parents cannot agree on a parenting plan, existing parent–child relationships will continue after separation; that is, the relative proportion of time that children spend with each parent after divorce would be equal to the relative proportion of time each parent spent performing child caregiving functions before divorce. Children's needs regarding maintaining relationships with each parent, and stability and continuity in regard to their routines and living arrangements, would thus be addressed; and parents' needs for a fair, gender-neutral criterion would also be accommodated.

The third stage involves a rebuttable legal presumption of equal parenting time in cases where both parents were primary caregivers before divorce and are in dispute over the relative proportion of time each parent spent performing child caregiving functions before divorce. Because some parents will dispute each other's estimates of past time devoted to child care, with 'mathematizing' time a focus of conflict, in the interests of shielding children from ongoing conflict, an equal parenting time division would be the legal norm in cases where both parents were primary caregivers before divorce. The fourth stage involves a rebuttable legal presumption against equal parenting in cases where it is established that a child is in need of protection from a parent or parents. This presumption would develop clear and consistent guidelines for child custody determination in family violence and child abuse cases, consistent with those for children in two-parent families, with the safety of children the paramount consideration.

To ensure success, a shared parental responsibility presumption would constitute only the first of four needed pillars of a new approach to child custody determination. The second pillar would be that of treatment, including programmes assisting in the development of parenting plans, family mediation, specialized support and intervention in high conflict cases, as well as parenting coordination, parallel parenting and reunification programmes for children and parents separated from each other as a result of parental alienation. Prevention programmes would constitute the third pillar, involving shared parenting education programmes, within the high school system, in marriage preparation courses, and upon divorce as an essential component of a more comprehensive programme of parent education and support. Finally, the enforcement pillar would provide for judicial determination of child custody in cases of established child abuse and family violence, as well as enforcement of shared parental responsibility orders.

A presumption of shared parental responsibility would provide a powerful symbol of the importance of continuing parent–child relationships and their immunity to the termination of the spousal relationship, and have immediate and beneficial consequences for children of separation and divorce.

Challenges for social work

The main challenges for social workers working with families in conflict over parenting after divorce arrangements are again related to the context of their practice: an adversarial legal system in which sole custody or primary residence orders are the norm. Again, social workers find themselves as part of a highly litigious and adversarial system, in which children are being removed from the care of one of their parents and placed with an already burdened parent solely responsible for their care and well-being. Primary residence arrangements are associated not only with the loss of a primary attachment for children, but also with an increased risk of being caught in the midst of ongoing parental conflict and family violence. In some cases, parental alienation results, a form of abuse with particularly devastating consequences for children.

The disconnection between child custody law, policy and practice in Canada and empirical research supporting a shared parenting approach as affording children more stable relationships with both of their parents is striking. Social workers have thus started to adopt new roles that promote the active involvement of both parents in children's lives after divorce: as divorce educators, family mediators (including high conflict mediation), post-divorce family therapists, and parenting coordinators. In each of these roles, social workers aim to assist parents in separating (and setting aside) their previous marital conflicts from their ongoing parenting responsibilities. In high conflict cases, parallel parenting plans are established, with the goal of more cooperative parenting plans being put in place when the dust settles. Social workers are also beginning to address the post-traumatic stress experienced by parents and children who have been disconnected from each other by family court systems and alienating parents. They are also adopting new roles in regard to establishing reunification programmes for these children and parents.

Child care policy

The 2002 *National Work Life Conflict Study* (Higgins and Duxbury 2002), a Health Canada-sponsored project examining work–life balance with a sample of 33,000 Canadians across the country, noted a 'precipitous decline' in the amount of time that parents are spending with their children over the ten-year period 1991 to 2001. The decline was most marked among mothers; in ten years, mothers' time with their children had declined by 33 per cent, primarily the result of increased time spent in paid work outside the home. Fathers' time in paid employment also increased, and their time with their children also declined, by 15 per cent. Statistics Canada's (2005) study of time usage revealed that in 2005, Canadian workers spent 45 minutes less per day with family members than families spent in 1985.

According to Bibby (2003), although 90 per cent of Canadian adults report that a two-parent home in which parents are able to raise their children is the ideal child care arrangement, they believe that a broad array of child care options should be available within a society of diverse values and heterogeneous family forms. Most parents of dependent children would prefer part-time paid work to the full-time arrangements they actually have in order to allow them the time they would like for the care of their children. In the Bibby study, after at-home parental care, parents' second child care preference was grandparent care, then care by another relative; and fourth, child care in a home setting. Yet the child care debate in Canada has focused almost entirely on financially supporting the out-of-home regulated day-care option. As a result, many Canadian parents feel derailed in regard to achieving their ideal child care arrangement, as despite their best intentions, they find themselves having to subcontract that care to third parties outside the home.

Preferential funding for third party regulated day-care at the expense of direct benefits to parents has had a significant impact on increasing the labour supply of parents with preschool children, but has also contributed to the disengagement of parents from children's lives (Lefebvre and Merrigan 2008). In Canada, the proportion of two-parent families with both parents in the paid labour market grew from 25 per cent in 1971 to 78 per cent in 2006; parental time with children declined from 4.2 hours per day in 1986 to 3.4 hours in 2005 (Lefebvre and Merrigan 2008).

The province of Quebec has been held up as a model jurisdiction with respect to child care provision, with substantial subsidies for day-care centres but reduced direct financial benefits to parents themselves. With the introduction of the Quebec day-care programme in 1997, the provincial government removed many of its universal benefits for children, including its generous family allowance which, in 1997, was $8,000 after the birth of a third child. The non-refundable credit for dependent children under 18 and the tax reduction for low-income families have both been eliminated. Instead, the day-care programme provides over $32 per day per child in day-care (paid to providers), so that parents need only pay $7 a day. The imbalance between those getting the financial help and those not has been a common criticism by home care activists in Quebec, as only 48 per cent of the province's children use subsidized day-care, though all parents are obliged to pay for it: parents of day-care children get an $8,000 per year subsidy while others get nothing. Anti-poverty groups argue that the state's subsidy of day-care is unfair, since the wealthy get the same tax break as do the poor, as long as they use day-care. The current cost of the Quebec day-care plan is $1.5 billion per year.

In addition to the concerns of child care activists and anti-poverty groups, Baker *et al.*'s (2005) analysis of the Quebec day-care system found the impact on children to be dramatic: on a variety of behavioural and health outcomes, ranging from aggression to motor skills to social skills to illness, day-care children fare far worse than stay-at-home children. Kozhaya's (2006) study underlined the concerns of anti-poverty groups, finding that the families who benefited most from the Quebec subsidized day-care system were those of higher income: 58 per cent of the children who got subsidized day-care were from homes with incomes over $60,000, although only 49 per cent of the population are from that income sector. Lefebvre (2002) also found that children who attended day-care in Quebec were more likely to come from privileged backgrounds than children who did not, with only 22 per cent of the very poorest children in the province being in day-care. Both Lefebvre and Kozhaya concluded that administratively, day-care is very costly, with the expense to the state being $11,600 per child in Quebec, not including fee subsidies, below market/free rent at public buildings such as universities and schools, administration costs, regulatory costs, wage subsidies, research, training costs, grants, capital expense subsidies and grants, equipment subsidies and grants, non-profit treatment, charitable status tax treatment, promotion, lobbying and advertising. In the United States, the Rand Corporation (Datar 2005), which along with the World Bank has strongly supported preferential government funding for day-care, surveyed day-care facilities about costs. Excluding capital, rent, major repairs and food, costs averaged $15,217 per year for infants, $11,827 for two-year-olds, and $9,678 for three- to five-year-olds.

In the child care debate in the last two Canadian federal elections, both the Liberal and NDP proposals would have created a two-tier system of child care in Canada, with only children in licensed or regulated day-care settings (currently less than 25 per cent nationally) qualifying for state support. The Conservative plan, while providing only $1,200 per year per child directly to parents, is a universal programme, whereby money 'flows with the child'. Insofar as it respects parents as responsible for making their own child care choices, it is recognized by parental child care advocates as a step in the right direction, but unlikely to promote more parental involvement, as $100 per month per child is only a token amount of support.

Non-taxable universal child benefit payments to parents

A child care programme that funds only one option of care – the regulated day-care sector – overlooks the needs of families who provide or wish to provide more in-home, family-based care for their children, and is a disincentive to parental care of children. The establishment of a national day-care programme, providing a network of accessible, high-quality, non-profit day-care centres across the country, is the culmination of a policy trend that has steadily decreased and removed direct child care benefits to parents, such as universal child benefit payments, a significant factor in reduced parental child care involvement.

A national strategy with parental child care involvement at the centre would proceed in a very different fashion to a national day-care programme, as it would seek to provide incentives for parents to spend more time with their children. It would give parents autonomy over their child care options and allocation of parenting expenses, providing a universal benefit inclusive of a broad array of parenting choices: children in regulated day-care settings, children in informal family day homes or with trusted neighbours, children in the care of relatives such as grandparents, and children raised at home by their parents.

Lefebvre's (2002) analysis of the costs and benefits of state funding of various arrangements for care of children concluded that the most efficient system would be a non-taxable universal child benefit, suggesting annual amounts of $2,500 per child aged 0–3 years, $2,000 per child aged 4–5 years, and $1,500 per child 6–17 years. A figure many child care advocates are now holding out as a baseline is a direct parental subsidy of $4,000 per year per child (suggested by the National Association of Women and the Law, Citizens for Public Justice, and Campaign 2000), more in keeping with Scandinavian nations' funding patterns. Finland, for example, has a long flat-rate child allowance given to all children up to age three who are not in the day-care system, amounting to $4,300 per year. An additional $238 per month is given to low-income families, totalling $595 per month or $7,104 per annum. Sweden's government has announced funding changes for child care: parents who use day-care will continue to receive state funding of $1,600 a month; those who use home-based care and did not get any government benefits before will now get funding of $570 per month, or $6,840 per year.

Other needed reforms have been identified: higher maternity and parental leave benefits for a period sufficiently long to ensure parental bonding with infants, birth allowances to parents paid on a flat basis and mandatory job security provisions. Support for shared parental responsibility for child care is important, as maintaining traditional gender roles replicates gender differences in labour market outcomes, including the gender gap in wages and foregone earnings. Programmes that support paternal involvement in child care such as paternity benefits will encourage women to remain attached to the labour force, rather than dropping out for prolonged periods (Lefebvre 2002).

Challenges for social work

Canadian social workers are particularly challenged in the arena of child care, as social and economic policies have placed increasing pressure on parents to prioritize their work over their family responsibilities. Social workers have been largely silent on the issue of supporting parents in their stated desire to spend more time with their children, in favour of advocating for a national early childhood education and day-care programme that supports those who choose third-party care over parental care in the lives of young children. As parents themselves challenge government retrenchment of programmes and benefits and seek to extend the new Universal Child Care Benefit (a $100 a month payment to parents of all children aged 0–6) to allow them greater choice in care options, social workers are slowly becoming allies in this effort.

Discussion

The neo-liberal agenda privileges the role of the state as one of facilitating the market-based economy over that of taking responsibility for the welfare of its citizens. As Teeple (1995) notes, child care, child custody and child protection policy and practice in Canada have dramatically changed within the social and economic context of neo-liberalism, which supports both the expansion of transnational corporate interests and the concomitant retrenchment of national welfare structures in the interests of facilitating corporate agendas. The past 20 years has witnessed a dramatic retrenchment of welfare services and programmes in Canada – a wholesale dismantling of the welfare state in the context of a growing globalization of the economy.

Programmes designed to assist parents have been particularly hard hit, with an array of legislative and policy changes designed to reduce social spending and to dismantle programmes aimed to support parents in addressing their children's needs. Since the mid-1990s, in the child protection realm, with declining resources, social workers are increasingly pressured to concentrate on the fulfilment of their statutory obligations via standardized risk assessments rather than attending to the root causes of child neglect, and child removal rates have skyrocketed. In the child custody realm, the overriding concern of government is the reduction of social assistance expenditures, and thus rather than promoting shared parental responsibility, traditional sole custody arrangements prevail, in which one parent is removed as a primary caregiver and relegated to the role of providing financial support. In the child care arena, the Family Allowance programme and other direct benefits to families have been eliminated in favour of funding third-party caregivers, with the consequence of forcing parents to spend the bulk of their time in paid employment at the expense of time spent with their children.

Thus Canadian child protection, child custody and child care policies and systems represent significant barriers to parental involvement in children's lives. In a free market society, family ties are not only undervalued but actively discouraged, as loyalty to the free market takes precedence. Family responsibilities are a major encumbrance to free market societies. Thus it is no surprise to find, in the Preamble to Bill C-303, a federal day-care funding initiative, that the primary objective of Canadian child care policy is neither maximizing parental involvement nor the well-being of children, but to 'support the participation of parents in employment or training and community life'.

Does reducing the social safety net, and focusing on ensuring that parents are in paid employment and away from children, serve the best interests of children, and is this a universal principle the public endorses? Survey results reveal the opposite. Most parents want to see the current federal grant of $1,200 per child per year enriched to the point where it is 'sufficient to have an impact upon parents' (child care) choices' (Ipsos-Reid 2007: 6). Parents want to spend more time with their children, and to share their paid employment and child care responsibilities. With increased direct financial support to parents for child care, it becomes possible for both parents to continue their participation in paid employment and increase their investment in their parenting roles.

The key to improving children's well-being is ensuring that social institutions support parents in the fulfilment of their parenting responsibilities. Such a 'parental-responsibility-to-children's-needs' approach would, first and foremost, clearly acknowledge the central place of parents in children's lives. It would provide, in the realm of child care, direct family allowance payments to parents, and other incentives for parents to spend more time with their children; in the child custody arena, legislative reform in the direction of shared parental responsibility, and parental reunification for children estranged from one of their parents via sole-custody decrees; in the child protection realm, family preservation and support programmes, and greater family reunification efforts for children in government care.

The forced disengagement of parents from children's lives is a contributing factor to decreased child well-being, and steps must be taken to reverse this trend. The unasked questions in current Canadian debates in child care, child custody and child protection policy remain: how are current federal and provincial child and family policies undermining parental involvement in children's lives? What are the responsibilities of government institutions to support parents in the fulfilment of their parental responsibilities? Although research supports the importance of parental care for optimal child development, without adequate state support for such care, it cannot be said that Canadian social structures truly value the importance of parents in their children's lives and the well-being of children.

In Canada, the child welfare system, including child protection, child custody and child care, is decentralized, governed by both federal and provincial/territorial jurisdictions. This has resulted in uneven policies and programmes for children in relation to geography and age. Regular and systematic child impact assessments of federal and provincial legislation, policies and programmes are needed to monitor the status of children's well-being across the country, particularly as children are the segment of the population most vulnerable to changing social and economic policies. The establishment of a National Children's Commissioner to monitor and protect children's rights and well-being, coordinate the efforts of all levels of government, and resolve gaps and disputes in service responsibility between federal and provincial governments has been recommended by several bodies, including the UN Committee on the Rights of the Child.

Conclusion

If the true measure of a nation's standing is the degree to which it values its most vulnerable citizens, then it is imperative that the parental care of children is institutionally supported. A national child and family policy with parental care at the centre of a network of care would be a powerful symbol of the sanctity of parent–child relationships.

If incentives, not disincentives, are provided for parents to remain actively involved in their children's lives, children will benefit; all policies that undermine rather than support responsible parental care will lead to negative outcomes. It is thus the responsibility of communities, social agencies and institutions to support parents in the fulfilment of their parental responsibilities to their children's needs.

In Canada, much needs to be done by way of fulfilling this collective social responsibility. Funding parenting and supporting shared parental responsibility, so that children can spend more time in parental care, and so that fewer children are removed from the care of either or both of their parents, is critical. As representatives of state institutions, social workers have a duty of care to support children and families. No less than the well-being of children is at stake.

The main challenge for social work within the social and economic context of neo-liberalism is to directly challenge the continuing retrenchment of national welfare structures in the interests of facilitating corporate agendas. The maintenance and promotion of a social work role that first and foremost supports parents in the fulfilment of their parenting responsibilities offers a means to achieve this objective. New developments in social work practice in the fields of child protection, child custody and child care in Canada signal that a paradigm shift in this direction has already begun.

References

Baker, M., Gruber, J. and Milligan, K. (2005) *Universal Child Care, Maternal Labor Supply, and Family Well-Being*, National Bureau of Economic Research, Working Paper No. W11832. Online. Available at www.nber.org/papers/w11832 (accessed 9 August 2013).

Bauserman, R. (2002) 'Child adjustment in joint custody versus sole custody arrangements: A meta-analytic review', *Journal of Family Psychology* 16: 91–102.

Bianchi, Suzanne, Robinson, John and Milkie, Melissa (2006) *Changing Rhythms of the American Family*, New York: Sage.

Bibby, R. (2003) *The Future Families Project: A Survey of Canadian Hopes and Dreams*, Ottawa: Vanier Institute of the Family.

Bonach, Kathryn (2005) 'Factors contributing to quality coparenting: Implications for family policy', *Journal of Divorce and Remarriage* 43(3/4): 79–103.

Cameron, G., Coady, N. and Adams, G.R. (2007) *Moving Toward Positive Systems of Child and Family Welfare*, Waterloo: Wilfrid Laurier University Press.

Datar, A. (2005) *Delaying Kindergarten: Effects on Test Scores and Child Care Costs*, Rand Corporation research brief, Santa Monica: Rand Corporation.

Eamon, M.K. and Kopels, S. (2004) 'For reasons of poverty: Court challenges to child welfare practices and mandated programs', *Child and Youth Services Review* 26(9): 821–36.

Ellis, Desmond and Wight-Peasley, Loretta (1986) *Wife Abuse Among Separated Women*. Paper presented at the Meeting of the International Association for the Study of Aggression, Chicago.

Fabricius, W. (2003) 'Listening to children of divorce: New findings that diverge from Wallerstein, Lewis, and Blakeslee', *Family Relations* 52(4): 385–96.

Fabricius, W.V., Braver, S.L., Diaz, P. and Velez, C.E. (2010) 'Custody and parenting time: Links to family relationships and well-being after divorce'. In Michael E. Lamb (ed.) *The Role of the Father in Child Development*, 5th edn, pp. 201–40. Cambridge: Wiley.

Farris-Manning, C. and Zandstra, M. (2003) *Children in Care in Canada*, Ottawa: Child Welfare League of Canada.

Higgins, C. and Duxbury, L. (2002) *The 2001 National Work-Life Conflict Study*, Ottawa: Health Canada. Online. Available at https://workfamily.sas.upenn.edu/wfrn-repo/object/la2oq4co18ii2n1p (accessed 9 August 2013).

Hotton, Tina (2003) 'Childhood aggression and exposure to violence in the home'. Crime and Justice Research Paper Series. Catalogue No. 85-561-MIE2003002. Ottawa: Statistics Canada, Canadian Centre for Justice Statistics.

Ipsos-Reid (2007) *Focus Groups on Issues Surrounding Child Care: Final Report*, Ottawa: Human Resources and Skills Development Canada.

Kaspiew, Rae, Gray, Matthew, Weston, Ruth, Moloney, Lawrence and Qu, Lixia (2009) *Evaluation of the 2006 Family Law Reforms*, Melbourne: Australian Institute of Family Studies.

Kelly, J. (2000) 'Children's adjustment in conflicted marriage and divorce: A decade review of research', *Journal of the American Academy of Child and Adolescent Psychiatry* 39(8): 963–73.

Kozhaya, N. (2006) *$7-a-Day Child Care: Are Parents Getting What They Need?*, Montreal: Montreal Economic Institute. Online. Available at: www.iedm.org/249-7-a-day-childcare-are-parents-getting-what-they-need- (accessed 9 August 2013).

Kruk, E. (2011) 'A model equal parental responsibility presumption in contested child custody', *American Journal of Family Therapy* 39: 375–89.

Kruk, E. (2012) 'Arguments for an equal parental responsibility presumption in contested child custody', *American Journal of Family Therapy* 40(1): 33–55.

Lefebvre, P. (2002) 'The effect of child care and early education arrangements on developmental outcomes of young children', *Canadian Public Policy* 28(2): 159–85.

Lefebvre, P. and Merrigan, P. (2008) 'Child care policy and the labor supply of mothers with young children: A natural experiment from Canada', *Journal of Labor Economics* 26(3): 519–48.

Marshall, K. (2006) 'Converging gender roles', *Perspectives on Labour and Income* 7(7). Statistics Canada. Online. Available at www.statcan.gc.ca/pub/75-001-x/10706/9268-eng.htm (accessed 9 August 2013).

Melli, Marygold S. and Brown, Patricia R. (2008) 'Exploring a new family form: The shared time family', *International Journal of Law, Policy and the Family* 22: 231–69.

Nanos Research (2009) *Stat Sheet, National Omnibus 200903, Parenting*. Online. Available at: www.nanosresearch.com.

Office of the Public Advocate of New York (2002) *Families at Risk: A Report on New York City's Child Welfare Project*, New York: Child Welfare Fund. Online. Available at http://publicadvocategotbaum.com/policy/pdfs/Risky_Care_for_Foster_Kids.pdf (accessed 12 August 2013).

Pivot Legal Society (2008) *Broken Promises: Parents Speak About B.C.'s Child Welfare System*, Vancouver: Law Foundation of British Columbia. Online. Available at: http://d3n8a8pro7vhmx.cloudfront.net/pivotlegal/legacy_url/310/BrokenPromises.pdf?1345765642 (accessed 9 August 2013).

Statistics Canada (2005) *General Social Survey – Time Use*, Ottawa: Minister of Industry.

Statistics Canada (2007) *Crime Statistics*, Ottawa: Minister of Industry.

Statistics Canada (2014) *Family Violence in Canada: A Statistical Profile*, Ottawa: Minister of Industry.

Swift, K. and Callahan, M. (2009) *At Risk: Social Justice in Child Welfare and Other Human Services*, Toronto: University of Toronto Press.

Swift, K. and Parada, H. (2004) 'Child welfare reform: protecting children or policing the poor?' *Journal of Law and Social Policy* 19: 1–17.

Teeple, G. (1995) *Globalization and the Decline of Social Reform*, Toronto: Garamond.

Trocme, N., Fallon, B., MacLaurin, B., Daciuk, J., Felstiner, C., Black, T., Tonmyr, L., Blackstock, C., Barter, K., Turcotte, D. and Cloutier, R. (2005) *Canadian Incidence Study of Reported Child Abuse and Neglect 2003: Major Findings*, Ottawa: Minister of Public Works and Government Services Canada. Online. Available at: www.phac-aspc.gc.ca/cm-vee/csca-ecve/pdf/childabuse_final_e.pdf (accessed 12 August 2013).

United Nations Children's Fund (UNICEF) (2007) *Child Poverty in Perspective: An Overview of Child Well-Being in Rich Countries*, Florence: UNICEF Innocenti Research Centre. Online. Available at www.unicef.org/media/files/ChildPovertyReport.pdf (accessed 12 August 2013).

Chapter 6

Politics as social work

The micromanagement of behaviour in the new millennium

Kenneth McLaughlin

Introduction

The political aspect of the contemporary social work role is clear to see. Much of it is prescribed by statute and related guidance which set parameters on the role and scope of any intervention. Duties can include, *inter alia*, the assessment and application for detention of someone under mental health legislation, intervention into family life which can result in the removal of a child from its carers, the allocation of scarce resources to those deemed to meet the department's eligibility criteria (which also entails refusing resources to those deemed ineligible) and the assessment of prospective adoptive or foster parents.

In addition, the policy and practice framework in which social work operates invariably reflects the prevailing ideology of the day. This can be seen in the United Kingdom context where, since the post-Second World War period, we have seen the rise and decline of the state social welfare model and its replacement with a neo-liberal, mixed economy model of care, which has placed free market economics into the fabric of health and social care. This development heralded a more business-oriented approach to social welfare and social work, with the imposition of such things as financial accountability mechanisms, processes of managerialism and performance indicator frameworks (Rogowski 2010). This is not to suggest that the direction and role of social work goes uncontested; on the contrary there is often heated debate over such things as whether social work is about the maintenance of the status quo or a vehicle for progressive social change, with both positions advocated by some, and a combination of both advocated by many (Payne 1996; Pritchard and Taylor 1978).

In this chapter I do not wish to detail the socio-political history of social work, which has been extensively done elsewhere (e.g. McLaughlin 2008a; Payne 2005; Rogowski 2010). My aim here is to highlight the way that the overt politicization of social work coincides with a trend whereby Politics (with a capital P) has given way to a more micro-political agenda in the sense that government is increasingly concerned with the micromanagement of individual behaviour. The paradox is that as social work came to be seen as an inherently political endeavour, Politics, in the broader sense of being concerned with structural and ideological matters, became more akin to social work, seeking to mould, manage, manipulate and coerce those sections of the population not considered to meet contemporary social mores. In this respect, I wish to look at the extent to which ever more human interaction is micromanaged. First, this is discussed in relation to social work's relationship to politics, with both neo-liberal and radical policies implicated as influencing such a development. Second, I consider how such micromanagement operates at the level of civil society, a sphere that is now increasingly 'manufactured' from above as opposed to forming organically from below. Third, what has been termed the 'politics of behaviour' or 'politics of nudge' are considered not as new developments but as a further aspect of politics as social work.

Whilst the focus of my analysis is on the UK context, the trends identified will be of interest to practitioners, activists and policymakers in the international sphere. The detailed overview of developments in one locality can be compared and contrasted with those in other countries that have broadly similar welfare practices, and for those countries which have, or aspire to have, a similar level of state or other form of professionalized welfare provision, the tensions and pitfalls of the politicization of behaviour and its concomitant micromanagement that are highlighted here can serve as a reminder that, all too often, the rhetoric of care can become a means of control.

Politics and social work

Given its role and function within modern society, it would be absurd to deny the political role of social work. Yet it is worth considering that such a position is, in historical terms, a relatively recent one. As social work developed in the nineteenth century within the Charity Organisation Society (COS), it sought to portray itself as different from both religious and political organizations. Whilst it may have shared much with both, it nevertheless attempted to claim an identity distinct from them. Such a 'non-political' nature was seen as being of benefit to it in fulfilling its societal role. In this respect:

> Social work was differentiated from politics in so far as it was less interested in the distribution of power than in the resolution of social conflict. Its goal was a social ideal, not a political system. As such, it was seen by its exponents as something better than purely political activity ... The differentiation of social work from religious movements was not always clear. In the Settlements, in particular, the social gospel was sometimes entangled with the religious gospel. The Charity Organisation Society solved this problem by seeing itself as an alternative to religious evangelism.
>
> (Seed 1973: 39–40)

This positioning of itself between two dominant spheres allowed social work to portray itself as non-political whilst simultaneously rationing services and differentiating between the 'deserving' and 'undeserving' poor. By presenting itself as apolitical and therefore above political argument and conflict, it attempted to portray itself as a philanthropic enterprise. In addition, as separate from the church, its moral stance could be presented from a humanistic perspective untainted by the decline in religious authority and tradition (Jones 1997).

Of interest here is the way politics, social work and wider social change interact, with perspectives differing as the world itself changes, new ideas and values replacing those that can no longer hold society together in the traditional way. For example, an emerging socialist movement denounced the moral righteousness of the COS, with Attlee (1920), for one, insisting that social workers should seek broader social and political change and not view their clients' problems as due to individual inadequacy. Attlee, of course, became Labour Prime Minister from 1945 to 1951, presiding over the formation of the welfare state.

The twentieth century saw various competing perspectives as to both the causes of individual and social problems and the role of both the state and social work in either alleviating or contributing to such a situation (e.g. Payne 2005; Pritchard and Taylor 1978), a debate that continues to this day, for example in discussions over the United Kingdom coalition government's proposed reductions to the welfare bill. Arguably though, it was the radical social work movement of the late 1960s and early 1970s that brought to the fore the overtly political nature of the post-war social work role, with the welfare state and social workers being implicated as props for the maintenance of capitalist relations of exploitation and social inequality (Bailey and Brake 1975). The argument that the problems of social work's clients are rooted in society and not due to individual inadequacies also resonated with many social work students, who had been influenced by the radical civil rights movements of the late 1960s (e.g. Jones 2011). This initial class-focused critique was soon followed by other groups who brought to the fore the way in which dominant and oppressive ideologies and practices concerning race, gender, sexuality and disability were embedded within much social policy discourse, social work education and social work practice. The social work profession, including social work education, was charged with being in denial over the political aspect of its role in maintaining the status quo and perpetuating discrimination in the mistaken belief that it was an apolitical activity (e.g. Dominelli 2002; Thompson 2006).

Whilst there have been many important ideological insights and practical benefits of the highlighting of the political aspect of social work, it is important to note that the trajectory of the radical tradition was not only influenced by optimism for wider social change but also by political defeat, the worker-role rather than worker–capital relationship gradually taking on more importance in pursuit of the radical agenda, a micro-political outlook gradually replacing a belief in broader structural change (McLaughlin 2008a). For both the Left and Right of the traditional political divide, there was an increasing focus on individual behaviour, the Right viewing problematic behaviour as due to individual weakness, the Left viewing it as a manifestation of oppressive ideological constructs. In each case, though, there was a tendency to police and manage ever more realms of human interaction.

The micromanagement of social work

As neo-liberalism and free market economics have become more pervasive, there is a sense amongst many that social work is at a crossroads (Lavalette 2011). The period of consecutive Conservative governments from 1979 to 1997 is seen as being pivotal in the implementation of a more individual, market-oriented approach to welfare provision. Clarke's (1996) essay from the penultimate year of this period of Conservative hegemony is titled 'After Social Work?', and is concerned with how the marketization of social work and welfare provision will affect social work and social workers. The coming to power of New Labour in 1997 with its 'modernization' agenda continued the process that the previous incumbents of government had pursued, with social work becoming, if anything, even more business-like than during the period of Conservative rule (Harris 2003).

One consequence of the opening up of welfare provision to the market was the influx of private, voluntary and charitable organizations to provide direct services to social work's clientele, a move designed to promote user choice and deliver cheaper, more cost-efficient services. Whilst there is nothing wrong per se in the provision of choice or the break-up of local authority domination of the provision of care services, they have led to some adverse consequences. First, the allocation of services can be primarily based on cost rather than need. In addition, as more and more services are outsourced, statutory or local authority social work begins to be primarily around the more coercive aspects of the role, for example in the implementation of child protection or mental health act proceedings. Indeed, with social work being left to deal with those with the most complex needs at a time of growing inequality and declining community resources, in many respects social work today is often about little more than managing the deterioration of clients' lives (Jones et al. 2004).

Increasingly, the 'professional' social worker is focused on delivering outcomes that have been set by government and social policy advisors. For example, the rise in performance indicators and assessment schedules that detail what is to be asked and what answers are to be noted, are prescribed in advance. Failure to adhere to such guidelines could see the social worker's fitness to practise being called into question by the Health and Care Professions Council (HCPC), which has the power to remove the social worker's professional registration, thereby preventing the individual from working as, or calling themselves, a social worker. We have a paradox here, in that measures to increase the professional status and social esteem of social work, for example in the registration and regulation of social workers, take place simultaneously with ones that undermine the autonomy and discretion of the worker. This has led some to question whether following the rise of social work as a profession in the 1970s we are now witnessing its fall (Rogowski 2010).

Such criticisms provide a detailed and accurate account of the way in which political interference into the day-to-day working of social work can lead to a more prescriptive and authoritarian relationship between social workers and their clientele. However, the narrow focus on such developments tends to ignore or downplay other aspects of the way the politicization of social work manifests itself in such interactions, and many of these political interventions were encouraged from within the social work profession.

The micromanagement of language

One aspect of the politicization of social work concerned the use and role of language. Language is active, not passive; it does not merely reflect reality but plays a role in its construction and maintenance. It therefore follows that language is a powerful medium for either perpetuating oppression or resisting a non-egalitarian social system. The use of language was embedded within a complex system of power relations, its use seen as either perpetuating or challenging patterns of oppression; it could not be neutral (Dominelli 2002; Thompson 2006).

If language is such a powerful medium, then aspects of it that play a role in the oppression of people do require challenge. The problem was that there became a reification of language, with certain words being elevated to an all-powerful force, removed from the material circumstances within which they arise. For example, the discourse of race emerged as a way of justifying existing inequality, in particular the reality of the slave trade. So whilst it is certainly correct that language can provide a means to naturalize and consolidate existing racist social relations, the roots of racism do not lie in language (Malik 1996).

Nevertheless, when terminology is held to not only construct but also oppress people, it can be accorded high political significance, with much effort being spent on attempts to control and censor those who utter words that offend the current moral sensitivities of society, or a particular group within society. In the process, a censorious climate can emerge in which the authorities are able to dictate the boundaries of acceptable discourse. For example, there is now widespread political control over what is regarded as acceptable speech. In December 2011, the Scottish government passed the Offensive Behaviour at Football and Threatening Communications (Scotland) Act 2012, which, among other things, outlaws 'sectarian' speech (Scottish Government 2012). In England, 2011 saw high publicity over the alleged racist language of several football players, most notably Chelsea's John Terry and Liverpool's Luis Suarez. Meanwhile, 34,000 schoolchildren a year are reported to their Local Education Authority for 'hate-speech incidents' (Hart 2011). There are numerous other instances of the policing and criminalizing of speech deemed offensive (Liberty 2012), which in effect amounts to the state management of public discourse.

Such measures allow the authorities to draw the boundaries of acceptable speech and debate, and social work is not immune to endorsing such censorship of the masses. For example, the anti-oppressive credentials of professional and student social workers frequently take the form of chastising their clientele and the wider public for using 'inappropriate' or 'offensive' language (Collins *et al.* 2000). This is far removed from the original intentions of the proponents of anti-oppressive practice, who saw it as a model to 'understand and tackle the structural problems and address their consequences by changing social relations at all possible levels' (Rogowski 2010: 72–3). Whilst such aims are indeed laudable, and there has been much work done by social work in challenging and changing the more meso and macro elements affecting service users' lives, even at the height of its political ambitions Anti-Oppressive Practice often focused more on the more micro aspects of life. This was exemplified in the 'political correctness' debate, which often took the form of deciding what was, and was not, appropriate language for social discourse. Ironically, the intensity of the reaction to a focus on language highlights the importance of language. After all, getting so irate over 'mere words' highlights that words are not trivial at all (Cameron 1995). However, there was legitimate concern that such a focus downplayed more relevant aspects of the problems facing social work's clientele, exemplified in the following quote:

> I used to think I was poor. Then they told me I wasn't poor I was needy. They told me it was self-defeating to think of myself as needy, I was deprived. They then told me deprived was a bad image, I was underprivileged. They told me underprivileged was over used, I was disadvantaged. I still haven't got a dime. But I sure have a great vocabulary.
>
> (Quoted in Philpot 1999: 13)

There can also be more subtle ways in which state/professional power is enhanced over those subject to social work. This can be illustrated in the way that the concept of 'empowerment' has undergone a conceptual shift, one very much influenced by wider political change. During the 1970s when there was a strong working-class affiliation, certainly when compared to the present period, radical activists had a commitment to the 'self-activity' of the working class (Langan 2002). In such a climate of collective working-class action, the notion of social workers 'empowering' their clients did not hold much resonance; the belief was that the working class, who, as now, form the majority of social services' clientele, were capable of organizing themselves, of gaining power from below by virtue of their collective strength, not having it handed down to them from above by some philanthropic social worker. In this respect, the rise of the concept of empowerment and its institutionalization within social work theory and practice is reflective of both the decline of working-class collective power and the changing conception of 'empowerment'; from something to be taken, by force if necessary, to something to be handed down by the state, here in the guise of the social worker.

The contemporary notion of empowerment as a process that allows service users to have more control over their lives can also prove illusory, becoming a mechanism for drawing people into participating in processes and decisions over which they have little control. As Langan (2002) notes:

> Parents are said to be empowered by being invited to attend child protection case conferences; they thus become complicit in measures of state intervention in their family life decided on by professionals and the police. Applicants for community care are empowered by the fact that their designated social worker is also the manager of a devolved budget which is limited by criteria quite independent of the applicant's needs. Too often, empowerment means reconciling people to being powerless.
> (Langan 2002: 215)

In other words, the power that is given is bound within certain parameters, and these can lead to a lowering of expectations as well as being predicated on the client ultimately being submissive to those who, in reality, wield power. In other words, if language can construct reality, it can also obscure it. That is why it is important to look behind seemingly benign terms such as 'empowerment' and 'anti-oppression', and also to be aware of the implications for interpersonal interactions and citizen–state power relations as the boundaries of public discourse are subject to increased regulatory control.

The micromanagement of civil society

If the left-wing drive to highlight the political aspect of social work was influenced by the decline of a belief in wider societal change, the academy and the worker's professional role replacing grassroots political organization and the worker's relationship to capital, in many respects a similar loss of belief characterizes the more right-wing, neo-liberal turn towards viewing politics as a form of social work, which is also an attempt at managing many of the problems of the late twentieth century in a changing political climate. For example, Lorenz (1994) sees social work as having a vital part to play in enabling the integration of European states as they attempt to manage both integration and differentiation as people migrate from country to country. Such interaction happens at the level of civil society, an area in which, according to Lorenz, social workers are well placed to manage social concerns and problems. He sees social work values around difference, human dignity and fairness as being able to create a space where a 'communicative community' can discuss and debate over issues at the micro, meso and macro levels.

The problem with this approach is that it fails to grasp the extent to which civil society, certainly in the United Kingdom, has been colonized by the state and its proxies. It thereby risks exacerbating this encroachment into community life and in the process undermining community co-operation of the informal, organic kind. Increasingly, civil society, if conceived as that realm of free association between individuals outside of the spheres of family, market economy or state intervention to engage in voluntary activity, does not exist. It is difficult to think of an example of contemporary life that is not subject to state scrutiny. From the proliferation of closed-circuit television cameras in public spaces to the gaze and powers of state-sanctioned bodies that regulate the behaviour of their members, both inside and outside work, the individual is closely monitored. The expansion of Criminal Record Bureau (CRB) checks further increased governmental and bureaucratic control over both civil society and the workplace. With many volunteering roles and a wide array of jobs now subject to official scrutiny via the Disclosure and Barring Service (DBS), civic engagement increasingly requires sanction by the state (Appleton 2012).

In effect, we have what Hodgson (2004) has termed a 'manufactured civil society', whereby civil society is not what it once was but has become composed of 'groups that look like civil society, but are in fact a mixture of state/voluntary sector organizations' (Hodgson 2004: 139). Hodgson notes the way in which government-sponsored groups reframe the communities' defined needs into those that fit the remit of the group/government. Using the example of Sure Start, she notes that, 'while the rhetoric of manufactured groups might be about providing what the community wants, the practice is more concerned with adapting perceived community needs to the criteria set by the state – criteria that the group itself has to address' (2004: 149). As one Sure Start worker explained, 'you have to *make them feel that what we are doing is what they would like us to do*' (quoted in Hodgson 2004: 139, emphasis in original). In essence, the community is lulled into accepting the group and in the process community 'wants' are adapted to fit in with the remit of the group/organization.

In other words, such organizations are not organic to the community but are manufactured outside it. Even those local community groups that are more rooted in the locality can find that the criteria for receiving external funding necessitates them agreeing to use their position to implement initiatives and develop procedures around awareness of cultural diversity, domestic violence, safeguarding children and vulnerable adults, the effects of bullying, and health campaigns around such things as 'safe drinking', 'healthy eating', smoking cessation and the recycling of waste. So, rather than responding to locally identified needs, they end up instituting government policy by proxy and endorsing a form of behavioural politics.

Politics as social work

The New Labour government pursued policies that were termed the 'politics of behaviour' (Field 2003), with a wide range of organizations charged with monitoring and intervening in the management of public interaction. For example, housing associations and local authorities not only provide accommodation, but take an increasing role in the moral policing of their tenants' behaviour as they police 'anti-social' behaviour. Sure Start children's centres have been criticised for being more concerned with offering therapeutic guidance with regard to parenting styles than with the material effects of poverty on the life experiences and future chances of their clientele (Melhuish *et al.* 2004). In a similar vein, general practitioners are increasingly co-opted by government to promote a certain way of living (Fitzpatrick 2001).

The regulation of lifestyle is now entrenched in British society. Perhaps the most high profile of such initiatives has been the ban on smoking in enclosed public places, initially applicable to the workplace, pubs and restaurants, but which some campaigners now want to extend so as to stop people smoking in their own cars (Triggle 2011). The draconian nature of such measures is perhaps most clearly illustrated by the extension of the smoking ban to include those detained in secure psychiatric hospitals who are unable to leave the hospital grounds, and who are therefore prevented from enjoying a cigarette (McLaughlin 2008b).

The trend towards the micromanagement of behaviour continued under the 2010–2015 Liberal-Conservative coalition government as it embraced what has been called *the politics of nudge*. Influenced by the 'libertarian paternalism' advocated by Thaler and Sunstein (2008), the coalition government set up a 'Behavioural Insight Team' to explore ways in which it could nudge us towards making the correct choices in life as decreed by those in power (Lawrence 2010). Of course, governments have always tried to shape the way their citizens think and behave, but the politics of nudge represents the negation of Politics (with a capital P) in the sense of being concerned with the battle of ideas over how best to organize society and allow people to realize their full potential. The politics of nudge focuses not on social vision but on individual cognition, and is also duplicitous in that by nudging the electorate towards acting in certain ways, the government attempts to implement policy by deception. Rather than having a public debate about what the people think is the best course of action, the decision is made by a small group of people and attempts are made to impose this on the electorate by stealth.

Conclusion

Social work, as an activity concerned with the behaviour of individuals within society, sought to try to modify 'problematic' behaviour. The particular form such intervention took was invariably influenced by the moral, religious and political ideals of the respective bodies that undertook such endeavours. The setting up of the welfare state and the establishment of social services departments following the Seebohm report of 1968 are held by some as heralding a period that represented the heyday of social work as a progressive and flourishing profession. The state took responsibility for the provision of welfare but also gave professionals a significant degree of professional autonomy, not only in the identification of need and prioritization of services, but also in the nature that any intervention should take (Rogowski 2010). Whilst recent decades have indeed seen a shift away from such state welfare provision to the extent that the state, in the guise of the local authority and social workers, is less involved in the provision of services and/or direct care other than with those deemed 'high risk', to a significant degree, the state is actually more involved in the minutiae of the lives of its citizens than before.

So, it is certainly the case that social work remains a political activity. However, in essence, the debate over the extent to which social work is, or should be, political, misses the fundamental problem, the extent to which, in contemporary society, politics has become social work. Intervention into the minutiae of people's lives is a key aspect of social work, whether in the guise of community, charity or social worker. Increasingly, however, the state, in various guises, is encroaching ever further onto this terrain.

It is a mistake to exclusively locate the drive towards the increased regulation of both professional and public interaction with the neo-liberal political establishment. Whilst such observations contain much truth, they fail to account for the role of many on the Left, including within social work, who also influenced a situation in which both professional and interpersonal relationships have become subject to scrutiny and censure. If we are to challenge this state of affairs and avoid the mistakes of the past, we need to have as accurate an account of its development as possible.

For those concerned with the current trajectory of social work and the wider political agenda, there is a need to challenge the colonization of the life-world by political and professional interventions into both the private sphere and civil society. If instinctively this does not sit comfortably with social workers, this is due to the fact that they work with many people who do require professional intervention, and such intervention is often against their will but is permitted by statute. However, encouraging a climate in which personal autonomy and responsibility is assumed, where the vast majority of the population is treated as capable moral agents, where political state-sanctioned intervention in the minutiae of people's lives is kept to a minimum, would free up social workers to work with those who are most in need/at risk and would also pressure government to focus on the wider socioeconomic political agenda rather than dwell on the minutiae of its citizens' lives.

In many countries, social work is still rooted in community development activities, with the penetration of the state and professionalization not as developed as in the United Kingdom. However, this is likely to change as they develop economically. For those working in such countries, the developments highlighted above can alert them to the dangers that can flow from the encroachment of the state and the drive towards professionalism whereby political action is reduced to the realm of interpersonal relationships and the micromanagement of people's lives.

References

Appleton, J. (2012) *Vetting Tree Surgeons: CRB Checking and Local Authorities*, London: Manifesto Club. Online. Available at: www.manifestoclub.com/files/mc%20report_vetting%20tree_screen.pdf (accessed 12 August 2013).

Attlee, C.R. (1920) *The Social Worker*, London: Bell and Sons.

Bailey, R. and Brake, M. (eds) (1975) *Radical Social Work*, London: Edward Arnold.

Cameron, D. (1995) *Verbal Hygiene*, London: Routledge.

Clarke, J. (1996) 'After social work?' in N. Parton (ed.) *Social Theory, Social Change and Social Work*, London: Routledge.

Collins, S., Gutridge, P., James, A., Lyn, E. and Williams, C. (2000) 'Racism and anti-racism in placement reports', *Social Work Education*, 19(1): 29–43.

Dominelli, L. (2002) *Anti-Oppressive Social Work Theory and Practice*, Hampshire: Palgrave.

Field, F. (2003) *Neighbours From Hell: The Politics of Behaviour*, London: Politicos.

Fitzpatrick, M. (2001) *The Tyranny of Health: Doctors and the Regulation of Lifestyle*, London: Routledge.

Harris, J. (2003) *The Social Work Business*, London: Routledge.

Hart, A. (2011) *Leave Those Kids Alone: How Official Hate-Speech Legislation Interferes in School Life*, Manifesto Club. Online. Available at: http://tommower.co.uk/manifestoclub/MC%20Report_Leave%20those%20kids%20alone02.pdf (accessed 13 August 2013).

Hodgson, L. (2004) 'Manufactured civil society: counting the cost', *Critical Social Policy*, 24(2): 139–64.

Jones, C. (1997) 'Poverty' in M. Davies (ed.) *The Blackwell Companion to Social Work*, Oxford: Blackwell.

Jones, C. (2011) 'The best and worst of times: Reflections on the impact of radicalism on British social work education in the 1970s' in M. Lavalette (ed.) *Radical Social Work Today: Social Work at the Crossroads*, Bristol: The Policy Press.

Jones, C., Ferguson, I., Lavalette, M. and Penketh, L. (2004) *Social Work and Social Justice: A Manifesto for a New Engaged Practice*, Social Work Action Network. Online. Available at: www.socialworkfuture.org/about-swan/national-organisation/manifesto (accessed 13 August 2013).

Langan, M. (2002) 'The legacy of radical social work' in R. Adams, L. Dominelli and M. Payne (eds) *Social Work: Themes, Issues and Critical Debates*, Hampshire: Palgrave.

Lavalette, M. (ed.) (2011) *Radical Social Work Today: Social Work at the Crossroads*, Bristol: The Policy Press.

Lawrence, F. (2010) 'First goal of David Cameron's "nudge unit" is to encourage healthy living', *Guardian*, 12 November 2010. Online. Available at: www.guardian.co.uk/politics/2010/nov/12/david-cameron-nudge-unit (accessed 13 August 2013).

Liberty (2012) *Speech Offences*, London: Liberty. Online. Available at: www.liberty-human-rights.org.uk/human-rights/free-speech/speech-offences/index.php (accessed 13 August 2013).

Lorenz, W. (1994) *Social Work in a Changing Europe*, London: Routledge.

McLaughlin, K. (2008a) *Social Work, Politics and Society: From Radicalism to Orthodoxy*, Bristol: The Policy Press.

McLaughlin, K. (2008b) *A Cruel and Unusual Ban*, London: spiked Ltd. Online. Available at: www.spiked-online.com/index.php/site/article/5177/ (accessed 13 August 2013).

Malik, K. (1996) *The Meaning of Race*, London: Macmillan.

Melhuish, E., Belsky, J. and Leyland, A. (2004) *The Impact of Sure Start Local Programmes on Child Development and Family Functioning: A Report on Preliminary Findings*, London: Birkbeck University. Online. Available at: www.ness.bbk.ac.uk/impact/documents/397.pdf/ (accessed 13 August 2013).

Payne, M. (1996) *What is Professional Social Work?* Birmingham: Venture Press.

Payne, M. (2005) *The Origins of Social Work: Continuity and Change*, Hampshire: Palgrave.

Philpot, T. (1999) 'Editor's introduction: The modern mark of Cain' in T. Philpot (ed.) *Political Correctness and Social Work*, London: IEA Health and Welfare Unit.

Pritchard, C. and Taylor, R. (1978) *Social Work: Reform or Revolution*, London: Routledge and Kegan-Paul.

Rogowski, J. (2010) *Social Work: The Rise and Fall of a Profession?* Bristol: The Policy Press.

Scottish Government (2012) *Offensive Behaviour at Football and Threatening Communications (Scotland) Act 2012*. Online. Available at: www.scotland.gov.uk/Topics/Justice/law/sectarianism-action-1/football-violence/bill (accessed 13 August 2013).

Seed, P. (1973) *The Expansion of Social Work in Britain*, London: Routledge and Kegan-Paul.

Thaler, R. and Sunstein, C. (2008) *Nudge: Improving Decisions About Health, Wealth and Happiness*, New York: Penguin.

Thompson, N. (2006) *Anti-Discriminatory Practice* (2nd edn), Hampshire: Palgrave Macmillan.

Triggle, N. (2011) 'Ban smoking in cars, says British Medical Association', *BBC News*, 17 October 2011. Online. Available at: www.bbc.co.uk/news/health-15744352 (accessed 20 February 2012).

Part III

Vulnerability and social work response in a global context

George Palattiyil, Dina Sidhva and Mono Chakrabarti

We live in a society characterised by risk and vulnerability, which have assumed a significant position in the contemporary social work literature. As Stalker (2003) puts it, risk has become a major preoccupation in social work (p. 211). The media and Internet constantly remind us of the dangers of life in the twenty-first century. In the UK, for example, historic child abuse cases (the Jimmy Savile sexual abuse enquiry, Rotherham child sexual abuse case, etc.) have led to a moral panic discourse underpinning social work intervention with children, exemplified in the activities of the UK's Child Exploitation and Online Protection Centre (Clapton *et al.*, 2013). Similarly, there have been significant changes over the last decade in the legislative and policy context in which social workers operate with regard to vulnerable adults who are at risk of harm (McKeough and Knell-Taylor, 2002; Brammer, 2007; Penhale and Parker, 2008). These changes have led to newer legislation in the field of adult care services (Department of Health, 2000; Patrick and Smith, 2009), with the aim of affording maximum protection to those who are vulnerable and marginalised in our society.

Globally, individuals and families are exposed to numerous vulnerabilities resulting from new challenges such as heightened inequality, forced migration and refugees, increased threat of terrorism and emerging pandemics and natural disasters, entailing a sustained social work response. For example, the advent of HIV and AIDS saw a greater social work involvement in prevention and care efforts, in addition to campaigning against stigma and discrimination. Social work continues to respond to HIV and other emerging public health concerns, especially in the area of protecting the human rights of those affected by these illnesses. Similarly, social work has been at the forefront, supporting asylum seekers, refugees and other forced migrants whose lives have been unimaginably disrupted due to the inhumane treatment and multiple adversities they have been exposed to. They have complex needs and are likely to require a wide range of social services; many may be unaware of their entitlements and how to access services. A major problem asylum seekers encounter is post-traumatic stress disorder, which impacts heavily on their ability to tell their stories in a coherent way to immigration officials in the host countries (Palattiyil and Sidhva, 2011). Failure to provide a coherent story of their journey renders their cases less valid, thus increasing the likelihood of such cases being rejected. Social work has been playing a key role in responding to these challenges globally, by promoting human rights-based approaches, trying to ensure asylum seekers and refugees are treated with dignity, equality and respect.

Part III provides an opportunity to critically examine some of these issues and the role of social work in responding to these challenges.

As the dynamics of abuse have been revealed by research and through the documentation of day-to-day practice, it has become clear that managing vulnerability without empowering children and adults is a challenging area of social work that requires advanced knowledge, managerial skills and face-to-face skills. Chapter 7 explores and discusses the challenges and opportunities for social work in this context.

Incidents of violence and discrimination against immigrants and religious communities demand the attention of social work practitioners and the international social work community. Chapter 8 provides a case study of responsive and integrative social work practice in the aftermath of the 9/11 attacks in the United States.

Chapter 9 describes the emerging field of childhood studies and its approaches to understanding childhood and children in contemporary society. This emerging field will continue to challenge social work to reshape professional knowledge and practice.

The bio-medical-social framework for practice does not address the structural issues of poverty, gender inequality, stigma and discrimination, and cultural norms which drive the HIV/AIDS epidemic. Professional social work can build upon the work done in the arena of HIV to evolve a framework for anti-oppressive or structural practice that impacts policy in this important arena. Chapter 10 describes the issues faced by social workers in Botswana, who play a vital role in working with issues related to HIV and AIDS. Social and economic hardship present great challenges for social workers in this context, and the need for additional support and resources is highlighted.

Chapter 11 provides a critical examination of these issues and the role of social work in challenging the ever pervasive stigma and discrimination that people living with HIV and AIDS continue to experience.

References

Brammer, A. (2007) New abuse laws in Scotland. *The Journal of Adult Protection*, 8(4), 39–43.

Clapton, G., Cree, V.E. and Smith, M. (2013) Moral panics and social work: Towards a sceptical view of UK child protection. *Critical Social Policy*, 33(2), 197–217.

Department of Health (2000) *'No Secrets': Guidance on Developing and Implementing Multi-Agency Policies and Procedures to Protect Vulnerable Adults from Abuse*. London: Department of Health.

McKeough, C. and Knell-Taylor, E. (2002) Protecting vulnerable adults where they may be both victim and perpetrator. *Journal of Adult Protection*, 4(4), 10–16.

Palattiyil, G. and Sidhva, D. (2011) *They Call Me 'You are AIDS': A Report on HIV, Human Rights and Asylum Seekers in Scotland*. Edinburgh: University of Edinburgh.

Patrick, H. and Smith, N. (2009) *Adult Protection and the Law in Scotland*. Haywards Heath: Bloomsbury Professional.

Penhale, B. and Parker, J. (2008) *Working With Vulnerable Adults*. Oxford: Routledge.

Stalker, K. (2003) Managing risk and uncertainty in social work: A literature review. *Journal of Social Work*, 3(2), 211–33.

Chapter 7

What kinds of violence and abuse affect vulnerable people?

Reflections on the evolving context of adult protection and safeguarding in the United Kingdom: legislation, regulation and professional practice

Hilary Brown and Susan Hunter

Introduction

Personal violence and abuse are facts of life for all adults to some extent, but research suggests that risks loom larger for less advantaged groups whether on the basis of class, poverty, gender, sexual orientation, disability and/or mental ill-health. But it seems as if while these adults face considerably more risk, they are often less able to draw on personal or community resources or to seek remedies through mainstream helping agencies or the civil or criminal justice systems.

Local authorities in England and Wales have been required, since 2000, to put systems in place that coordinate the input of these agencies when vulnerable people are harmed. 'Vulnerable adults' (Department of Health 2000), that is, those who meet the criteria for assessment to receive social services on account of learning disability, mental ill-health, older age, physical impairment or sensory impairment, can be offered additional supports when seeking justice or protection from violence. But vulnerability is a difficult concept and can be used to infantilize as well as to empower or protect. A social model of vulnerability locates vulnerability in the way that people who are perceived to be different are isolated and overlooked rather than as a property of them as somehow 'weak' individuals. The research literature suggests that people who are labelled as having an impairment, or who are older, are often placed in, or left in, situations of risk that others would find intolerable, for example in crowded hospital wards, crumbling neighbourhoods or isolated institutions. When they are harmed, others respond as if it does not matter; their complaints go unheeded and even serious crimes against them are downplayed, and when things do come to light, they are not properly supported or recompensed and the sanctions that would be applied to someone who had harmed another are not brought to bear on their abusers, because it is as if people characterized as having impairments do not count enough to warrant a robust response.

Agencies are expected to work together to prevent abuse and to provide prompt and consistent responses, designed to augment, not replace, the remedies available to all citizens. Mainstream statutory agencies are thereby being asked to 'go the extra mile' in relation to these groups and to coordinate their efforts in receiving reports, managing investigations, conducting assessments, ensuring safe provision of services and in advocating for justice and redress.

Many disabled and older people are well able to manage these matters without additional input, in the same way as other adults would cope with such events: they make their own decisions about reporting crime, accessing refuges, making complaints about poor professional practice and challenging harassment. But if they wish to use the 'safeguarding adults' system, they should find that their concerns are met with a streamlined and human rights approach and that crimes against them are taken seriously. The professional networks that underpin these arrangements serve to counter attitudes that might otherwise minimize harms done to them, downplay the long-term consequences of such harms or set aside their civil and human rights. However, the responsibilities of statutory agencies, in relation to these at-risk groups, do not override the person's wishes in regard to their own safety unless the person is deemed to lack capacity to make his or her own decisions.

The potential for reducing choice and empowerment in the name of vulnerability is a dilemma with which social workers are well familiar (Hollomotz 2012; Stalker and Harris 1998). The role of mainstream agencies in all these cases is to make multi-disciplinary decisions with, or on behalf of, the person in respect of their accommodation, relationships, risk-taking, health care and personal safety. Additional supports can also be offered in respect of the court system with the potential for special measures that consist of safeguards such as screens or live video-feeds to give evidence, use of intermediaries in court, additional penalties that can be applied when harm has been done deliberately to someone on the basis of their disability, and sanctions through regulatory systems where individual workers or services have failed in their duty of care. Hence these particularly vulnerable groups are offered additional case coordination, signposting and supports, both in court and in accessing welfare services, so that they can be protected from violence and future harm.

Types of abuse

This identification of high-risk groups and the terminology of vulnerability is contentious, as are the definitions of *abuse* and *abusing* used to trigger these responses. So what kinds of abuse are covered within these statutes and what are the dynamics that fuel violence to disadvantaged and marginalized people?

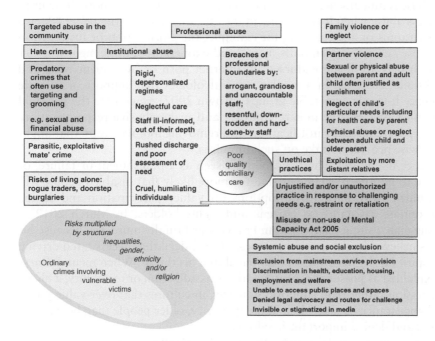

Figure 7.1 Map showing constellations of abuse and heightened risk to vulnerable groups.

The simplest way of defining abuse is to name discrete types of abuse, for example physical, sexual, psychological or financial abuse or neglect, and this is the framework that has been used in many research and policy evaluation programmes. More complex understanding contextualizes these acts, taking into account the relationship between the person abusing and the person who has been victimized, the setting in which such abuse has occurred and been allowed to continue, the motivation of the perpetrator and the dynamics that have created opportunities for them to abuse, or lacunae within which harm could not be prevented. Figure 7.1 sets out the types of abuse that emerge from this research literature, showing the overlaps with other forms of hate crime and predatory abuse, the additional sources of abuse that can occur in institutional settings and professional encounters, the common ground in relation to domestic violence and intergenerational abuse made more prevalent as a result of longer periods of familial care and the particular ethical issues that can arise where exceptional decisions are taken to use coercive solutions.

All of these forms of abuse represent violations of human rights. Some could reasonably be framed as hate crimes, while others are acts of ignorance, cruelty or desperation. Understanding motivation and patterns is essential to good prevention and to proportionate responses.

Abuse is fundamentally fuelled by inequality, and it is far more difficult to address abuse when it is endemic in the culture and/or in the belief systems and customs of a society. So, for example, the glorification or justification of abuse against women both shapes and exonerates abusive men, whether their beliefs are being endorsed by Internet porn or by ancient texts and traditional customs. In a similar vein, ideologies that support or tolerate violence towards vulnerable groups (Brown 2002) exacerbate the personal dynamics that emerge in care contexts and make abusive responses more likely, providing ready justifications and removing moral censure that might otherwise provide a brake on such impulses.

Hence in cultures where disability is seen as a punishment or failure, or linked to notions of shame or sin, it is more likely that disabled people will be hidden away, barred from options for valued participation and denied appropriate assistance as citizens and rights holders. In March 2012, a young man visiting relatives from France was brutally murdered because his hosts believed he was a witch, possessed by a devil that necessitated driving the spirit out by inserting an iron bar down his throat. When mental illness is explained as possession, or it manifests as addiction or instability, it elicits oppression rather than support. Similarly, in cultures that over-value youth and appearance over wisdom and experience, older people may be marginalized and denied important freedoms.

Hence the personal dynamics that get played out in relationships between people with unequal power may be legitimized in the social customs, criminal codes or religious beliefs of a community, offering simplistic and victim-blaming explanations for difference and providing a mandate for control and punishment.

What systems are growing up to address these situations?

Characteristic of the evolution of social work practice in the United Kingdom (and more widely in Western countries since the middle of the twentieth century), has been an increase in the professionalization of support offered to people unable to care for themselves for whatever reason, and in the extent of interventions by the state in family life, especially in relation to child protection and abuse. The dominance of the child protection agenda within social work is well documented (Lonne *et al.* 2008; Munro 2011), and the legal provisions well developed since the 'battered child syndrome' was first described in the 1960s (Kempe 1971). The evolution of adult safeguarding is more recent, more fragmented and more contentious within the professional literature and public debate, but it dates from the identification of 'granny bashing' in the 1980s, the exposure of conditions in large institutional settings throughout the 1970s and 1980s, and the uncovering of widespread sexual abuse of people with intellectual disabilities (Brown *et al.* 1995).

At the heart of this discourse is a debate about the nature of adulthood and autonomy in Western philosophical traditions and a tug of war between these principles and a more paternalistic concern with welfare, safety and containment. The tension between the rights of adults to make autonomous decisions and the necessary exceptions that are sanctioned in law have a long history in legal and moral debate.

Making decisions with or on behalf of people who are struggling

All jurisdictions in the United Kingdom have enacted legislation that relates to decision-making under either 'capacity' or 'incapacity' acts, and these prescribe strict conditions for compulsory detention in hospital of individuals for their own safety or that of others under various Mental Health acts. Furthermore, all jurisdictions have recently modernized this legislation to ensure that the concept of capacity is decision-specific, time-limited and conditional on efforts having been made to provide accessible information and assistance with communication. Contentious, serious or irreversible decisions are subject to scrutiny by the courts and should be transparent and open to appeal (Hammerburg 2009). The concept of incapacity cannot then be used as a pretext for removing or compromising civil rights but is judged as multi-faceted and circumstance-specific. The legislation serves to strengthen participation and rights to independent advocacy.

There are different models of proxy decision-making, but in the United Kingdom, the concept of 'best interests' has been adopted as the benchmark and the legislation starts from a presumption of capacity that has to be shown, on the balance of probabilities, to be unfounded. This legislation is underpinned by a range of principles such as that formal decisions should reflect the least restrictive alternative, that they should be of benefit to the individual, and that they should take into account the current and past preferences of the individual where these are known and where this is possible. The model of decision-making itself is predominantly cognitive and focuses on deficits in reasoning and weighing up of options. This leaves unexamined the issues that arise when a person's emotional withdrawal or lability undermines any consistent decision-making. Decisions are also made in social force fields, and where there is heightened dependency of one person on another and/or where a person is under undue influence or duress, that person's decision-making may be curtailed or manipulated (see Brown 2011). It is the debate to address this shortfall that has generated the most contention and that runs the most risk of inadvertently breaching civil rights.

But whereas proxy decision-making has been enshrined in new legislation, the need for intervention in situations characterized by abuse has, with the exception of Scotland, been met by lower-level professional guidance working within existing professional networks and statutory agencies. In England *No Secrets* and in Wales *In Safe Hands* require social services departments at the local level to set up the conditions for partnership working, appropriate sharing of information and multi-agency governance through local Safeguarding Boards. Their success is measured through regulatory bodies and by the national monitoring of referrals, investigations and outcomes. Structures for commissioning serious case reviews are in place to audit cases that have either had particularly harmful outcomes and/or have revealed weaknesses in the system of cross-agency working or professional judgments (Brown 2009; Manthorpe *et al.* 2009; Manthorpe and Martineau 2012).

In Scotland, however, the Parliament at Holyrood decided to give professionals a proper legal mandate to intervene in the lives of individuals whose best interests are seen to be compromised, to provide assessment, support and protection and to provide it without those individuals' consent when certain conditions are met. Scotland for the moment is unique in Europe in having decided to legislate on this matter, and the Scottish legislation therefore merits some detailed discussion of its intent, safeguards and outcomes.

The Adult Support and Protection (Scotland) Act 2007 (ASPA) establishes the duty for 'council officers' (usually social workers) to investigate the circumstances of adults who can be shown to be 'at risk of harm'; it sets out a *duty* on public bodies to collaborate, including by the creation of adult protection committees, and makes available new intervention powers in the form of assessment banning and removal orders. The combined impact of longer life expectancy amongst older and disabled people together with welfare policies of de-institutionalization reinforced the arguments for establishing these powers to intervene in the private lives of individual citizens and gave these powers statutory force. This was intended to ensure access by professionals to vulnerable adults, as a minimum for the purposes of assessment and, where concerns are confirmed, to ensure that relevant bodies in health, social care and the police in particular, address the issue and implement protective measures.

Particularly controversial but thought unlikely to be widely used is the power to override the wishes of a person 'with capacity' who is at risk of significant harm but who can be deemed to be under 'undue pressure' without which the individual would make different decisions about their lives (Patrick and Smith 2009). The case to intervene in these controversial circumstances has to be made in court before a sheriff and, as yet, there is little case law, in part because the challenges of mounting robust proofs in court are considerable.

In line with proper concerns about privacy and self-determination, the Act contains a number of measures to counterbalance some seemingly unrestrained powers. First of all, and in order to be referred, the individual about whom there is concern must meet the three-point test of being at risk of harm, being unable to safeguard his or her own well-being or interests, and being more vulnerable to being harmed as a consequence of his or her disability, infirmity, etc. than individuals 'not so affected'.

This means that disability alone is not a sufficient criterion for consideration under the Act. Once access has been gained, professionals can only proceed with the adult's consent and do not have powers of detention, although banning and removal orders can be sought where the risk of significant harm is present. Even though checks on the scope of professional intervention are intended to support autonomy and self-determination, the conduct of adult protection investigations (though not necessarily referrals) has been of concern to people with learning disabilities (Learning Disability Alliance 2011). Furthermore the Human Rights Act of 1998 requires that all interventions should be legal, fair and proportionate. Nonetheless practitioners have reported satisfaction with the ASPA legislation, which despite its weaker powers compared with the in/capacity and mental health legislation, has enabled engagement with some very vulnerable individuals where none was feasible previously, and firmer partnerships with other agencies essential to the support as well as the protection of vulnerable individuals (Mackay *et al.* 2011). Some of these measures may also be included in legislation that is going forward in England and Wales in the Care and Support Bill that is currently under discussion. Moreover, European countries are moving away from policies based on institutional and restrictive care and the Ten Year Action Plan of the European Union, launched in St Petersburg in 2006, provides a framework to underpin moves towards provision based on rights and citizenship rather than on isolation and protection.

Models of and mechanisms for prevention

In 2002, the Council of Europe had brought together a model of prevention that works at all these levels: informing and empowering individuals, making sure individual services are alert to sites of abuse and creating clear routes for reporting, building the capacity for specialized investigation, and creating an infrastructure for supporting people through legislation and national awareness raising. At each of these levels, the intent was to tackle primary prevention by building safe communities and services that stop abuse in its tracks; secondary prevention by ensuring that any abuse that does occur is promptly recognized, referred on and stopped; and tertiary prevention that ensures that there are remedies that prevent long-term harm and that help people to recover, get justice and move on.

Mainstreaming care provision has been seen as a solution to some of these dynamics but even in those countries that prioritize community living, independent budgets and individualized services, protective agencies have been called upon to intervene when vulnerable people have been preyed on by individuals outside the purview of statutory service provision. So as state-run and institutional care has ceased to be the norm and as the work-force has become more casualized, this border-control model of safeguard-ing that policed recruitment to professions and regulated their qualifications and professional standards has become more porous, contentious and dif-ficult to uphold within and across professional and national boundaries. In some countries, service provision is dominated by non-governmental organ-izations (NGOs) and commissioned or policed by civil authorities, whereas in others the roles are reversed. What is important is that there are robust and independent checks and balances in place.

In England and Wales, when a vulnerable adult is thought to have been abused, all workers and agencies are expected to make a referral into the adult social services system to alert the system to the possibility of abuse and to trigger an investigation that takes place across all the relevant agen-cies on behalf of the individual. If a crime has been committed, then police take the lead, but behind them the health and social care services conduct their own inquiries and try to ascertain what can be done to keep this per-son safe in the immediate and longer term future; apply sanctions to, and / or control the whereabouts of a perpetrator (this might involve them losing their liberty through the criminal justice system, or their having their liveli-hood impinged through losing their job or having their professional licence withheld, or their access to this individual or to vulnerable people as a group restricted); and/or determine how this service should improve its practice (for example, in relation to managing challenging individual service users, or in relation to recruitment and training of staff) so that any lessons that have been learned from this case can be applied across the board and used to make service provision safer and abuse-proof for other vulnerable people.

What is global about abuse of people with disabilities?

We have seen that, as citizens, people with disabilities are not immune to but disproportionately affected by the pressures that economic austerity puts on people, including loss of their jobs, failure to regenerate their neigh-bourhoods, more extreme forms of isolation and exclusion and cuts in the public services upon which they depend. Family members and paid carers are also under increased strain, and that may exacerbate the difficulties of caring for disabled relatives or clients. So this is a pincer effect; disabled people are more likely to be at risk, while services are less likely to be able to respond to early warning signs or to disclosures and allegations. In hard times people are asked to fend for themselves, and that is not helpful for people who necessarily rely on others on a day-to-day basis. Against this backdrop what do we know about the way these pressures are manifest in disabled people's lives?

Policy decisions are usually presented as 'reform', with the structure of provision glossed over as an irrelevance to the face-to-face interactions that occur between service users, their families and networks of professional helpers. But there is plenty of evidence that organizational factors have both direct and indirect impacts on the likelihood of abuse and neglect (Wardhaugh and Wilding 1993). Reducing the role of the state in politics usually starts by attacking 'dependence' on state benefits or services, but this distorts the fact that state provision allows women, especially women with children or extra caring responsibilities, to achieve *more* independence, not less. State services allow women to return to work, to maintain an independent income, to leave relationships that have broken down or turned violent. They provide a platform that allows individuals to cope and to feel supported. Tomita (1990) posited a model of abusive behaviour that is rooted in internalized deprivation, and she showed how lack of resources cascades down through the absence of supportive structures to create an internal dialogue of entitlement and hard-done-by-ness that can be turned upside down into a justification for abuse.

Hence it is no surprise that older people are treated differently when they form a relatively small sub-group of the population – one needing to be supported by a larger pool of working-age adults – but when the demographics are thrown into reverse or where economies contract, then older people's welfare comes to be seen as an unsupportable burden on the middle generation. Several authors have suggested that rates of elder abuse increase under this pressure, becoming more prominent as a social problem (Brogden and Nijhar 2000). In a similar vein, where populations are increasingly migrating from rural to urban communities, traditional responsibilities for caring are eroded or displaced, and this creates gaps that have to be filled by professional networks or volunteer organizations.

So-called 'economizing' usually involves reducing investment in the induction and development of a professionalized workforce, but it may also involve failing to see vulnerability or hiding behind a myth of disappearing family care. Recruiting staff from poor, disadvantaged and discriminated against communities may leave people who feel themselves to be deprived looking after a group of people whom they see as undeserving; for example, poor black staff looking after older people who do not belong to their communities and whose own families are seen not to care for them. This leads to unhelpful and uncomfortable dynamics of exploitation, with shadows left over from the difficult heritage of 'servant-hood'.

Sexual transactions also take place against these backdrops, and in many cultures women and men with disabilities are disadvantaged in the market for economically viable partners, leaving them at risk in hostile encounters or economically led marriage arrangements. Young women with intellectual disabilities, for example, may be married to older men or young able-bodied women may be married to intellectually disabled men for the sake of immigration status or economic gain, without their full or informed consent. Sexual minorities are doubly disadvantaged, with

disabled gay men being put at more risk of both homophobia and abusive transactions and finding themselves unable to protect themselves from
sexually transmitted diseases or HIV. Women with disabilities are often
caught in partnerships characterized by poverty and unequal power, where
they are at risk of domestic violence or unwanted pregnancy. And women
who become disabled later in their adult lives are more likely to be abandoned than cared for by their partners. The material conditions of a person's life cannot be disregarded just because they have a disability, because
a person's disability is managed within the limitations set by such matters.

But the particular forms of organized care services also create specific
patterns of risk. In the United Kingdom, these 'protection' systems had
their roots in the closed world of state-funded services but now struggle to
cohere in relation to the multiplicity of not-for-profit and for-profit agencies
that currently make up the market for care in the United Kingdom and the
United States. And while Western countries that provided state-run services
struggled to prevent abuse in their institutions, those countries relying on
care from church and faith-based organisations have also seen high levels
of abuse behind closed doors and their governments and civil authorities
have been penalized for failing to monitor and hold these organizations to
account. Meanwhile in countries with a market in care provision, satellite
services tend to drift away from standard practices and are able to evade
regular scrutiny, sometimes leaving individual service users at the mercy of
poor or unscrupulous providers. Each country needs to design checks and
balances, regulation and scrutiny, specific to the structure of care provision
in its own jurisdiction.

Nor is abuse confined behind borders, because the ubiquity of trafficking in the sex trade and of economic migration means that these difficulties
move across our countries, with painful traumas being re-enacted in new
countries. United Nations troops occupying the roles of peace-makers have
been convicted of sexual abuse, and international charity workers in impoverished settings have been convicted of sexually abusing children, which
demonstrates how international these issues have become. Internet porn
and child pornography presents one of the most challenging exceptions to
rights of free expression and the unrestricted circulation of material via the
Internet, prompting European countries to launch shared protocols allowing websites to be closed down so the abuse of children is not repeated in the
virtual world once they have been restored to safety. These protocols have
culminated in an international agreement to take robust measures against
these new forms of exploitation (Council of Europe 2007).

What are the practice issues?

Faced with abusive practices, workers need a particular skill set and motivation towards integrity. They often need to feel able to stand up to their

own community's devaluing of disabled or other vulnerable groups, for example to challenge homophobia or to assert the rights of women who have suffered domestic violence. In going against the grain, they often put themselves at risk in myriad ways, from being ostracized by a work group to being made the target of hate crimes themselves. Independent bodies to support 'whistle-blowing' may go a little way towards mitigating these risks, but even they cannot make reporting abuse a comfortable or easy matter.

Skills in assessing and working with vulnerable people need to be augmented to include investigative and quasi-legal skills, alongside independent advocacy (both legal and non-legal) and to include skills in counselling and acknowledging trauma. Professionals need to be 'elastic' so that they can move from working collaboratively and supportively with families, colleagues in sister organizations and state bodies, into a position of challenging and policing them when this is called for. Making this switch is very difficult for individual workers and is often delayed or undermined by lack of confidence or the absence of a clear mandate in situations where facts are hard to come by or explanations are ambiguous.

Much effort is currently being invested in training at a range of levels, in the light of radically changing demographics, service design and legislation. At one end of the scale there is a clear need for highly trained practitioners, able to exercise professional judgment in both complex legal and personally sensitive situations, skilled in recognizing the signs of abuse and vulnerability in adults, possessing the communication skills to establish working relationships in fraught situations in services and families. Particular training needs have emerged in relation to assessing capacity to make informed decisions, understanding the complexity of judging the severity of harm, and developing a multi-faceted view of the thresholds of becoming an 'adult at risk'. One study with a sample drawn from three authorities pointed out that referrals were split evenly between those who lived at home and those in residential care, which reminds us of the training needs amongst this staff group and that institutional care itself is not necessarily the safeguard it is sometimes assumed to be (Mackay *et al.* 2011).

However, the requirement for awareness and training, broadly defined, goes beyond the professional sphere. Building community capacity to support individuals is crucial to the protection of vulnerable people, as is the promotion of public awareness agenda and what might be termed 'zero tolerance' for abuse of vulnerable people. Professionals alone cannot keep individuals safe – real protection is 'co-produced' by individuals, communities and professionals (Hunter and Ritchie 2007; Schwartz 1992), meeting the need for an increasingly sophisticated and knowledgeable work force alongside community awareness raising, initiatives and resourcing.

Leadership is complex in these settings. It needs to meld supervision as oversight with supervision as reflection and debriefing. Working with abusive individuals and just knowing about abuse that has been done to a vulnerable person can create a kind of vicarious traumatization, because as one worker explained, 'You cannot unknow' what you have faced. Managers also need to be skilled in diagnosing the root of problems and the extent to which abuse has been intentional or driven by personal pathology, or situational and a product of service structures, staff shortages, knowledge gaps or a bullying peer group. For example, screening the workforce makes sense as a way of reducing the chances of paedophiles or serial sexual offenders entering the workforce in order to exploit children or vulnerable adults (although it can never do so completely), but if a service is set up without enough, or appropriately skilled, staff, then individuals will be punished for organizational failures and a worker removed from the workforce will be simply replaced by someone else who is put into the same untenable situation. Moreover, because the workforce is so mobile, it is unlikely that whole systems regulation can be managed across borders and/or that professional registers can tell the whole story.

Concluding remarks

As the dynamics of abuse have been revealed by research and through the documentation of day-to-day practice, it has become clear that managing vulnerability without disempowering children and adults is a challenging area of social work that requires advanced knowledge, managerial skills and face-to-face skills. The legislative frameworks in our different countries have to balance autonomy with a mandate to step in when a vulnerable person is under duress, or when a vulnerable group is being unacceptably hidden away or singled out for bullying and harassment. Ensuring that positive accounts and images of disability and older age are put into the public domain can create a positive story about difference and help to create a public mandate for respectful treatment. Community leaders need to counter any suggestion that these are people who can be abused with impunity, and expressing positive regard for people who might otherwise be marginalized is an essential bulwark against the tolerance of abuse and exploitation, whether this takes place in institutions, behind the closed doors of family life or in public places. We have strong international bodies and instruments such as the United Nations Convention on the Rights of Disabled People to guide us in creating proportional safeguards and upholding individual rights. We can no longer afford to work alone on these agendas; we must learn from the people who rely on our services and on our support, and because abuse crosses borders, we must learn together how to be effective in preventing it.

References

Brogden, M. and Nijhar, P. (2000) *Crime, Abuse and the Elderly*, Cullompton: Willan Publishing.

Brown, H. (2002) *Safeguarding Adults and Children With Disabilities Against Abuse*, Strasbourg: Council of Europe Publishing.

Brown, H. (2009) 'The process and function of serious case review', *Journal of Adult Protection*, 11(1): 38–50.

Brown, H. (2011) 'The role of emotion in decision-making', *Journal of Adult Protection*, 13(4): 194–202.

Brown, H., Stein, J. and Turk, V. (1995) 'The sexual abuse of adults with learning disabilities: Report of a second two-year incidence survey', *Mental Handicap Research*, 8(1): 3–24.

Council of Europe (2007) *Convention on the Protection of Children against Sexual Exploitation and Sexual Abuse*, CETS Publication No. 201, Strasbourg: Council of Europe Publishing.

Department of Health (2000) *No Secrets: Guidance on Developing and Implementing Multi-Agency Policies and Procedures to Protect Vulnerable Adults from Abuse*, London: HMSO. Online. Available at: www.gov.uk/government/uploads/system/uploads/attachment_data/file/194272/No_secrets__guidance_on_developing_and_implementing_multi-agency_policies_and_procedures_to_protect_vulnerable_adults_from_abuse.pdf (accessed 14 August 2013).

Hammerburg, T. (2009) *Persons With Mental Disabilities Should Be Assisted But Not Deprived Of Their Individual Human Rights*, Strasbourg: Council of Europe Publishing.

Hollomotz, A. (2012) 'Are we valuing people's choices now? Restrictions to mundane choices made by adults with learning difficulties', *British Journal of Social Work*, doi: 10.1093/bjsw/bcs119.

Hunter, S. and Ritchie, P. (2007) *Co-production and Personalisation in Social Care. Changing Relationships in the Provision of Social Care*, Research Highlights 49, London: Jessica Kingsley.

Kempe, H. (1971) 'Paediatric implications of the battered baby syndrome', *Archives of Disease in Childhood*, 46(245): 28–37.

Learning Disability Alliance (2011) 'More protection for adults at risk', *LDA Newsletter*, issue 34. Oct. Dalkeith.

Lonne, B., Parton, N., Thomson, J. and Harries, M. (2008) *Reforming Child Protection*, London: Routledge.

Mackay, K., McLaughlan, C., Rossi, S., McNicholl, J., Notman, M. and Fraser, D. (2011) *Exploring How Practitioners Support and Protect Adults At Risk Of Harm in the Light Of The Adult Support and Protection (Scotland) Act 2007*, Stirling University Research Report. Online. Available at: https://dspace.stir.ac.uk/handle/1893/3524 (accessed 14 August 2013).

Manthorpe, J. and Martineau, S. (2012) '"In our experience": Chairing and commissioning serious case reviews in adult safeguarding in England', *Journal of Social Work*, 12(1): 84–99.

Manthorpe, J., Stevens, M., Rapaport, J., Harris, J., Jacobs, S., Challis, D., Netten, A., Knapp, M., Wilberforce, M. and Glendinning, C. (2009) 'Safeguarding and system change: Early perceptions of the implications for adult protection services of the English individual budgets pilots – a qualitative study', *British Journal of Social Work*, 39(8): 1465–80.

Munro, E. (2011) *The Munro Review of Child Protection: Final Report. A Child Centred System*, Department for Education Publication Cm 8062, London:

Stationery Office Ltd. Online. Available at: www.gov.uk/government/uploads/system/uploads/attachment_data/file/175391/Munro-Review.pdf (accessed 14 August 2013).

Patrick, H. and Smith, N. (2009) *Adult Protection and the Law in Scotland*, Haywards Heath: Bloomsbury Professional.

Schwartz, D. (1992) *Crossing the River: Creating a Conceptual Revolution in Community and Disability*, Northampton, MA: Brookline Books.

Stalker, K. and Harris, P. (1998) 'The exercise of choice by adults with intellectual disabilities: A literature review', *Journal of Applied Research in Intellectual Disabilities*, 11(1): 60–76.

Tomita, S.K. (1990) 'The denial of elder mistreatment by victims and abusers', *Violence and Victims*, 5(3): 171–84.

Wardhaugh, J. and Wilding, P. (1993) 'Towards and explanation of the corruption of care', *Critical Social Policy*, 13(37): 4–31.

Chapter 8

Social work in a post-9/11 context

Integrative practice with immigrants and refugees in the United States

Amelia Seraphia Derr and Biren (Ratnesh) A. Nagda

A *few days after 9/11, a 16-year-old Somali girl was attacked and stabbed at a gas station ... About four days later six Somali women were fired for wearing the hijab. Soon after, the hawalas were raided. Then three grocery stores were targeted by the USDA. Our whole community was suffering. First, we couldn't send money to our families and then we couldn't even do our shopping for food. Our children were suffering from not being able to eat our halal meat. Even the school nurses testified that our children were weak because of this. Still now, a lot of cab drivers are getting harassed from the police and clients. They are afraid to come out and stand for their rights. People are getting calls from FBI agents who are asking questions about relatives and other personal questions ... America is our new home. It could have been any of us in that building. After September 11th, it didn't matter if you were a U.S. citizen. It didn't matter if you were a U.S. resident. It didn't matter anymore. Once again we had no rights. We have no voice.*

(Testimony of a Muslim woman quoted in Derr 2002)

Once I stayed after school to play basketball, two boys came up and one boy had boxing gloves on. One boy took my basketball and he started punching me until the teacher came and gave me my basketball back and I was on the ground crying. I have been hit so many times. I don't even know why the point I came to America for ... I thought things would get better. Ever since I have come to America I have gone to a different school at the end of every school year. So I was tired of moving around and trying to make friends. When I moved ... I thought it might go away 'cause nobody knew me here so I thought maybe I could be different ... I tried to fit in. Then September 11th happened and people started being mean to me again. Calling me Habib, towelhead, diaperhead. People called me Osama and Osama's son ... It made me feel very bad when they called me diaperhead because I love my hair, it is part of my religion and I never want to cut my hair ... It hasn't gone away since September 11th and people still call me those names. I wish kids who bully would just quit. Can't they see it hurts people? Even if they don't show it? I know teachers know it goes on in school and they just ignore it. Please don't ignore it.

(Testimony of a Sikh boy quoted in Derr *et al.* 2005)

The testimonies of the Muslim woman and the Sikh boy give voice to the dramatic changes in the public, community and personal lives of immigrants in the United States after the terrorist attacks of 9/11. Hate crimes, school bullying, employment discrimination, racial profiling and detention and deportations without charges all increased immediately and in the years after the attacks. Policies such as the USA PATRIOT Act, the National Security Entry-Exit Registration System (NSEERS), and the Alien Absconder Apprehension Initiative singled out Arabs, Muslims, Sikhs and South Asians and made profiling and targeting institutionally justified (Rodriguez 2008). Policymakers legitimized civil rights violations in the name of personal and national security. The tenor of public sentiment shifted to an aggressive and intolerant view towards immigrants. Many communities experienced religious, ethnic and racial violence with little recourse to justice.

This chapter focuses on the changing nature of social work practice with immigrants and refugees in the United States in a post-9/11 context. We begin with a discussion of the nature of the backlash after 9/11 and illustrate its impact on immigrant and refugee communities at the macro-, meso- and micro-levels. Next, we highlight how the national social work bodies responded to the aftermath of 9/11. We follow this by presenting an integrative practice model with corresponding practice principles that we illustrate with a case example from our work with immigrants in the Pacific Northwest of the United States. We conclude the chapter with practice and policy recommendations.

Post-9/11 backlash

The tragic events of 9/11 left a lasting scar on the United States. Never before in the memory of most of the population had there been such a dramatic assault on US soil.[1] For some, the feelings of hatred and desire for retaliation against those who were responsible for the attacks manifested as heightened anti-immigrant sentiment. Individuals and communities who were mistakenly associated with the Taliban were victims of overt backlash. Muslim and Sikh Americans, many of whom were immigrants, were most often targeted with violence and discrimination. Although the backlash was heavily directed towards these two religious groups, a process of what Joshi (2006) calls racialization of religion occurred in which anyone 'looking' Muslim was also targeted. Thus, the reach of the backlash extended into many communities of colour and religious groups.

Macro-level backlash: institutionalized targeting of immigrants

At the macro level, the backlash involved wide-sweeping policy changes that restricted the rights of immigrants within the United States. For example, the USA PATRIOT Act, passed on 26 October 2001, allowed for detentions and deportations without charge (Besthorn 2008). Prior to this legislation, detainees were informed of charges against them and given an opportunity to access legal counsel. The new law made that right obsolete; many detainees were held for months without knowing why and were then deported. In another example, the NSEERS Special Registration programme required all non-citizen men from 24 Arab and/or Muslim countries[2] who were 16 years of age or older to report to immigration control, where they were photographed, fingerprinted, interrogated and sometimes deported (Martin and Martin 2004). Within approximately two years, over 80,000 men registered. Of these, 13,799 were placed in deportation proceedings, and 2,870 were detained (Asian American Legal Defense and Education Fund 2004). Other policy changes after 9/11 increased local law enforcement capacity to enforce federal immigration laws, made it more difficult for immigrants to obtain driver's licences and delayed family reunification (Constitution Project 2008; Penn State University Dickinson School of Law Center for Immigrants Rights 2009; Rodriguez 2008).

Muslim and Sikh immigrants also faced increased discrimination in the workplace. The Equal Employment Opportunity Commission (EEOC) recognized that post-9/11 employment discrimination based on religion and national origin was a distinct phenomenon and tracked and reported it separately from other categories. In the first few months after 9/11, the EEOC reported a 250 per cent increase in this type of discrimination and in the 15 months after 9/11 it handled 705 reports of people fired or harassed due to post-9/11 discrimination (EEOC 2011; Ibish 2003). Local immigrant organizations reported that people were fired from their jobs for refusing to remove religiously-mandated headwear or for needing to pray at certain times of the day (Hate Free Zone Washington 2002). Government efforts to combat terrorism meant a shifting policy landscape that often targeted immigrants with racial and religious profiling. These policy changes served as institutional justification for acts of hatred and violence that occurred on meso and micro levels.

Meso-level backlash: intergroup conflict and violence

At the meso level of social interactions, intergroup conflict erupted between angry Americans and those they saw as representations of terrorists simply because of their accent, skin colour or religious practices. An 'us versus them' mentality pervaded on borders and in schools, neighbourhoods and workplaces. Anti-immigrant groups became more organized and vocal.

For example, the Minutemen Project took the law into their hands and began patrolling the US borders, armed and looking for migrants, including those they suspected as terrorists (Navarro 2009). Muslim, Sikh and Jewish places of worship were sites of xenophobic vandalism and violence. In Seattle, for example, a man drove his car into a mosque, poured gasoline on the mosque and shot off a gun (Kamb 2001). In an effort to protect themselves from growing violence, immigrants owning stores or providing public services attempted to assert their 'Americanism' by displaying US flags in their cabs or business windows and wearing patriotic clothing. Similarly, mosques and gurdwaras also deployed signs of patriotism to stem the tide of backlash, and some members of religious communities felt the need to hide their religious identity (Abu El-Haj and Bonet 2011; Shammas 2009; Singh 2002).

Micro-level backlash: hate crimes and bullying

At the micro level, individuals and families faced increasing psychological trauma. Hate crimes against Muslims rose by a staggering 1,600 per cent after 9/11, according to the Federal Bureau of Investigation (2002). Bullying and harassment of Muslim and Sikh students skyrocketed (Britto 2011; Singh 2011). Children were scared to go to school because they were mistakenly associated with terrorists. For example, devout Sikhs are required to keep their hair unshorn and covered. This head covering became an easy target for abuse. Many families made the difficult decision to cut their children's hair in an attempt to hide their religious identity and shield them from threatened violence. Some families decided to move back to their country of origin and give up on the dream of living in the United States (Asian American Legal Defense and Education Fund 2004). Not surprisingly, this type of discrimination and abuse after 9/11 has been shown to be associated with increased distress and negative health and mental health outcomes (Padela and Heisler 2010; Rousseau *et al.* 2011).

Social work's response to 9/11

Oftentimes, the micro, meso and macro levels of the post-9/11 backlash overlapped; individuals and families commonly experienced more than one form of attack. However, the profession of social work's public response to the events of 9/11 focused only on micro-level intervention. Social workers comprised 50 per cent of the onsite crisis counsellors and were at the forefront of promoting healing in response to experiences of trauma at the World Trade Center in New York City, at the crash site of Flight 93 in Pennsylvania, and at the Pentagon in Washington, D. C. (Tosone *et al.* 2011). The social work response after 9/11 addressed two aspects of micro-level intervention: victim care and clinician self-care.

Providing services for the victims of 9/11 – those who lost loved ones or witnessed the terrorist attacks – was the primary focus of social work organizations. National social work organizing bodies issued guidelines for grieving and bereavement care (Clark 1997), for providing crisis counselling for disaster victims (O'Neill 2001a), and for talking with children about the horrific events of 9/11 (NASW 2002; Rosenfeld 2001). Normalizing the help-seeking process was another priority for the National Association of Social Workers (NASW); its official statement on 9/11 included a reminder that 'asking for help is a sign of strength, not weakness' (NASW 2001a: 1). Social workers contributed financially through the 911 Fund: A Social Workers Response, an effort to support disaster relief work and victim care (O'Neill 2001b).

Social workers were also concerned with secondary trauma and compassion fatigue within the workforce. The events of 9/11 had lasting effects on social workers involved in the disaster relief (Bauwens and Tosone 2010). NASW documented the symptoms of clinician trauma such as anxiety, sleep disturbance and hyper-vigilance (O'Neill 2002). Social work scholars found that clinicians with prior exposure to traumatic life events were more resilient after 9/11 (Tosone *et al.* 2011), and those with secure attachment were more able to cope with secondary trauma while working with victims (Tosone *et al.* 2010).

Despite the field's prominent role in advocating for healing for victims and service providers after 9/11, when it came to the violent targeting of US residents who were perceived to be 'the enemy', national social work groups were slow to respond and seemingly unaware of events occurring in immigrant communities. Although the social work values of social justice, dignity and worth of the person and empowerment should compel efforts to change oppressive situations such as the post-9/11 backlash, national social work organizations, practitioners and scholars were relatively silent and apolitical. The NASW issued a statement after 9/11 urging social workers to be aware of prejudice against Arabs and Muslims (NASW 2001b), but offered no guidance for working with victims of the backlash. This lack of a nationally organized and public response to the backlash against immigrants in the wake of 9/11 belies the field of social work's commitments to social justice and human rights, and serves as the impetus for further reflection in our case study regarding social workers' response to the emerging needs of immigrants and refugees in the United States.

Case example: integrative response to the post-9/11 backlash

Although the predominant public social work response to 9/11 was at the micro level, some scholars advocated for a more integrated approach in order to effectively respond to emerging issues of the backlash. One study that documented the effect of the 9/11 backlash on Muslims highlighted a 'need to work across levels of practice, from individual to institutional, to promote effective change' (Barkdull *et al.* 2011: 151). Our case example showcases just such an integrated practice approach.

In contrast to national social work organizations, many immigrant organizations mobilized quickly to stop the backlash. Groups like the Sikh Coalition, the Council of American-Islamic Relations (CAIR), South Asian Americans Leading Together (SAALT), and the American-Arab Anti-Discrimination Committee worked to educate the general public and provide legal and advocacy services to backlash victims. In some areas of the country, such as in our case example, social workers who were closely tied to these grassroots community efforts became aware of the backlash events before larger mainstream social work organizations, and thus were able to be partners in a broader movement.

The Pacific Northwest of the United States is home to a large number of Sikh and Muslim immigrants. Though far from the attack sites, the area saw numerous events after 9/11 that targeted these local communities, leading to widespread fear and isolation. One local non-profit organization, whose mission addressed domestic violence in the South Asian community,[3] mobilized its volunteer base to respond to this alarming increase in violence towards immigrants. These early volunteer efforts quickly morphed into a separate non-profit organization[4] with a mission to combat the trend of hate and discrimination. Its strategy addressed the backlash on three levels: advocacy for victims, education programmes and community organizing. Social workers from a local university[5] were involved in these initial efforts and became an integral part of the emergent organization. They provided advocacy services, led educational campaigns and facilitated community dialogues. As the organization developed, a social worker was hired on staff, which allowed for a permanent practicum placement for MSW students at the agency. The first author of this chapter, Amelia Seraphia Derr, was employed as a social worker in this agency for five years, and co-author Biren 'Ratnesh' Nagda collaborated on community outreach and education efforts as part of his service activities at the local university.

A model for integrative practice

In the rest of this chapter, we draw on our work with the non-profit agency to discuss an integrative practice model of working with the targeted immigrant and refugee communities. In responding to the backlash, we addressed the macro, meso and micro levels through an integrative model that recognized and acknowledged the realness of violence and disempowerment and sought to mobilize the individual, social and structural resources for empowerment. Working with immigrant and refugee communities, we needed to attend to issues of identity and social position in home and host countries, to honour the strength of specific religious and ethnic identities but dissolve the insularity of the communities, and to work with the complementarity of informal social support networks and the newness of formal social services.

To develop an integrative practice model that did not compartmentalize interventions solely at the micro, meso or macro levels, but harnessed the potential of interventions at each level to leverage change at all levels, we drew upon our extensive practice with structural and critical social work (Moreau 1990; Mullaly 2007) and intergroup dialogue (Gurin *et al.* 2013; Nagda and Gurin 2007; Nagda *et al.* 1999). Structural social work (Mullaly 2007) and critical social work (Moreau 1990) scholars advocate for an approach to social work practice that contributes in all ways to social change. However, such an approach does not focus solely on structures as targets of social change, but also provides care to those targeted by supremacist ideologies and institutions (Mullaly 2007).

> [Structural social work] situates seemingly individual problems within social and material conditions and alienating social structures while at the same time emphasizes the importance of human agency ... [It] attempts to bridge the duality of the personal and the social, the individual and community, and offer social workers an understanding of diverse populations in the context of social structures and social processes that generally support and reproduce social problems.
>
> (Lundy 2004: 55–7)

Moreau (1990) particularly has underscored the processes of critical thinking, consciousness-raising and empowerment as part of structural social work. Intergroup dialogue extends these processes to a critical-dialogic approach that calls for (1) an attention to consciousness raising, an awareness of structural inequalities and individual social identities; (2) building relationships within and across differences; and (3) envisioning change and taking action (Zúñiga *et al.* 2007). These processes are centred on respectful and reciprocal dialogic, face-to-face engagement that honours group identities while forging relationships across difference and mobilizing relationships for social change. Informed by these practice theories and approaches, and working directly with immigrants post-9/11, we developed three practice principles: (1) awareness of insider-outsider status; (2) work within and across communities; and (3) agency through struggle and hope. Figure 8.1 illustrates the relationship between these practice principles and the post-9/11 backlash. It shows the comprehensive context of our work: the impact of the backlash on immigrant and refugee communities at the macro, meso and micro levels, the agency responses to the backlash and the emerging practice principles that highlight an integrative practice approach. In what follows, we discuss each principle and highlight examples of key practices.

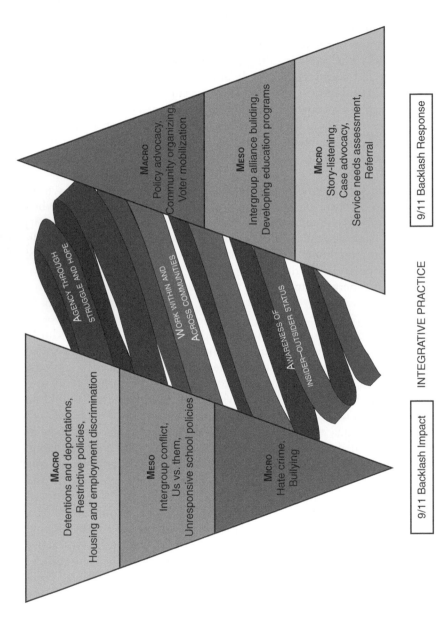

| 9/11 Backlash Impact | INTEGRATIVE PRACTICE | 9/11 Backlash Response |

Figure 8.1 Principles for integrative practice: connecting micro, meso and macro levels.

Practice principle one: awareness of insider-outsider status

Social work ethics and practice with marginalized communities calls for building meaningful relationships with communities and a critical awareness of how power dynamics of insider-outsider status affect the relationship. Professional privilege can render social workers outsiders and separate from the community. Even when the social worker is a member of that community, professional status can create barriers. In contrast, the community has epistemic privilege, which is insider knowledge of the lived realities of daily experiences (Narayan 1988). To build trust and work meaningfully together, social workers need to bridge the community's lived experiences with their own professional identity without enforcing an expert role. Building relationships by creating a space for story-telling and story-listening is crucial to break down the fear and silence related to the targeting.

Social workers at our agency provided one-on-one services for victims of the backlash, including conducting assessments, creating action plans and connecting to other agencies or counsellors as necessary. The advocacy staff, supervised by a social worker and staffed by MSW students, served people experiencing hate crimes, bullying, detentions and deportations, job discrimination and a variety of other concerns. An important part of this work was to listen intently to the stories of the backlash.

The testimony of a young Sikh boy at the beginning of the chapter shows how 9/11 magnified intolerance and continuing harassment of the boy. His plea to teachers to 'please don't ignore it' could apply equally to social workers. By listening to his story and validating his experiences, social workers at the agency were able to build trust with the young boy and his family.

The social worker spent time with the family of the boy to process their experience and move forward with action. The boy had faced years of abuse at school with no intervention, and the abuse escalated after 9/11. A peer who was throwing things at him during class threatened the young boy. After asking him to stop to no avail, he struck out to defend himself from oncoming attacks. He was then charged and convicted of assault. The social workers connected the family to advocacy staff, who worked to prevent the young boy from going to jail. They met with school officials to create a safety plan and organized members of the Sikh community to support him as he faced his court date. With the permission of the family, a story ran in a regional newspaper and members of the community filled the courtroom at his sentencing. In part due to these advocacy efforts, his sentence was reduced from 30 days in juvenile jail to two days of incarceration and the remainder of the time on home arrest. Later, the young boy told his story publicly in front of legislators to raise awareness of the post-9/11 backlash. This led to policy changes regarding bullying at his school and policy changes regarding religious practices at the juvenile jail. The young boy's movement from silence and shame to speaking publicly about his experiences was a testament to his courage, cultivated through a supportive relationship with the agency staff.

It is important that social workers listen and learn from the community and work towards bridging professional privilege with the community's lived experiences. Such bridging can be productive in providing access to resources the community may not be privy to, may not feel entitled to, or may be barred from.

Although the staff from our agency presented themselves as advocates for victims of the post-9/11 backlash, they were often approached for help with other issues such as domestic violence, healthcare needs and substance abuse. The social worker who worked closely with the Sikh community began to notice there was a great need for direct social work services but no agency to which people could be referred. She conducted a community-wide needs assessment and worked in partnership with a local immigrant mental health agency to write a grant and gain funding for a Sikh staff member to be hired to provide culturally responsive social services for that community. Being attuned to the insider-outsider dynamics for both social workers and community members enabled the social workers to practice intentional relationship building through listening, brokering resources within and outside the community, and advocating with school officials.

Practice principle two: work within and across communities

Just as social workers are brokers between individuals and agency/community resources and services, they can also serve as bridges between affected communities. We came to learn that the various ethnic and religious communities targeted in the aftermath of 9/11 were not connected to others who were also experiencing similar backlash. We continuously strived to break down this isolation by creating new relationships. Social workers at our agency led the education programme and efforts to promote intergroup dialogue and connection across communities. The education team, composed of members of communities targeted after 9/11 and allied communities, led training programmes in K-12 and college classrooms, with teachers and law enforcement and at social service agencies.

By working with care and humility to honour the specific experiences of different communities, social workers can mobilize the voices within communities as well as build bridges across communities. Through this active collaboration, for example, the education team at our agency realized a need for more substantive educational material in schools and at trainings. The team organized partners to create a curriculum documenting the backlash after 9/11. The education team thus became a coalition of many of the targeted communities and their allies.

The team, along with partners in the Arab, Muslim, Sikh, Somali and South Asian communities, worked together to define their priorities and write the content of the curriculum. Social work faculty with an expertise in intergroup dialogue and social justice education turned the content into lesson plans with learning goals, structured activities, readings, reflection assignments and dialogue questions (see Derr et al. 2005). The curriculum was used in 11 local school districts and at the university level to provide students with tools to engage across differences in healthy ways and to interrupt post-9/11 backlash happening in their communities. It also led to policy changes regarding bullying at several school districts.

Unexpectedly yet positively, developing the curriculum became a vehicle of collaboration for communities who had not previously been in contact, enabling them to work on a common goal and relate through shared circumstances. Thus, for example, members of the Sikh community became aware of the struggles of the Somali community and vice versa. Through this shared experience, each was able to act as advocates for the other.

Many communities that were not directly affected by the backlash also wanted to build alliances with those who were directly targeted. Such commitment arose from a realization of injustices and, more often, from the lessons of history. This historical connection was critical because many of the affected communities were recent immigrants to the United States, who may not have known or understood the historical precedents and replication of events.

The education team built connections with the local Japanese American community through the Japanese American Citizens League (JACL). The local JACL chapter had a long-standing education programme to teach about the Japanese American internment during the Second World War. As an act of alliance and unwavering support, the JACL invited the team to participate and share a 'then-and-now' perspective linking the issues of Second World War internment to the exclusion efforts post-9/11.

The Japanese American internment of 1942 served as a stark parallel to the detention of Muslims and others post-9/11. The similarity of orders issued by the federal government, demonization of racial, ethnic and religious groups, and fear-mongering all exemplified the historical parallels that illuminated the structured and legitimated nature of violence and exclusion. Thus, by working within and across communities, social workers were able to mobilize previously unforged alliances among those similarly targeted by the 9/11 backlash and those who had deep experiential empathy because of their own history.

Practice principle three: agency through struggle and hope

The necessity for social work intervention post-9/11, as conveyed in the testimonies at the beginning of the chapter, was due to the structural and direct violence on communities. A structural analysis of oppression can sometimes cause social workers to essentialize the affected communities only in terms of marginalization and struggle. Yet these very communities have survived and, in many instances, thrived precisely because of their strong ethnic, racial and/or religious identity and community support. Thus social workers must carry a twin consciousness – to recognize and validate the struggle of structural marginalization and its impact on communities and to mobilize hope embodied in the strengths of communities.

The staff at our agency encouraged individuals coming to the agency through the advocacy or education programmes to use their personal stories to advocate for policy and societal change. People who were victims of the backlash participated in lobby days at the state capitol and met with legislators. They marched in rallies and led voter registration drives.

The personal stories and experiences of victims, therefore, became bridges for connections with others and to the political process on a path of becoming empowered to make change. Learning about the communities' strengths, survival and success can help mobilize communities and connect their personal voice to a political voice.

Our agency, in coalition with many local and national immigrant, peace, religious and community groups, organized a public forum on the first anniversary of 9/11. Victims of the backlash came forward to share their stories in this public hearing. A panel of elected and appointed government officials bore witness to their testimonies and responded afterwards via a panel discussion. The event was modelled after the hearings held during the 1980s regarding redress for the Second World War Japanese American internment.

Many identities – ethnic, religious, national origin – that were the basis for targeting actually serve as strong sources of strength for communities. As narrated in the Muslim woman's quote at the beginning of this chapter, their strength was drawn from being connected to their home countries as well as desiring, but being denied, that connection with the United States. Speaking out on lived experiences of being targeted as a result of these identities seemed to validate not only the individual speaker's experience but also that of fellow community members and allies. The individual stories resonated with the community's stories. The pain in the story was integrally tied to the hope felt when the community's reality was recognized publicly and responded to by public officials and political leaders. In weaving the stories of different communities together, the political voice simultaneously made visible the injustices suffered by many and mobilized alliances towards justice for all.

Concluding thoughts

Integrative social work practice refers to working at the intersections of macro, meso and micro levels of practice. In many ways, as we have shown, these areas are not distinct, especially in the immigrant and refugee experience post-9/11. The experiences of societal marginalization and marking as the 'enemy' as instituted through securitization and criminalization in federal policies parallels reinforcement or reinstatement of outsider status within residential, occupational and educational settings. What may have been previously perceived to be integrated settings because of social, academic or economic achievement now become more clearly exclusionary (Bhatia and Ram 2009). The forced or compelled assimilation (hair cutting, removing religious items such as the *hijab* or *patka*, wearing the American flag) all reinforces 'otherness' and the pressures to give up racial/ethnic/religious identification in order to fit in and maintain the status quo.

Growing out of our practice with immigrants facing backlash after 9/11, we came to appreciate the importance of harnessing the power of relationships for social justice. At the micro level, the relationship cultivated by bridging immigrant epistemic privilege and social worker professional privilege can serve for greater community empowerment. At the meso level, harnessing the power of social relationships within and outside the communities to break down isolation and to examine similar processes of social exclusion and empowerment is crucial. At the macro level, harnessing political consciousness and political voice while affirming religious and cultural identities and complexities serves to validate private experiences in public forums. While change at each separate level can be effective and important, the integrative approach helps reinforce change at all levels. Thus community mobilization, for example, helped legitimize individual voices and sense of belonging, propelled identity development in newer realities, informed immigrant communities of rights and responsibilities, and brokered access to community and political leaders who in turn could affect change at the local and federal levels. Most importantly, the three practice principles – awareness of insider-outsider status, work within and across communities and agency through struggle and hope – compel social workers to understand the complexity of experiences of immigrant and refugee communities, and to challenge essentialization into either/or dualities and compartmentalization of interventions into singular levels.

Incidents of backlash against Muslims, Sikhs and immigrants after acts of terrorism are not isolated to the United States. Similar situations have occurred around the world. For example, after the London bombings on 7 July 2005, Muslims in Britain were targeted with violence, harassment and discrimination (Shibli 2010). More recently, attacks against Muslims rose in response to the vicious killing of a British soldier on 22 May 2013 (Siddique and Jones 2013). Incidents of violence and discrimination against immigrants and religious communities such as those described in this chapter demand the attention of social work practitioners and the international social work community. Successful and responsive integrative practice approaches, such as the one presented in this case study, can be strengthened through the support of international social work organizations. Policy statements from such agencies that specifically address hate crimes, employment and education discrimination, racial profiling and detentions and deportations without charge could compel national social work organizations to take a stronger stance on these issues and bring awareness to continuing incidents of backlash occurring around the world.

Notes

1 Some people who had been alive during the Second World War likened 9/11 to the devastation felt after the attack on Pearl Harbor. But most people had never experienced such a vicious attack with so many casualties.
2 Men from these Arab and/or Muslim countries (plus North Korea) were required to register: Iraq, Iran, Libya, Syria, Sudan, Afghanistan, Algeria, Bahrain, Eritrea, Lebanon, Morocco, North Korea, Oman, Qatar, Somalia, Tunisia, United Arab Emirates, Yemen, Pakistan, Saudi Arabia, Bangladesh, Egypt, Indonesia, Jordan, Kuwait.
3 Chaya.
4 Hate Free Zone Washington.
5 University of Washington.

References

Abu El-Haj, T.R. and Bonet, S.W. (2011) 'Education, citizenship, and the politics of belonging: Youth from Muslim transnational communities and the "War on Terror"', *Review of Research in Education*, 35(1): 29–59.

Asian American Legal Defense and Education Fund (2004) *Special Registration: Discrimination and Xenophobia as Government Policy*, New York: Asian American Legal Defense and Education Fund. Online. Available at: www.aaldef. org/docs/AALDEF-Special-Registration-2004.pdf (accessed 15 August 2013).

Barkdull, C., Khaja, K., Queiro-Tajalli, I., Swart, A., Cunningham, D. and Dennis, S. (2011) 'Experiences of Muslims in four western countries post-9/11', *Affilia*, 26(2): 139–53.

Bauwens, J. and Tosone, C. (2010) 'Professional posttraumatic growth after a shared traumatic experience: Manhattan clinicians' perspectives on post-9/11 practice', *Journal of Loss and Trauma*, 15: 498–517.

Besthorn, F.H. (2008) 'Post 9–11 terror hysteria: Social work practice and the US Patriot Act', *Advances in Social Work*, 9(1): 17–28.

Bhatia, S. and Ram, A. (2009) 'Theorizing identity in transnational and diaspora cultures: A critical approach to acculturation', *International Journal of Intercultural Relations*, 33(2): 140–9.

Britto, P. (2011) *Global Battleground or School Playground: The Bullying of America's Muslim Children*, Washington, DC: Institute for Social Policy and Understanding. Online. Available at: www.ispu.org/Getpolicy/34/2294/ Publications.aspx (accessed 15 August 2013).

Clark, E. (1997) *Bereavement Care for the Adult*, Washington, DC: NASW. Online. Available at: www.socialworkers.org/pressroom/events/911/clark.asp (accessed 21 July 2012).

The Constitution Project (2008) *The Use and Abuse of Immigration Authority as a Counterterrorism Tool: Constitutional and Policy Considerations*, Washington, DC: The Constitution Project.

Derr, A.S. (ed.) (2002) *Struggles in Our Democracy: The Aftermath of September 11th*, Seattle: Hate Free Zone Washington. Online. Available at: www.docstoc. com/docs/101616812/STRUGGLES-IN-OUR-DEMOCRACY (accessed 15 August 2013).

Derr, A.S., Nagda, B.A., Pringle, R. and Gomez, S. (2005) *Justice and Democracy: Challenges and Opportunities in the Aftermath of September 11th, 2001*, Seattle: Hate Free Zone Washington.

Equal Employment Opportunity Commission (EEOC) (2011) *EEOC Remembers September 11, 2011*, Washington, DC: EEOC. Online. Available at: www.eeoc. gov/eeoc/events/9-11-11.cfm (accessed 15 May 2013).

Federal Bureau of Investigation (2002) *Uniform Crime Reports 2001 Hate Crimes Statistics*, Washington, DC: FBI. Online. Available at: www.fbi.gov/about-us/cjis/ ucr/ucr#cius_hatecrime (accessed 12 July 2012).

Gurin, P., Nagda, B.A. and Zúñiga, X. (2013) *Dialogue Across Difference: Practice, Theory and Research on Intergroup Dialogue*, New York: Russell Sage Foundation.

Hate Free Zone Washington (2002) *Justice for ALL: The Aftermath of September 11th. Report from the Public Hearing September 21, 2002*, Seattle: Hate Free Zone Washington.

Ibish, H. (ed.) (2003) *Report on Hate Crimes and Discrimination Against Arab Americans: The Post-September 11 Backlash*, Washington, DC: American-Arab Anti-Discrimination Committee.

Joshi, K.Y. (2006) *New Roots in America's Sacred Ground: Religion, Race, and Ethnicity in Indian America*, New Brunswick: Rutgers University Press.

Kamb, L. (2001) 'Community answers targeting of mosque', *Seattle Post-Intelligencer*, 14 September 2001. Online. Available at: www.seattlepi.com/default/article/ Community-answers-targeting-of-mosque-1065909.php (accessed 15 August 2013).

Lundy, C. (2004) *Social Work and Social Justice: A Structural Approach to Practice*, Peterborough, Ontario: Broadview Press.

Martin, S. and Martin, P. (2004) 'International migration and terrorism: Prevention, prosecution and protection', *Georgetown Immigration Law Journal*, 18(2): 329–44.

Moreau, M. (1990) 'Empowerment through advocacy and consciousness-raising: Im plications of a structural approach to social work', *Journal of Sociology and Social Welfare*, 17(2): 53–67.

Mullaly, R.P. (2007) *The New Structural Social Work*, Don Mills, Ontario: Oxford University Press.

Nagda, B.A. and Gurin, P. (2007) 'Intergroup dialogue: A critical-dialogic approach to learning about difference, inequality and social justice', *New Directions for Teaching and Learning*, 111: 35–45.

Nagda, B.A., Spearmon, M., Holley, L.C., Harding, S., Balassone, M.L., Moise-Swanson, D. and de Mello, S. (1999) 'Intergroup dialogues: An innovative approach to teaching about diversity and justice in social work programs', *Journal of Social Work Education*, 35(3): 433–49.

Narayan, U. (1988) 'Working together across difference: Some considerations on emotions and political practice', *Hypatia*, 3(2): 31–47.

NASW (2001a) *Statement on the September 11th Tragedies in New York, Pennsylvania, and Washington D.C.*, Washington, DC: NASW. Online. Available at: www.socialworkers.org/pressroom/events/911/statement/asp (accessed 7 June 2012).

NASW (2001b) *Defending Our Freedom, Defending Our Values: Ethnic and Religious Diversity*, Washington, DC: NASW. Online. Available at: www.social-workers.org/pressroom/events/911/defend/asp (accessed 7 June 2012).

NASW (2002) *Social Workers Remember September 11 – One Year Later*, Washington, DC: NASW. Online. Available at: www.socialworkers.org/pressroom/events/911/default/asp (accessed 23 May 2012).

Navarro, A. (2009) *The Immigration Crisis: Nativism, Armed Vigilantism, and the Rise of a Countervailing Movement*, Lanham: AltaMira Press.

O'Neill, J.V. (2001a) *New York Turns to Oklahoma for Guidance*, Washington, DC: NASW. Online. Available at: www.socialworkers.org/pressroom/events/911/news/two/asp (accessed 7 June 2012).

O'Neill, J.V. (2001b) *NASW Responds to Terror Attacks*, Washington, DC: NASW. Online. Available at: www.socialworkers.org/pressroom/events/911/news/terror/asp (accessed 7 June 2012).

O'Neill, J.V. (2002) *Facing Clients' Fears, and Their Own: Sept. 11 Anxiety Makes Hard Job Harder*, Washington, DC: NASW. Online. Available at: www.social-workers.org/pressroom/events/911/news/facing_fears/asp (accessed 7 June 2012).

Padela, A.I. and Heisler, M. (2010) 'The association of perceived abuse and discrimination after September 11, 2011, with psychological distress, level of happiness, and health status among Arab Americans', *American Journal of Public Health*, 100(2): 284–91.

Penn State University Dickinson School of Law Center for Immigrants Rights (2009) *NSEERS: The Consequences of America's Efforts to Secure its Borders*, Washington, DC: American Arab Anti-Discrimination Committee.

Rodriguez, R.M. (2008) '(Dis)unity and diversity in post-9/11 America', *Sociological Forum*, 23(2): 379–89.

Rosenfeld, L.B. (2001) *Children's Response to Terrorism*, Washington, DC: NASW. Online. Available at: www.socialworkers.org/pressroom/events/911/rosenfeld.asp (accessed 7 June 2012).

Rousseau, C., Hassan, G., Moreau, N. and Thombs, B. (2011) 'Perceived discrimination and its association with psychological distress among newly arrived immigrants before and after September 11, 2001', *American Journal of Public Health*, 101(5): 909–15.

Siddique, H. and Jones, S. (2013) 'Attacks on Muslims spike after Woolwich killing: Community answers targeting of mosque', *Guardian*, 23 May.

Shammas, D. (2009) 'Post 9/11 Arab and Muslim American community college students: Ethno-religious enclaves and perceived discrimination', *Community College Journal of Research and Practice*, 33: 283–308.

Shibli, M. (2010) *7/7: Muslim Perspectives*, Northolt: Rabita, Ltd.

Singh, A. (2002) '"We are not the enemy": Hate crimes against Arabs, Muslims, and those perceived to be Arab or Muslim after September 11', *Human Rights Watch Report*, 14(6): 1–41.

Singh, R. (2011) 'Bias-based bullying against Sikh children in the post-9/11 environment'. Testimony of Rajdeep Singh before the U.S. Commission on Civil

Rights Briefing on Federal Enforcement of Civil Rights Laws Protecting Students Against Bullying, Violence and Harassment May 13, 2011. New York: The Sikh Coalition.

Tosone, C., Bettmann, J.E., Minami, T. and Jasperson, R.A. (2010) 'New York social workers after 9/11: Their attachment, resiliency, and compassion fatigue', *International Journal of Emergency Mental Health*, 12(2): 103–16.

Tosone, C., McTighe, J.P., Bauwens, J. and Naturale, A. (2011) 'Shared traumatic stress and the long-term impact of 9/11 on Manhattan clinicians', *Journal of Traumatic Stress*, 24(5): 546–52.

Zúñiga, X., Nagda, B.A., Chesler, M. and Cytron-Walker, A. (2007) *Intergroup Dialogues in Higher Education: Meaningful Learning about Social Justice*, San Francisco: Jossey-Bass.

Chapter 9

The making of childhood in a post-modern age

Challenges and possibilities for social work in the United States

Mekada J. Graham

Introduction

Since the mid-1980s, sociologists have fashioned a change of approaches to the social study of children. This wave of scholarly activity, sometimes referred to as the 'new' social study of children, or more recently *childhood studies*, has reframed childhood as a historically and socially specific phenomenon that reflects the particular socio-cultural context of children's lives. The new social study of childhood takes the study of children, located in socialization and development paradigms in multi-disciplinary contexts, to engage with childhood in a variety of interesting ways.

From this perspective, attention is given to children's agency as they construct their own perspectives on daily lived experiences, with recognition that these social experiences are mediated through the social categories of gender, race and disability, unseating universal conventions of sameness and generality. In the context of child welfare, this general interest in children's everyday lives is closely tied to international trends in promoting children's rights and their participation in developing policies regarding the welfare services they receive.

Providing children with opportunities to have a greater say in decision-making processes has been central to discussions about governance in recent years. The backdrop to these developments in promoting children's rights is the United Nations Convention on the Rights of the Child (UNCRC; UN 1989) in shifting attitudes towards children regarding participation in the public sphere and the services they use. Much of the literature surrounding this revised thinking about children and their agency is confined to countries taking up the challenge of the UNCRC (1989).

Although the United States signed the UNCRC document, it failed to ratify the treaty (together with Somalia) in 1989, and since that time little debate or discussion has taken place in the United States about the treaty and its implications for policy and child welfare (Nybell *et al.* 2009).

Matthews (2007: 330) suggests that the absence of these discussions may be linked to a different focus in research where 'children's rights do not resonate in the United States in the same way they do in other countries [and] compared to peer relationships, children's relationships with adults have received relatively little attention in the United States'. Nevertheless, albeit with a different focus on research, childhood studies is a growing field of study in the United States, with an established body of literature outside of child welfare, and in this context has contributed much to improving the status of children.

Even though there is a lack of interest in children's rights in the context of child welfare, children are among the highest users of state services in the United States. The recent economic downturn and retreat of public services has pushed some children and their families on the margins into deep poverty (Sherman 2009). Increasing inequities across the developed world have heightened disparities between rich and poor, and children have taken the burden of these inequities. Finn *et al.* (2010) argue that universal commitments to children have been eroded, citing unequal access to educational resources and public disinvestment in children's welfare in poor and working-class neighbourhoods. As a result of these retrenchments in public welfare, a recent comprehensive study of child well-being placed the United States at the bottom among economically advanced nations (UNICEF 2007).

The purpose of this chapter is to first outline the key elements in the development of the field of childhood studies and outline its broader understanding of children in contemporary society. The next goal is to explore both sociological and psychological approaches at micro and macro levels that underpin models of current practice. The final goal is to identify ways in which childhood studies can contribute to a child well-being model of practice, based upon strengths rather than deficits, taking account of lived experiences and social contexts. This child-centred approach opens up children's lived experiences in public care settings and engages with them as recipients of welfare services.

Revising childhood: an integrated approach to children's lives

Several scholars have recorded the social and economic changes which have taken place over several decades in advanced industrial nations (Beck 1998; Smart *et al.* 2001). These changing conditions have been identified generally as late modernity or globalization and are a common feature of contemporary life. In the same way societal change has altered adult lives in different ways, children are equally affected, with new patterns of consumption and modes of family relationships. Based on Prout (2003), demographic trends including a declining birth rate, smaller families, fewer siblings, together with increased longevity and changing intergenerational relations, have combined to transform the experiences of many children within childhood (UNICEF 2000).

The field of childhood studies has grown rapidly, drawing upon different disciplines such as history, anthropology, psychology and geography to bring about understandings of childhood that construct a more integrated approach – a joined up view of children in context. Kehily (2009), in her introduction to childhood studies, draws attention to the material culture of childhood and the creation of cultural products and practices that separate children from adults. These aspects of childhood bring together social sciences and cultural studies in order to untangle the different ways of being a child and different kinds of childhood in contemporary society. Perhaps the most important feature of this research is the awareness that childhood is not universal; instead, it is a product of culture that varies across time and space.

Childhood studies has taken a critical stance in questioning the taken-for-granted categories offered in established academic discourses by employing post-modern paradigms to consider new cultural patterns of childhood in contemporary society (Alanen 2011). The development of childhood studies, with its focus on children as social beings in their own right, capable of making sense of and affecting their societies, draws attention to the hidden aspects of children's lives and the multiple ways that childhood is socially constructed. This shift brings to the fore the political nature of childhood in conveying the perspectives of children into knowledge production. Opening up these spaces resonates with several hitherto silenced groups and their experiences through stratification and other oppressive practices in many academic structures (Matthews 2007).

As childhood studies advances as an interdisciplinary field, it provides an opportunity to create new spaces for children to convey their perspectives and a better understanding of the complexities of childhood. Children are now re-positioned so that 'children's interrelationships and interactions with others – children as well as adults – as equally important. In doing so, it has allowed a focus on the work that children themselves do to socialize each other (including the way they socialize adults) and how these activities contribute to, and produce, change' (Christensen and Prout 2005: 41).

Alongside these developments, childhood studies is grappling with its definition as a new area of scholarship and the difficulties of drawing clear boundaries and contours, a problem which has troubled other interdisciplinary fields such as women's studies, encouraging questions about their legitimacy and status. By attending to the multiplicity of childhoods from a range of disciplines, it is difficult to weave a unified body of knowledge, since diverse contributions appear to be based upon only a shared interest in children and childhood. At the same time, these various perspectives widen our understanding of childhood and the multidimensional aspects of children's lives. Even though childhood studies is grappling with these issues as it reaches a critical stage in its development, the field has had a major impact in the children's rights movement and the UNCRC in uncovering social and political practices that undermine children's welfare (James 2010).

In response to these developments, the field of children's rights has become a priority, as it translates into the public sphere through the frame of children's anticipated participation in policy and practices that affect their everyday lives. Similarly, this revised way of thinking about children and their participation has begun to enter the social professions, including education, social work and professional training, in reshaping traditional accounts of children in contemporary society. It is to this discussion that I now turn.

Changing paradigms of childhood: key issues and themes for social work

One of the challenges ahead is connecting social workers to changing social, political and economic conditions in relation to the everyday practices in child welfare systems and children's lives. Finn *et al.* (2010) argue that the process of globalization is directly shaping children's everyday experiences and the meanings of childhood. For example, the movement of people across the globe and migration of families and individuals has important implications for children as they come to terms with living in new locations. Finn *et al.* (2010: 248) draw attention to this phenomenon, reflecting that 'more and more children have "travelling lives" as they negotiate complex circuits of migration and changing meanings of identity and belonging'. These features of social change shaping contemporary society provide the context for child welfare practice. Indications are that UNCRC documents are a good starting point in outlining internationally a set of rights for children.

In both the United States and the United Kingdom, social work education has been somewhat reluctant to engage with childhood studies, as its underpinning knowledge is based upon post-modern concepts that are troubling to deep-seated assumptions and ideas in the profession, including social work education (Graham 2011; Nybell *et al.* 2009). Emerging discourses in childhood studies unsettle established discourses, as they recognize children as new 'knowing subjects', who have the capacity to act upon and interact with the social world. These revised paradigms of childhood follow key social changes in Western societies, where conditions of childhood have been re-conceptualized to unlock the 'real' everyday experiences of children and youth in order to understand their position in contemporary society. According to Christensen and Prout (2005: 47), 'children become the direct focus of the analysis rather than necessarily being seen through their link to other social institutions such as family and schooling. This both re-conceptualizes childhood and broadens the range of its referents, context and meanings'.

The approach that applies the socially constructed characteristics of childhood has become increasingly important in shifting a sense of universal childhood to embrace childhood's broader political dimensions. This means that children are viewed in context, and in a place where the social divisions of gender, class and race that frame children's experiences in contemporary social life are considered.

Social work is deeply embedded in the care, well-being and protection of children at risk, and the profession draws upon sociological and psychological theories to shape practice at the macro and micro levels. One of the key pointers of the profession is its commitment to social justice and the well-being of individuals, families, groups and communities. This task was articulated in 2000 by the International Federation of Social Workers as follows:

> The social work profession promotes social change, problem solving in human relationships and the empowerment and liberation of people to enhance well-being. Utilising theories of human behaviour and social systems, social work intervenes at the points where people interact with their environments.
>
> Principles of human rights and social justice are fundamental to social work.

These statements also articulate the idea of person-in-environment in developing a multidimensional understanding of human behaviour, and the field of childhood studies has developed a way of looking at structural oppressions and the link between socio-economic disadvantage and life opportunities of young people leaving care, including low levels of well-being (Goodyer 2013).

Child development theories are among the main theories regarded as particularly significant for professionals because they provide universal benchmarks for setting standards in child welfare. Social workers draw upon these models to inform assessments of children, family relationships, parenting styles and attachment. Although developmental perspectives offer tools in assessing what is 'normal' and assisting in identifying behaviours that may give cause for concern, they also operate within a deficit paradigm, which focuses on limitations and lack of competence, shaping policy and practice interventions (Taylor 2004). These epistemological explanations of childhood are set as a neutral distinct stage in the human life cycle, which offers a scientific account of the 'normal' child as a means of identifying and classifying the 'abnormal child' (Moss *et al.* 2000). The underlying central mode of thought behind universality and movement through stages has been the subject of intense critique, because this powerful discourse leaves out the idea of childhood as a product of history, society and culture.

Moreover, although developmental psychology holds many diverse and competing perspectives, some of which are more attentive to children as subjects, it tends to produce a mainstream model with a vision of childhood as a natural, largely biological process that unfolds through stages in the life course. Taylor (2004) considered these approaches to developmental psychology to ascertain their relevance and importance for practice. Although developmental markers are acknowledged in child development,

Taylor (2004: 228) critically evaluated some key assumptions. First, universal claims are often made about children and the family 'as though children and childhood can be understood trans-historically and trans-culturally, [in other words], children are the same across time and place and there is something static and essential about childhood'. As Burman (1994) explained, these established discourses should be understood within the social and political context in which they emerged, because culture-specific descriptions are all too easily translated into universal prescriptions (Woodhead 1999). These critiques and concerns have encouraged the developmental psychologists to adopt a cultural approach in studying children's development as a socio-cultural process.

In a similar way, sociological perspectives in childhood have been critiqued through the study of socialization and how children become social. Socialization takes the form of a complex set of social processes in which children internalize cultural values through learning and development. During childhood, children acquire the knowledge and skills to become adults and are heavily influenced by their parents, schooling, peers and the guidance of significant others. The social institutions of education, families and material environments are the focus of research, which tends to perceive children in passive roles and as representatives of the future generation. As Graham asserted:

> [C]hildren do not simply internalize the social world, but also interact with structures and strive to make sense of their culture. In this respect, the social context of children's lives becomes accentuated as they are accorded agency as social persons in the fullest sense. As the agency of children evolves, they construct their own perspectives of daily lived experiences, changing notions of children as 'adults in the making'.
>
> (Graham 2011: 1537)

The dominant discourses around childhood framing professional practice have created a deficit model of children and one in which the ages and stages of children as future adults are prioritized, rather than investigating what it means to be a child in contemporary society (Hogan 2005; James *et al.* 1998). Alanen (2004) captured the essence of these discourses by explaining:

> [C]hildren were typically treated as 'dependent variables' of various categories adults, professionals and institutions who 'have' children, take care of them, work on them, are responsible for organizing their living conditions, or are responsible for organizing their living conditions, or in any other way relate to them. Consequently, children were looked upon from the viewpoints of adults, professionals, agencies and institutions.
>
> (Alanen 2004: 2)

As these approaches extend our understanding of childhood in Western societies, underpinning knowledge drawn from developmental psychology continues to be the linchpin in assessing the development of children and evaluating parenting standards. In social work practice, it is argued that without these universal benchmarks, it becomes impossible to set standards which are crucial to child welfare. It is these matters which underlie social work's reluctance to embrace social constructive approaches to childhood. In this context, the focus on the individual child draws attention away from changing social conditions and the ways in which children experience their lives through specific social arrangements based upon their social backgrounds. This model has been strongly criticized by several authors (Alanen 2011; Prout 2013) in seeking to uncover structures and practices that undermine the social standing of children and their agency, and at the same time these criticisms appear to offer few immediate alternatives in a climate of financial realignment and cutbacks in child welfare services.

The focus on children's social agency has important resonance with the profession's responsibility to listen to children and take their experiences and views seriously across a range of practice modalities. These long-standing practice approaches in therapeutic work with children have been taken into a wider context with interest in children's everyday lives. Some of the key features of childhood studies have begun to enter social work, particularly in regard to participation and children's everyday lives. The next section explores children in context and incorporates the idea of giving voice through participation.

Children in context: social conditions

Although children's rights have been central to several discourses in understanding children and childhood, there is a reluctance to discard socialization and peer relationships and instead focus on children's lack of power in relationships with adults. These differences in approach have implications for the way in which the 'child' is conceptualized in social welfare and the promotion of the child's well-being. Early professional practice has been framed within a wholly paternalistic perspective of children, through the lens and viewpoints of adults organizing and taking care of children, and this view has left little room for children to be involved or for their views to be taken seriously (Alanen 2004).

In the context of the general wealth of research about children's everyday lives, researchers are turning to children and youth in public care settings to uncover the living conditions and social circumstances of children who tend to be marginalized, and largely outside of mainstream agendas on children's perspectives (Berrick et al. 2000; Murray and Hallett 2000; Sandbaek 1999; Thomas and O'Kane 2000).

Although the methods used to understand children's lives have generated various theoretical approaches, existing literature tends to underplay the social categories of class, gender and race and how these forces impact upon lived childhoods. There is a pressing need to openly acknowledge the differential position of children in the broader social and political aspects that inform their lives. Goodyer (2013: 398) identifies the ways in which looked-after children's experiences are often neglected. For example, children and young people have often expressed dissatisfaction with social work services that they receive, saying that many social workers are unavailable and unresponsive and are preoccupied with negative issues. Reports of children's views of social work services have consistently expressed similar dissatisfaction (Butler and Williamson 1994; Goodyer 2013; Thomas and O'Kane 1998). Children are also concerned that social workers dwell on negative aspects of children and ignore the good things. Because the childhood studies approach places emphasis on the everyday experiences of children, their capabilities and agency, and values their views, this approach steers away from a deficit model, which often underpins social work with children as 'children with problems'. Using approaches enshrined in childhood studies would consider how a stable education, community membership and the maintenance of supportive social networks might contribute to the well-being of looked-after children and young people.

Clearly, there is growing awareness of different kinds of childhood experiences, where social inequalities and marginalization shape the lives of children and youth from oppressed groups. These complexities of contemporary childhood highlight the respective differences in the quality and character of different childhood experiences. The silence of children from minority communities is often associated with their marginal social and economic status in society in general, and more specifically, this marginalization is exacerbated for those children who are in public out-of-home care settings. By infusing the social context of children's lives into different forms of participation, a more inclusive picture of childhoods can be revealed to fill gaps in knowledge about patterns of discrimination and their impact on the everyday lives of children from minority communities.

Bringing childhood studies into practice

Several authors have bemoaned the fact that we have very little information about children's everyday lives in child welfare institutions (Graham and Bruce 2006; Thomas and O'Kane 2000). Social work often deals with children in difficult circumstances, often away from their families and environments. What are the perceptions and views of children when they are involved in welfare institutions? In what ways can child welfare practice shift the idea of children in child welfare as 'problems' towards a positive view of children's capacities and recognize the importance to children of the physical places and social contexts in which they lead their lives (Hill *et al.* 2004)? These questions can draw upon the research and theoretical frameworks of childhood studies, bringing knowledge of lived experiences and their impact upon the quality of life.

Child welfare disparities among children from minority communities have been the subject of intense debate and discussion among child welfare professionals and policymakers for several decades (Courtney and Skyles 2003; Needell *et al.* 2003). These discussions have sought to account for the over-representation of African American children in child welfare. For example, it is suggested that disproportionate representation is linked to differential treatment ascribed within the child welfare system. Other explanations cite high levels of poverty, unemployment and single motherhood as contributory factors. There is a series of complex relationships between these factors, which requires a sophisticated understanding of the interlocking nature of discrimination and oppression (Bernard 2002). Some authors have pointed to childhood as an integral part of society that is shaped and prescribed by social forces which frame the 'complex relations between children and institutions and the formal and informal hierarchies that influence children's lives' (Christensen and Prout 2005: 58). The focus on individual children largely divorced from their social contexts not only disallows their collective identities, but also promotes processes of exclusion, historical neglect and differential treatment of them as irrelevant or non-consequential (Krieken 1999).

A social model of childhood that incorporates elements of childhood studies through a post-modern lens has been proposed to integrate children's agency and social competencies and diversity among children. In this model, children are seen as active participants, and for children in public care, this means having their views taken seriously and treated with respect. Sandbaek's (1999) innovative study took a participatory approach in engaging with children receiving welfare services. In this research, there was a focus on resources and the positive aspects of children's lives. The accounts of children's everyday lives offer a deeper understanding of their interests, successes and the important persons in their lives. Recognition of social achievements, in which children themselves voice what they regard as successes and positive experiences, help to shift professional practice away from children with problems to opening up spaces of experience and competence. Children in Sandbaek's study were given the opportunity to talk about their social workers and voice their views and perceptions about the welfare services they received.

Another innovative project based in California seeks to empower current and former foster youth, using their voices in training child welfare workers about their needs, desires and cultural experiences. In this way the foster youth perspective can be integrated into child welfare systems. With the assistance of project staff members, foster youth receive training in advocacy, leadership and presentation skills and go on to train child welfare workers, using their voices to explore experiences and their needs.

Conclusion

The general aim of this chapter has been to sketch out the emerging field of childhood studies and its approaches to understanding childhood and children in contemporary society. The growth of research literature, journals and textbooks is evidence that childhood studies is coming of age, joining the growth of 'studies' in academe in creating new spaces and social visions for intellectual work. This critical hub of knowledge about children includes a focus on their agency and everyday lives, together with awareness of new cultural patterns of childhood. These revised ways of thinking about children and childhood are gaining ground, with sustained critiques of traditional accounts of childhood pointing to patterns of social change, globalization and children's rights.

Although child welfare tends to be tied to 'old' conceptualizations of children that have shaped child-care institutions and services, social work generally is attempting to unravel theories and research to explore how this knowledge can be imported into theory and direct practice with children. This engagement is allied to policy considerations about the participation of children in the public sphere. The field of childhood studies has much to contribute to child welfare, particularly its concern about children's agency and their voices regarding social life and experiences.

Children in difficult circumstances are often marginalized, and their views and experiences of child welfare systems and the services they receive are sometimes not recognized. In the years to come, childhood studies will continue to challenge social work to reshape professional knowledge and practice as new thinking about children in contemporary society emerges in a changing world.

References

Alanen, L. (2004) '*Theorizing children's welfare*', paper presented at New Perspectives on Childhood, University of Leeds, UK, 12–14 November 2004.

Alanen, L. (2011) 'Editorial: critical childhood studies?' *Childhood*, 18(2): 147–50.

Beck, U. (1998) 'Politics of risk society', in J. Franklin (ed.), *The Politics of Risk Society*, Cambridge: Polity.

Berrick, J.D., Frasch, K. and Fox, A. (2000) 'Assessing children's experiences of out-of-home care: methodological challenges and opportunities', *Social Work Research*, 24(2): 119–27.

Bernard, C. (2002) 'Giving voice to experiences: parental maltreatment of black children in the context of societal racism', *Child and Family Social Work*, 7(4): 239–51.

Burman, C. (1994) *Deconstructing Developmental Psychology*, London: Routledge.

Butler, I. and Williamson, H. (1994) *Children Speak: Children, Trauma and Social Work*, London: Longman/NSPCC.

Christensen, P. and Prout, A. (2005) 'Anthropological and sociological perspectives on the study of children', in S. Greene and D. Hogan (eds), *Researching Children's Experience*, Thousand Oaks: Sage Publications.

Courtney, M. and Skyles, A. (2003) 'Racial disproportionality in the child welfare system', *Children and Youth Services Review*, 25(5–6): 355–8.

Finn, J., Nybell, L. and Shook, J. (2010) 'The meaning and making of childhood in the era of globalization: challenges for social work', *Children and Youth Services Review*, 32: 246–54.

Goodyer, A. (2013) 'Understanding looked after childhoods', *Child and Family Social Work*, 18(4): 394–402.

Graham, M. (2011) 'Changing paradigms and conditions of childhood: implications for the social professions and social work', *British Journal of Social Work*, 41: 1532–47.

Graham, M. and Bruce, E. (2006) 'Seen and not heard, sociological approaches to childhood: black children, agency and implications for child welfare', *Journal of Sociology and Social Welfare*, 23(4): 51–63.

Hill, M., Davis, J., Prout, A. and Tisdall, K. (2004) 'Moving the participation agenda forward', *Children and Society*, 18(2): 77–96.

Hogan, D. (2005) 'Researching "the child" in developmental psychology', in S. Greene and D. Hogan (eds), *Researching Children's Experiences*, Thousand Oaks: Sage Publications.

James, A., Jenks, C. and Prout, A. (1998) *Theorizing Childhood*, Cambridge: Polity.

James, A. (2010) 'Competition or integration? The next step in childhood studies', *Childhood*, 17(4): 485–99.

Kehily, M. (ed.) (2009) *An Introduction to Childhood Studies*, 2nd edn, Maidenhead: Open University Press.

Krieken, R. (1999) 'The "stolen generations" and cultural genocide: the forced removal of Australian Indigenous children from their families and its implications for the sociology of childhood', *Childhood*, 6: 297–311.

Matthews, S. (2007) 'A window on the "new" sociology of childhood', *Social Compass*, 1(1): 322–34.

Moss, P., Dillon, J. and Statham, J. (2000) 'The "child in need" and "the rich child": discourses, constructions and practice', *Critical Social Policy*, 20(2): 233–54.

Murray, C. and Hallett, C. (2000) 'Young people's participation in decisions affecting their welfare', *Childhood: A Global Journal of Child Research*, 7(1): 11–25.

Needell, B., Brookhart, M. and Lee, S. (2003) 'Black children and foster care placement in California', *Children and Youth Services Review*, 25(5/6): 393–408.

Nybell, L., Shook, J. and Finn J. (2009) *Childhood, Youth and Social Work in Transformation*, New York: Columbia University Press.

Prout, A. (2003) 'Participation, policy and the changing conditions of childhood', in C. Hallett and A. Prout (eds), *Hearing the Voices of Children*, London: Routledge Falmer.

Sandbaek, M. (1999) 'Children with problems: focusing on everyday life', *Children and Society*, 13: 106–18.

Sherman, A. (2009) 'Income gaps hit record levels in 2006: new data shows rich-poor gap tripled between 1979 and 2006'. Available at: www.cbpp.org.

Smart, C., Neale, B. and Wade, A. (2001) *The Changing Experience of Childhood: Families and Divorce*, Cambridge: Polity.

Taylor, C. (2004) 'Underpinning knowledge for child care practice: reconsidering child development theory', *Child and Family Social Work*, 9: 225–35.

Thomas, N. and O'Kane, C. (1998) 'The ethics of participatory research with children', *Children and Society*, 12: 336–48.

Thomas, N. and O'Kane, C. (2000) 'Discovering what children think: connections between research and practice', *British Journal of Social Work*, 30: 810–35.

UNICEF (2000) *A League Table of Child Poverty in Rich Nations*, Florence: Innocenti Research Centre.

UNICEF (2007) 'Child poverty in perspective: an overview of child well-being in rich countries', Innocenti Report Card 7, Florence: Innocenti Research Centre.

United Nations (1989) Convention on the Rights of the Child. Available at: www.ohchr.org/en/professionalinterest/pages/crc.aspx (accessed 22 January 2015).

Woodhead, M. (1999) 'Reconstructing developmental psychology: some first steps', *Children and Society*, 13(1): 3–19.

Chapter 10

Social work and HIV/AIDS in Botswana

Issues, challenges and the way forward

Tapologo Maundeni and Poloko Nuggert Ntshwarang

Introduction

The HIV and AIDS pandemic is a major problem that Botswana is facing in the twenty-first century. Over the years, the situation has been so bad that in an emotional address to the UN in 2001, the then Botswana Head of State,[1] in talking about the impact of HIV and AIDS in the country, made this unusual admission: 'We are threatened with extinction. People are dying in chilling high numbers. It is a crisis of the first magnitude' (McGregor 2002: 1). Even though the country has a high prevalence of HIV infection, at 17.6 per cent (Government of Botswana 2009), recent statistics indicate that Botswana is one of the countries in sub-Saharan Africa that has managed to drastically reduce HIV incidence (new cases of HIV infection). According to UNAIDS (2012) Botswana's new infections decreased by 71 per cent compared to other neighbouring countries such as Zambia, Zimbabwe and South Africa, whose rates have dropped by 58 per cent, 50 per cent and 41 per cent, respectively.

Reduction in the incidence rate could be associated with an aggressive approach used by the government to deal with factors that increase the spread of HIV infection, such as inconsistent use of condoms, alcohol consumption, intergenerational sex, having sex with multiple concurrent partners and low levels of male circumcision. The government has developed educational and awareness-raising programmes, such as television programmes for youth designed to educate them about HIV and AIDS issues. In addition, the alcohol levy has been increased to discourage people from excessive alcohol consumption, and active radio, television and community campaigns have been instituted to encourage male circumcision. Furthermore, stiffer penalties entailing imprisonment of up to ten years have been put in place for those who sexually assault children under the age of 16 years.

In an attempt to deal with the social, economic and psychological consequences of HIV and AIDS as well as to identify prevention measures, the Government of Botswana embarked on a comprehensive approach to HIV and AIDS, including prevention, treatment and care (CSIS Task Force 2004).

Programmes that fall under the above-mentioned comprehensive approach include: a programme of free antiretroviral (ARV) treatment, which is the largest programme of its kind in sub-Saharan Africa; an innovative programme of routine testing for HIV – a step to break through the reluctance, lack of information and stigma that prevent people from acting against the disease (CSIS Task Force 2004); information, education and communication (IEC) initiatives; the creation of the Prevention of Mother to Child Transmission Programme (PMTCT); a home-based care programme that largely relies on volunteers; condom distribution and education (Population Services International 2004); as well as the establishment of the National Orphan Care Programme.

In spite of the various programmes in place, Botswana continues to have the highest rate of HIV prevalence in the world. Various factors have been associated with the rapid spread of HIV and AIDS in the country. One of them is the mobility of Botswana society. Existing literature shows that a typical Motswana (citizen of Botswana) moves among several homes – workplace, home village, cattle post and arable farm (Alverson 1978; Macdonald 1996). Government employees[2] are frequently transferred from one work place to another. Moreover, there is rapid construction of roads, hospitals and schools. Botswana straddles a major southern African trucking route, which has given rise to a booming commercial sex trade – a phenomenon that increases the tendency to have multiple partners, which increases the risk of HIV infection. Existing literature on sex work (Campbell 1997; Ntseane 2009) shows that commercial sex is a thriving industry in developing countries, in the midst of a hostile environment characterized by stigma, exploitation and violence against sex workers. Sex work in the context of Botswana has been linked to poverty and the social construction of masculinity.

The argument that poverty, among other things, contributes to the high rate of HIV prevalence in Botswana should be interpreted with caution, particularly taking into account that there are several African countries with higher rates of poverty than Botswana, yet they have lower rates of HIV and AIDS. Uganda is a good example of such countries. In a paper that analyzed HIV and AIDS policies in Uganda and Botswana, Allen and Heald (2004) argued that factors accounting for Botswana's failure to curb the rapid spread of HIV and AIDS include the prevalence of top-down approaches to HIV policies and strategies, which resulted in a certain level of community resistance to embracing such approaches; condom promotion that fuelled an alternative discourse on AIDS that linked condoms to HIV and AIDS; the widespread perception of HIV and AIDS as a manifestation of old Tswana illnesses acquiring new virulence because people are disrespecting traditional culture; the exclusion of diviners, healers and churchmen from the campaigns; and reluctance to talk openly about sex – partly due to rules of respect that lie at the heart of family and kinship structures. Allen and

Heald (2004) asserted that this unwillingness to openly discuss sexuality limits communication across generations and sexual divides. The authors contended that some of the factors that enabled Uganda to succeed in the war against HIV and AIDS included the emphasis on family values; campaign strategies that involved a wide range of institutions and individuals (both inside and outside of the government sector); the minimal emphasis on condoms; the diversity of Ugandan society that mitigated against cohesive alternative explanations of the disease; and the little resistance that society as a whole displayed towards health care approaches.

One other factor that fuels the spread of HIV and AIDS in the country is cultural beliefs. Botswana culture, for instance, demands that women must be subservient to their men-folk. Culturally, society expects men to control sexual relations within marriage, including decisions on contraception and on whether or not to use a condom. This societal expectation has implications for decision-making, and for women's health needs, particularly family planning, and the use of condoms.

Individuals and families affected by HIV and AIDS are faced with physical, psychological, social and economic challenges. The challenges are a result of the trauma and grief, social isolation, sense of shame and lack of emotional and financial support associated with HIV diagnosis and the death of a relative from AIDS (Nagler *et al.* 1995). Therefore, a wide range of professionals play a vital role in HIV interventions. These include social workers, social development practitioners, psychologists, nurses and medical doctors. This chapter focuses on social work in relation to HIV in the context of Botswana. Its purpose is three-fold: to explore the role of social workers in the area of HIV and AIDS, to highlight challenges that social workers who perform HIV-related work face, and to chart the way forward.

How HIV and AIDS affect people, particularly in the context of Botswana

In order to appreciate the role of social workers and the challenges they experience in the area of HIV and AIDS, it is important to highlight how HIV and AIDS affect people. Some people are themselves infected with the virus; some provide care to sick people; others have lost parents and loved ones due to the disease. The multiple impacts of HIV and AIDS affect people's cognitive functioning, physical functioning and general well-being.

A lot of children have been orphaned by HIV and AIDS. Consequently, they face challenges such as property-grabbing by relatives, inadequate care-giving and poor access to nutrition (Jacques 2010; Maundeni 2009; Mmonadibe 2009). HIV and AIDS have emotional and psychological impacts on people. The loss of relatives, significant others and parents as a result of AIDS often leads to anxiety, depression, fears and uncertainties about the future (Miller *et al.* 2007; Plattner and Meiring 2006).

Prior to the introduction of ARV therapy in Botswana, many families were left without bread-winners, due to the huge numbers of people who were dying. The situation escalated the number of orphans, needy children and destitute persons in the country. People who are HIV positive are often stigmatized and discriminated against. This is caused by lack of basic knowledge and understanding of HIV and AIDS. Stigma is socially constructed, because HIV and AIDS stigma is perceived as an individual's deviance from socially accepted standards of normality, in the form of immorality, promiscuity, perversion, contagiousness and death (Deng *et al.* 2007). According to Ntshwarang and Malinga-Musamba (2012), social stigma also prompts society's negative interpersonal responses towards individuals living with HIV and leads to flawed provenances of blame and responsibility. Some relatives and significant others do not want to be associated with people living with HIV and those suffering from AIDS. The stigma leads to the disintegration of the extended family, which used to be the backbone of support and care for families (Jacques 2003). Therefore the situation sometimes leaves those infected without care and adequate support.

The role of social workers in HIV and AIDS in Botswana

Health and illness are at one level a private or individual matter, while at another, they have implications for relationships and social functioning. For each person infected with HIV, there is also an affected family. Therefore, social workers not only work with people who are infected, they also work with those who are directly and indirectly affected. The government of Botswana employs social workers in various settings to provide services geared towards the alleviation of psycho-social problems experienced by people who are infected and affected by HIV and AIDS. They provide a wide range of services at institutional and community levels. Some of these services are discussed below.

Formation and facilitation of support groups

Social workers are at the forefront of the establishment and facilitation of support groups for people infected and affected by HIV and AIDS. Unlike in some developed countries such as the United States, which are using web-based electronic support, Botswana's technological status and culture still put more emphasis on face-to-face interactions. In most instances, when compared to face-to-face groups, electronic support groups are less effective because they are not moderated; hence unreliable information can be posted on the Internet (Eysenbach *et al.* 2004). Face-to-face support groups allow participants to have contact with social workers and allow continuation of support for issues other than HIV and AIDS. In Botswana social workers facilitate support groups in institutions such as hospitals and in communities at large. Such groups enable clients to get support and information from people with similar experiences. According to Kalichman *et al.* (1996) social support groups offer a means of addressing the support needs of people living with HIV. Findings of a study done in the United States to assess the effects of support groups on people living with HIV indicated that HIV-seropositive people who attended support groups reported less emotional distress and had more social contact than did non-attendees. There is a need to evaluate the effectiveness of existing psychosocial support groups for persons living with HIV and AIDS (PLWHAs) in Botswana.

Assisting clients to meet tangible needs

Social workers also play a role in assisting clients to meet their tangible needs. This role is particularly important, because people who are infected and those affected by HIV and AIDS, such as orphans and care-givers, often lose a source of income; therefore they need assistance in this area. As part of their role, social workers have to assess the individual's and family's capacity to provide basic needs and comprehensive care (Government of Botswana 2009). Where the client, family or the support system cannot provide the required needs, the social worker has to enrol the patient in any of the existing programmes for the needy, such as the destitute persons programme or food basket programme, and offer temporary assistance depending on the situation of the individual or family. For example, some HIV-positive people may have special daily nutritional needs which they are unable to meet; hence it is the responsibility of the social worker to enrol the person in the food basket package programme (Ministry of Local Government 2002). Social workers also have the responsibility to ensure that children who do not have reliable care-givers are taken to places of safety such as Child Line, Save Our Souls (SOS) residential facilities or foster homes.

Beyond the provision of shelter that takes place through the placement of orphans in residential facilities, social workers in the country also assist orphans with other tangible needs. The main document that is specifically tailored to meet the needs of orphans in Botswana is the Short Term Plan of Action (STPA) for the care of orphans. The overall goal of the STPA is to 'improve the socio-economic conditions of orphans by way of investing in human capital, within the broader context of sustainable human development' (Ministry of Local Government 1999: 9). It is worth noting that, to date, services aimed at meeting the basic needs of orphans (provided under the STPA) are uniform to all orphans. In other words, they do not take into account age-specific risks and protective factors that orphans confront on a daily basis. According to Dunn (2005), children develop at varying rates, and are impacted by gender issues due to cultural socialization. Therefore, intervention programmes must be sensitive to the diverse needs of children.

Social workers who are mandated to provide orphan care services engage in the following activities: identifying, assessing and registering orphans in need of general welfare support; identifying and assessing orphans in need of special care, such as HIV-infected, disabled and mentally handicapped orphans; providing food rations, clothing, blankets, toiletry items and shelter as the case may be; identifying local groups purchasing food, clothing and other necessities and distributing them to orphans; providing counselling; referring and registering terminally ill orphans for home-based care; providing skills training; identifying school drop-outs and helping them to go back to school; and training parents on orphan care.

Although the STPA stipulates that the provision of counselling is important, in reality, more often than not, orphans are provided with material assistance and other types of assistance are neglected. This is so because local authority social workers are overwhelmed with the volume of orphans,[3] while others have not received specialized training in child welfare. The few Orphans and Vulnerable Children (OVC) who receive counselling services from local authority social workers are largely assisted on a casework basis. Group work is not popularly used. This is so because of one or more of the following reasons: working hours of local authority social workers are rigid and therefore do not enable people who are free after hours to come for group sessions; some social workers are not thoroughly trained in group work; some issues confronting orphans are so deep and complex that they necessitate the utilization of case work because it takes time for clients to open up; and lastly, some clients lack resources that could enable them to pay for public transport to and from social service agencies on a regular basis.

Provision of education

Apart from addressing clients' tangible needs and providing psychosocial support through support groups, social workers also play the role of educators. The role of social workers as educators has been clearly articulated by the Government of Botswana (2009) which indicates that social workers work at family and community levels to build partnerships and network with stakeholders to pass on information to create awareness of HIV and AIDS. PLWHAs experience stigma, which colours their interactions with health care providers and the community due to the lack of information about HIV and AIDS on the part of the community. As a result social workers play a role in ensuring that the communities and society in general get accurate information about HIV and AIDS. Social workers help people overcome the biases that impede rational responses to the disease and the fears that surround HIV and AIDS by providing compassionate care and education (Ntshwarang and Malinga-Musamba 2012). Social workers do not play the role of educator alone; they sometimes perform that role with a team of multidisciplinary officers such as the police, medical personnel, teachers, psychologists and others who address issues related to their respective professions. A multidisciplinary approach is usually used because clients experience challenges that are diverse, complex and multi-faceted. A holistic or multidisciplinary approach challenges the prevailing trends that emphasize reductionist understandings of human behaviour and narrowly conceived bureaucratic responses to complex problems, affording social workers the ability to cope with the uniqueness of each individual's circumstances and the diverse knowledge sources required to make sense of complex and unpredictable problems (Ruch 2005). The multidisciplinary approach also helps to lighten the work of social workers and quicken ser-vice provision because other professionals and government authorities offer some services to meet the needs of clients.

The provision of education is done through various forums. Some of the forums are peculiar to Botswana, while others are not. One of the for-ums that is unique to Botswana is the *Kgotla*. The Kgotla is the highest public meeting, community council or traditional law court in a village (Moumakwa 2010). The forum is usually headed by the village chief. The spirit of the Kgotla promotes peace, harmony, unity and democratic values through uniting and building the social fabric of local communities in the country. The Kgotla is a forum for free exchange of ideas and views within a democratic environment. Therefore, it is a favourable place for empowering communities about different issues that affect them. Every member of the community is free to attend Kgotla meetings and comment or ask questions regarding issues that are presented. Moreover, the head of the Kgotla is a chief; therefore, he is well respected by the people. In addition, chiefs are custodians of culture, making it essential for them to be part of an audience that is empowered and sensitized in relation to sensitive issues such as HIV and AIDS. The Kgotla has proven to be an effective way of transmitting information on a wide range of issues to communities at grassroots level. One of the authors of this chapter was part of a team that addressed sev-eral Kgotla meetings on various psychosocial issues in December 2011. The attendance in such forums was excellent and the feedback that the team received from communities was very useful. Moreover, the communities also enlightened the presenting team about various socio-cultural issues that are crucial to the well-being of different groups, as well as what could be done to improve such issues.[4]

Other forums that social workers use to educate or sensitize people about HIV-related issues include hospitals and schools. In their outreach work, social workers visit schools on a periodic basis to educate school-going children on important issues that can put them at risk of contracting HIV, such as sexual abuse and engaging in sexual relationships at an early age. Botswana has not yet started the programme of school social work; there-fore the voluntary services offered by social workers add some value to the educational system and the country's efforts to combat HIV and AIDS.

Social workers also play the educational role even in their one-on-one contacts with clients in and outside of families.

In their role of raising the awareness of communities about HIV and AIDS, social workers act as role models through their behaviours. In that way, communities are more likely to embrace the messages conveyed to them. It should be noted that the population of Botswana is small, such that in most rural areas, people know each other. Community members may have high expectations of social workers' professional conduct outside their workplaces. Therefore, people would usually expect social workers to model what they educate them about, especially with regard to healthy sexual behaviour. Furthermore, the effectiveness of educational strategies used by social workers may be hampered by cultural beliefs. For example, older people usually do not expect younger people to talk to them about sensitive issues such as those related to sex. Therefore, messages disseminated by younger social workers may not be fully embraced by older people.

Counselling services

Social workers in Botswana are recognized as key players in promoting high levels of medication compliance in clients with HIV (Kgatlwane *et al.* 2006). For example, they are employed in hospitals to provide adherence counselling to clients who are enrolled on the ARV therapy programme (Ntshwarang and Malinga-Musamba 2012). HIV and AIDS are life threatening, and are likely to cause extreme emotional, cognitive and behavioural strife (Kalichman *et al.* 2007). The consequences of HIV and AIDS, such as depression, stigma, isolation and rejection, often require the infected person and the family to adjust to the HIV status. Thus the provision of counselling enhances the lives of both people infected and people affected, in the sense that it gives them the opportunity to accept their situations and develop measures to enhance their well-being.

Social workers offer various types of counselling, such as pre- and post-test counselling, PMTCT counselling, adherence counselling and grief and bereavement counselling.[5] During pre- and post-HIV test counselling, the social workers assess the clients' risks of exposure to HIV infection or re-infection and help them minimize attitudes and behaviours that increase risks of infection and maximize those that reduce HIV infection (Surface 2007). Social workers are liaisons who facilitate proper communication between the doctors and nurses to help clients fulfil medical orders and who provide a link between the hospital and other agencies and organizations in the community (Davidson 1990).

Community Home Based Care programme

Social workers in Botswana work actively with Community Home Based Care (CHBC) programme officers to ensure that people living with HIV or suffering from AIDS get the comprehensive care they deserve. The CHBC programme started in 1995 as a response to an increase in HIV and AIDS-related illnesses in Botswana (Ntseane and Solo 2007). CHBC is a method of care provided by health and non-health workers to people with terminal illness, including HIV and AIDS, in their homes (Uys and Cameron 2003). It embraces the family as the traditional unit of care and aims to promote the continuum of care to those infected and affected by HIV and AIDS (Government of Botswana 2009). At the hospital level, social workers, in consultation with the health care team, develop and implement a treatment plan that facilitates the patient's integration into home and community to reduce the trauma experienced by clients and care-givers after hospitalization as a result of unmet social and psychological needs (Ntshwarang and Malinga-Musamba 2012). Social workers work hand-in-hand with CHBC volunteers and health workers to ensure that patients in the CHBC programme and their care-givers have food and other items such as nappies and gloves.

Although CHBC eases congestion in hospitals, it has been criticized on the basis that clients are released from hospital to CHBC without proper discharge planning (Kang'ethe 2008). Inadequate discharge planning disadvantages both the clients and care-givers, in the sense that care-givers need to prepare themselves psychologically and economically for the arrival of the clients; hence failure to do so leads to improper care. Moreover, care-giving in the community is gendered, because most of the care-givers are female. The situation has a cultural influence because traditionally mothers and female children are expected to perform household-based chores, whereas men get more involved in chores outside the homes, such as cattle herding and ploughing. Therefore in the era of HIV and AIDS, women end up being overwhelmed by this role, leading to burnout and stress, hence the need to challenge the status quo by encouraging males to participate in CHBC programmes.

Other roles/services

Other roles that social workers play in relation to HIV and AIDS issues in Botswana include resource mobilization, administration and research, as well as acting as secretaries of various committees. In some agencies, social workers also assist in drawing blood samples from patients and sending them to laboratories for HIV testing. This role has received mixed reactions from some hospital social workers in Botswana. Some of the social workers perceive it as the nurses', doctors', lab technicians' and auxiliary staff's role. On the other hand, some view it as a risky activity, for which their employer should provide a risk allowance. In opposition to the negative views, other social workers see it as an activity that expands their scope of work, hence providing opportunity for other types of employment (Ntshwarang and Malinga-Musamba 2012).

So far, much attention has focused on social workers' role(s) in relation to assisting individuals, families and communities. It should be noted that the role of social workers in the area of HIV and AIDS in Botswana is not confined to work with ordinary community members. Social workers are also employed as HIV and AIDS coordinators in government ministries and departments. In their role as HIV coordinators, social workers organize and run workshops on HIV and AIDS, ensure equitable distribution of condoms, coordinate commemoration of World AIDS Day and ensure that HIV and AIDS youth clubs have adequate financial support for their activities at the district level. Coordination of HIV and AIDS work is a contentious issue for national planners. There have been concerns about duplication in planning for HIV and AIDS management, leading to competition between health service providers and organizations. For example, in Uganda, duplication of planning led to competition between the Ministry of Health and the Uganda AIDS Commission for control and funds. In Botswana the multi-sectoral approach to HIV and AIDS has allowed smooth coordination of HIV and AIDS activities through the National AIDS Coordinating Agency (NACA), which reports to the National AIDS Council (NAC).

Challenges faced by social workers in HIV and AIDS interventions

Social workers face several challenges in their efforts to contribute effectively to the fight against HIV and AIDS. These include training gaps, work-related stress, challenges related to disclosure of HIV status, challenges related to multidisciplinary work, difficulties in building sustainable support groups, challenges related to clients' cultural beliefs and practices, and challenges related to behaviour change. These issues are discussed below.

Training gaps

Most of the social workers in Botswana lack specialized training for working with PLWHAs. This is due to the fact that university training at the diploma and bachelor degree levels offers general training that equips them to work in any field.[6] Therefore, it is often a challenge to work in the area of HIV and AIDS without specialized training. Social workers struggle to deal with complex cases and feel incompetent to explain medical issues to clients (Ntshwarang and Malinga-Musamba 2012). Moreover, some of the circumstances in the field can be traumatizing, and if one did not have exposure to such issues during training, the situations can create serious psychological trauma for the social worker. Bamford et al. (2006: 45) emphasized that social workers working with PLWHAs must be culturally sensitive and possess relevant skills. They must also be knowledgeable about HIV infection and family community dynamics.

Work-related stress

Work-related stress is recognized as one of the most serious occupational health hazards in Botswana's health care facilities. The multiple negative impacts of work-related stress are manifested by health workers and reflected in work environments, and these may include physical and emotional symptoms, stress-related illnesses, and decreased well-being of workers, with accompanying negative impact on families. Such stresses may lead to reduced productivity, employee dissatisfaction, absenteeism, and high turnover, resulting in staff shortages and reduced quality patient care (Ministry of Health 2006).

Work-related stress experienced by social workers who work in the area of HIV and AIDS is exacerbated by several factors. One of them is that social work is one of the most overworked, underpaid, under-recognized and distressed professions (Rwomire and Raditlhokwa 1996: 12). The lack of recognition manifests itself in the low levels of remuneration and status accorded to social workers. As a result, social workers are more vulnerable to stress-generating situations, such as role-overload, role-conflict, role-ambiguity, over-responsibility and poor working conditions. By and large, social workers in Botswana provide generic social work services. For instance, social workers employed by local authorities deal with orphan and vulnerable children, destitution, disability, needy students, and marital instability cases and attend meetings in addition, relating to HIV and AIDS issues. They play multiple roles as advocate, broker, counsellor, teacher and liaison in the various cases they handle. This exposes them to heavy workloads and disgruntled service users, which in turn makes them more prone to trauma and burnout (Malinga and Mupedziswa 2009). Many social workers in Africa, and particularly in Botswana, find it difficult to handle work-related stress, resulting in frustrations and reduced efficiency (Rwomire and Raditlhokwa 1996: 12). The situation calls for the implementation of counselling services and on-the-job training for social workers. Ntshwarang and Malinga-Musamba (2012) have also recommended that social workers should engage in more specialized services to decrease burnout and work overload.

One other factor that contributes to stress among social workers is limited resources (both tangible resources such as transport and computers and non-tangible resources such as time). By and large, social workers barely find time to utilize strategies that are meant to help them cope with stress. For instance, as soon as a client passes on, the social worker will immediately move to another new case, and does not usually allow herself or himself time to mourn for the client. This can leave the worker with unresolved trauma. Providers who suffer from the death of more than one patient over a short period of time may experience symptoms of multiple losses.

Disclosure of status

Social workers face issues surrounding the disclosure of the client's HIV status. Social workers often face ethical dilemmas arising from clients' resistance to disclosing their positive status to care-givers. Social workers usually would want to act in the best interest of the client, but at the same time feel responsible for protecting care-givers from HIV infection. Therefore, they have to grapple with educating the clients about the importance of disclosing the positive status to care-givers to ensure maximum support and adequate care to the infected persons. Consequently, there is a need to intensify the education of patients and care-givers on the importance of disclosing HIV-positive status to significant others.

Disclosure is more challenging in cases of children. Insights from social workers around the country have shown that most parents and care-givers of children who are on ARV therapy face a tough time when it comes to disclosing the children's HIV status to them. Some care-givers give children false information about the ARV therapy drugs, and children often learn the truth about their conditions from outsiders. The situation leads to poor adherence to medication and lack of trust and often leaves the children traumatized and distressed about their HIV-positive status (Mmonadibe 2009).

Service provision gaps

In their intervention efforts, social workers work in cooperation and partnership with other sectors of the society (Potgieter 1998: 70). Schurink (1990: 20, 21) alludes to HIV and AIDS as involving professionals from different disciplines and voluntary organizations. This approach could go a long way in improving the success of HIV interventions. However, social workers who participated in a study of their experiences of HIV and AIDS intervention in Botswana pointed out problems with poor internal and external referral systems, poor discharge planning and lack of service provision as well as poor coordination and a low level of cooperation amongst service providers (Kesamang 2007). These sentiments are illustrated by the following quotes:

> But at times they fail to play their part [other hospital professionals]. Some just refer cases that are beyond the competency of social workers.
>
> My experience with the external referral is very bad. We usually refer to Social and Community Development [S&CD]. My experience is that they do not readily attend to patients in time.
>
> No, they do not refer to us neither give us any feedback on the cases that we refer to them [S&CD]. This sometimes makes it difficult to carry out our work.

The lack of feedback on cases that have been referred to social workers adversely affects service providers' ability to improve the welfare of their clients. Therefore, there is need for social workers employed in various organizations to design a referral system that will compel them to provide progress reports on referrals made between organizations.

Difficulties in building sustainable support groups

One other challenge that social workers working in the area of HIV and AIDS in Botswana experience relates to the formation and sustainability of psychosocial support groups. The authors' discussions with social workers between 2009 and 2011 revealed that although social workers are well equipped with knowledge and skills to facilitate psychosocial support groups, their ability to use this method of social work practice is hampered by factors such as lack of funds to meet transport needs of potential participants, as well as the rigid work schedule that they work under. For instance, the vast majority of social workers in the country are employed by the government, and they only work weekdays from 7:30 a.m. to 4:30 p.m. Consequently, they are unable to facilitate groups for working people, who are available largely after working hours. It is recommended that working hours for social workers who facilitate psychosocial support groups should be made flexible, or such workers should be paid overtime so that they can work outside the normal working hours.

Challenges related to clients' cultural beliefs and practices

A study conducted by Kesamang (2007) revealed that social workers who work in the area of HIV and AIDS in Botswana also experience challenges when working with clients whose personal beliefs may differ from the scientifically held understanding of HIV and AIDS. Cultural, sexual, religious and legal influences often make discussion about sexual practices, preferences, sexual desires, the number and type of sexual partners and the use of birth control difficult. Such subjects are taboo and are associated with embarrassment, shame, guilt and rejection. The same feelings may be experienced by care-givers as well. Moreover, some religious denominations and religious leaders do not encourage the use of condoms as a means to control birth and disease transmission (Ministry of Health 2006). This poses challenges and dilemmas to social workers, as they have to advocate for behavioural practices that prevent HIV transmission, such as condom use.

Challenges related to behaviour change

The last challenge discussed in this chapter relates to behaviour change. One would hope that with the introduction of ARV therapy, there would be a significant reduction in the numbers of people who die as a result of HIV-related illnesses, but the reduction has not been significant. Evidence that the country still has a mountain to climb in relation to achieving behaviour change is shown by the continued identification of new infections.

As noted elsewhere, Botswana has the largest ARV programme in the region. This is a step in the right direction; however, it is unfortunate to note that some people who are on ARV therapy continue to engage in risky behaviour (such as having multiple sex partners, non-adherence to treatment and alcohol and drug abuse) that complicates the treatment regime. Such people end up losing jobs as a result of illness and death related to HIV and AIDS. The situation increases the number of people requiring socio-economic services, further straining the existing limited HIV and AIDS resources, including those offered by social workers. These dynamics call for further research in the area of ARV therapeutic adherence, so that new mechanisms can be established to make it easier for people to keep up with the lifetime treatment regime.

Conclusion and way forward

The chapter has shown that social workers play a vital role in working with issues related to HIV and AIDS in Botswana. However, they face several challenges that impact the effectiveness of their services. Acting upon the following recommendations could go a long way to enable social workers to provide services of high quality to PLWHAs and their families.

First, there is a need to equip social workers with knowledge and skills to deal with stress and burnout. Second, social workers need to be adequately trained so that they can be equipped with the skills they need to adequately and effectively execute their duties in the field of HIV and AIDS. Third, in order for social workers to exercise their intervention role in HIV and AIDS effectively, there should be harmony among all concerned stakeholders and/or role-players. Fourth, there is a need to address myths and misconceptions that people have about HIV infection. It is crucial to develop an effective approach to address the breakdown of certain cultural norms that have been eroded by modernization without being replaced (Ministry of Education 2002). Fifth, more resources are needed to enable social workers who work with PLWHAs to discharge their duties effectively. For instance, transport should always be readily available, so that home visits could be conducted whenever the need arises. Moreover, the workload of social workers who work in the area of HIV and AIDS should be reduced so that they could have time to utilize stress-reduction strategies.

Sixth, CHBC tends to be centred on recovery; therefore social workers need to advocate for the establishment of hospice care facilities, because such facilities focus more on assisting people who are in end-of-life care so that they can die comfortably and peacefully. Integrating hospice care in the communities will not pose a major challenge, because both hospice care and CHBC in Botswana embrace community-centred care and empowerment of care-givers through education and supplementing existing health services. The introduction of hospice care has resource implications, but if a community approach is opted for, there will be minimal costs incurred for the implementation and running of the programme and this can give social workers an opportunity to learn more about end-of-life care and challenge them to develop other methods of care for the benefit of those who are infected with HIV.

Furthermore, there is a need to employ social workers in schools to address HIV-related psychosocial challenges experienced by students. Social workers should benchmark and network with private sectors and other countries to learn how service delivery can be improved. They should also continue to attend in-service training as well as international and local conferences that focus on HIV and AIDS, in order to broaden their knowledge and skills on the issues. Finally the Ministry of Local Government (the primary employer of social workers) should be given a higher budget, recognizing the magnitude of social and economic services offered by social workers.

Notes

1 President Festus Mogae, who retired in April 2008.
2 The Government of Botswana is the largest employer in the country.
3 It should be noted that some social workers are responsible for covering more than one village.
4 See Maundeni and Jacques (2012) for a detailed discussion of such issues.
5 Grief and bereavement counselling is not popular in Botswana. Most people who need this type of counselling seek support from informal support networks such as friends, churches and relatives.
6 It should be noted, however, that sometimes various organizations offer in-service training to social workers and other health care practitioners in areas such as HIV counselling, palliative care, CHBC, community capacity building, HIV and AIDS counselling, Kitso training, PMTCT, and couple HIV counselling. Moreover, the University of Botswana's Department of Social Work offers a few courses on HIV and AIDS.

References

Allen, T. and Heald, S. (2004) 'HIV/AIDS policy in Africa: what has worked in Uganda and what has failed in Botswana?', *Journal of International Development*, 16(8): 1141–54.

Alverson, H. (1978) *Mind in the Heart of Darkness: Value and Self-identity Among the Tswana of Southern Africa*, Johannesburg: Macmillan.

Bamford, M., Gaitley, R. and Miller, R. (2006) *HIV-AIDS: A Social Work Perspective*, Birmingham: British Association of Social Workers.

Campbell, C. (1997) 'Selling sex in the time of AIDS: the psycho-social context of condom use by sex workers on a Southern African mine', *Social Science and Medicine*, 50: 479–94.

CSIS Task Force on HIV/AIDS (2004) Botswana's Strategy to Combat HIV/AIDS Lessons for Africa and President Bush's Emergency Plan for AIDS Relief, Conference Report of the CSIS Task Force on HIV/AIDS. Available at: http://csis.org/files/media/csis/pubs/0401_botswanahiv.pdf (accessed 17 May 2012).

Davidson, K.W. (1990) *Social Work in Health Care: A Handbook for Practice*, London: Routledge.

Deng, R., Li. L., Sringernyuang, J. and Zhang K. (2007) 'Drug abuse, HIV/AIDS and stigmatization in a Dai community in Yunnan, China', *Social Science and Medicine*, 64: 1560–71.

Dunn, A. (2005) 'HIV/AIDS: what about very young children?', Bernard van Leer Foundation working paper. Available at: www.bernardvanleer.org/HIV_AIDS_What_about_very_young_children (accessed 24 July 2013).

Eysenbach, G., Powell, J., Englesakis, M., Rizo, C. and Stern, A. (2004) 'Health related virtual communities and electronic support groups: systematic review of the effects of online peer to peer interactions', *British Medical Journal*, 328(7449): 1166.

Government of Botswana (2009) *Botswana AIDS Impact Survey III: Statistical Report*, Gaborone: Central Statistics Office.

Jacques, G. (2003) 'The Oliver Twist Syndrome: orphans, HIV, and community drama in Botswana', in E. Biakolo, J. Mathangwane and D. Odallo (eds), *The Discourse of HIV/AIDS in Africa*, Francistown: University of Botswana, Department of English, 24–32.

Jacques, G. (2010) 'Parents without portfolios: the challenge to social work of child headed households in AIDS-stricken Africa', in B.Z. Osei-Hwedie, K. Osei-Hwedie and M. Rankopo (eds), *Issues in HIV/AIDS and Social Welfare*, Accra: Ghana Institute of Management and Public Administration, 107–132.

Kalichman, S.C., Sikkema, K.J. and Somlai, A. (1996) 'People living with HIV infection who attend and do not attend support groups: a pilot study of needs, characteristics and experiences', *AIDS Care*, 8(5): 589–600.

Kalichman, S.C., Klein, S.J., Kalichman, M.O., O'Connell, D.A., Freedman, J.A., Eaton, L. and Cain, D. (2007) 'HIV/AIDS case managers and client HIV status disclosure: perceived client needs, practices, and services', *Health Social Work*, 32(4): 259–67.

Kang'ethe, S. (2008) 'Inadequate male involvement in health issues: the cause of gender-skewed HIV and AIDS situations in Botswana', in T. Maundeni, B. Osei-Hwedie, E. Mukamaambo and P. Ntseane (eds), *Male Involvement in Sexual and Reproductive Health: Prevention of Violence and HIV and AIDS in Botswana*, Cape Town: Made Plain Communications, 7–27.

Kesamang, L. (2007) '*Social workers' experiences of HIV and AIDS intervention in Botswana', dissertation submitted in partial fulfilment of the requirements for the Master of Social Work degree, Faculty of Health Sciences*, Nelson Mandela Metropolitan University, Port Elizabeth, South Africa.

Kgatlwane, J., Ogenyi, R., Ekezie, C., Madaki, H.N., Moyo, S. and Moroka, T.M. (2006) 'Factors that facilitate or constrain adherence to antiretroviral therapy among adults at four health facilities in Botswana: a pre-intervention study', in S. Davey, T. Gerrits, A. Hardon and C. Hodgkin (eds), *From Access to Adherence: The*

Challenges of Antiretroviral Treatment, Geneva: World Health Organization, 71–164.

Macdonald, D.S. (1996) 'Notes on the socio-economic and cultural factors influencing the transmission of HIV in Botswana', *Social Science and Medicine*, 42(9): 1325–33.

McGregor, L. (2002) 'Botswana battles against "extinction"', *Guardian*, 7 July 2002, 2.

Malinga, T. and Mupedziswa, R. (2009) 'Hospital social practice in Botswana: yesterday, today and tomorrow', *Journal of Social Development in Africa*, 24(1): 91–117.

Maundeni, T. (2009) 'Children and HIV and AIDS in Botswana: challenges faced by the boy child', in C.M. Fombad, R. Mupedziswa, T. Maundeni and G. Mookodi (eds), *HIV and AIDS, Vulnerable Groups, Human Rights and Development in Botswana*, Gaborone: OSSREA Botswana Chapter, 135–53.

Maundeni, T. and Jacques, G. (2012) '"And a little child shall lead them": utilising Kgotla meetings to empower children and the communities that nurture them', in T. Maundeni and N.S. Nnyepi (eds), *Thari ya Bana: Reflections on Children in Botswana 2012*, Gaborone: University of Botswana and UNICEF, 74–80.

Miller, C.M., Gruskin, S., Subramanian, S.V. and Heymann, J. (2007) 'Emerging health disparities in Botswana: examining the situation of orphans during the AIDS epidemic', *Social Science and Medicine*, 64(12): 2476–86.

Ministry of Education (2002) *The Impact of HIV/AIDS on Education in Botswana*, Gaborone: Government Printers.

Ministry of Health, Botswana (2006) *Caring for Health Workers: A National Strategy for Botswana*, Gaborone: Department of HIV/AIDS Prevention and Care.

Ministry of Local Government, Social Welfare Division, Botswana (1999) *Short Term Plan of Action on Care of Orphans in Botswana, 1999–2001*, Gaborone: Ministry of Local Government.

Ministry of Local Government, Social Welfare Division, Botswana (2002) *Revised National Policy on Destitute Persons*, Gaborone: Ministry of Local Government.

Mmonadibe, P.N. (2009) 'Orphaned HIV-positive children in Botswana: challenges and prospects', in C.M. Fombad, R. Mupedziswa, T. Maundeni and G. Mookodi (eds), *HIV and AIDS, Vulnerable Groups, Human Rights and Development in Botswana*, Gaborone: OSSREA Botswana Chapter, 154–67.

Moumakwa, C.P. (2010) '*The Botswana Kgotla system: a mechanism for traditional conflict resolution in modern Botswana: a case study of the Kanye Kgotla*', Master's Thesis in Philosophy of Peace and Conflict Transformation, Faculty of Humanities, Social Sciences and Education, University of Tromso, Tromso, Norway. Available at: http://munin.uit.no/handle/10037/3211 (accessed 3 April 2012).

Nagler, S.F., Adnopoz, J. and Forsyth, B.W. (1995) 'Uncertainty, stigma and secrecy: psychological aspects of AIDS for children and adolescents', in S. Geballe, J. Gruendel and W. Andiman (eds), *Forgotten Children of the AIDS Epidemic*, New Haven: Yale University Press, 71–82.

Ntseane, D. and Solo, K. (2007) *Social Security and Social Protection in Botswana*, Gaborone: Bay Publishing.

Ntseane, P.G. (2009) 'The voices of sex workers: implications for adult education strategies', in T. Maundeni, B. Osei-Hwedie, E. Mukamaambo and P. Ntseane (eds), *Male Involvement in Sexual and Reproductive Health: Prevention of Violence and HIV and AIDS in Botswana*, Cape Town: Made Plain Communications, 131–48.

Ntshwarang, P.N. and Malinga-Musamba, T. (2012) 'Social workers working with HIV and AIDS in health care settings: a case study of Botswana', *Practice: Social Work in Action Journal*, 24(5): 287–98.

Plattner, I.E. and Meiring, N. (2006) 'Living with HIV: the psychological relevance of meaning making', *AIDS Care*, 18(3): 241–5.

Population Services International (2004) *Botswana Social Marketing Programme*, Gaborone.

Potgieter, M.C. (1998) *The Social Work Process, Development to Empower People*, South Africa: Prentice Hall.

Ruch, G. (2005) 'Relationship-based practice and reflective practice: holistic approaches to contemporary child care social work', *Child and Family Social Work*, 10(2): 111–23.

Rwomire, A. and Raditlhokwa, L. (1996) 'Social work in Africa: issues and challenges', *Journal of Social Development in Africa*, 11(2): 5–19.

Schurink, E. (1990) 'Social workers: AIDS, Acquired Immune Deficiency Syndrome, casework, group work, community work', *Social Work Practice*, 3: 20–1.

Surface, D. (2007) 'HIV/AIDS medication compliance: how social support works', *Social Work Today*, 7(5): 20.

UNAIDS Joint United National Programme on HIV/AIDS (2012) *Global Report: UNAIDS Report on the Global AIDS Epidemic 2012*, Geneva: UNAIDS.

Uys, L. and Cameron, S. (2003) *Home Based HIV/AIDS Care*, Cape Town: Oxford University Press.

Chapter 11

HIV/AIDS in India

Challenges for professional social work

Vimla V. Nadkarni and Anita Rego

Introduction

The HIV epidemic is symbiotically related to poverty and development, impacting individuals, families and communities, economically, socially, psychologically and politically. The social determinants that perpetuate and sustain the epidemic cannot be ignored. At the same time, tremendous medical progress has been made with the discovery and manufacture of antiretroviral therapy (ART). The inclusion of free ART in the Indian national programme has radically transformed the lives of people living with HIV/AIDS. On the other hand, the large scale prevention programmes have expanded their reach to the most at-risk sections of the population.

India's HIV programme is a success story. The incidence of new HIV infections in India is down by 57 per cent (National Institute of Medical Statistics and National AIDS Control Organisation (NACO) 2012). The success of the Indian HIV programme has demonstrated that greater sensitivity towards health disparities, heightened mobilization of political, financial and human resources and active engagement of affected communities are critical in containing the epidemic. HIV has also created an environment where people are no longer ready to accept inequality in health and economic status. No other development challenge has led to such a strong level of leadership and ownership by the communities and countries most heavily affected (Joint United Nations Program on HIV/AIDS (UNAIDS) 2009).

The social work profession has been an active partner in the response to HIV, with social work academicians and practitioners at the forefront of action. The mainstay of the profession has been practice, research, policy and capacity enhancement. The challenge ahead for the social work profession is to sustain and scale up prevention strategies, as well as to mainstream and enhance the life-sustaining impulse in people living with HIV despite economic and environmental barriers. The role entails increasing optimism and health actions among the affected and infected.

Social workers have to address the barriers that people living with HIV and AIDS face, and that impact on ART adherence, especially when they are deprived of a conducive environment, devoid of the basics of shelter, food, clean water and sanitation. Social work has to also respond to communities at risk and/or vulnerable people whose risks stem from structural inequalities and disempowered status. These vulnerabilities are reflected in their lack of access to information and services and their inability to use protection. What is demanded from the profession of social work is to promote protection and safe behaviour, generate an enabling environment and work towards policies grounded in equity and social justice. Social workers have to continue their struggle in pushing governments to be more inclusive and rights based.

This chapter will analyse some of these key issues and challenges that HIV has brought forth for social work (in policy, practice, research and training/ education), and link the debate with some of the structural issues of poverty, gender inequality and human rights.

Current scenario of HIV/AIDS in India

Though India is a country with low HIV incidence, it has the third largest number of people living with HIV/AIDS, because of the size of its population. The UNGASS 2010 report (Joint United Nations Program on HIV/ AIDS (UNAIDS), National AIDS Control Organisation, Ministry of Health and Family Welfare (India) 2010) affirms that the epidemic in India is showing an overall declining trend. Yet, India carries the major burden of HIV after South Africa and Nigeria. There are an estimated 23.9 lakh[1] people living with HIV/AIDS; the adult prevalence was at 0.31 per cent in 2009 (NACO 2010–2011: 1).

The HIV epidemic in India is largely a 'concentrated' epidemic, where infection is mostly localized among most-at-risk populations. The prevalence is reportedly 10 to 20 times higher among most-at-risk populations: female sex workers at 4.94 per cent; men who have sex with men (MSM) at 7.3 per cent; injecting drug users (IDUs) at 9.19 percent; sexually transmitted infection (STI) clinic attendees at 2.46 per cent; and single migrant men at 2.45 per cent. It spreads to the general population through the bridge populations, such as migrants and truckers (NACO 2010–2011: 6). Thirty nine per cent (9.3 lakhs) of all infections are among women (NACO 2010–2011: 5). There is an overall decline in HIV prevalence among antenatal care clinic (ANC) attendees, especially in high-prevalence states; however, there is an increase of new infections in low- and moderate-prevalence states as noted by the UNGASS India Report 2010 (Joint United Nations Program on HIV/AIDS (UNAIDS), National AIDS Control Organisation, Ministry of Health and Family Welfare (India) 2010: 11). Children under 15 years of age account for 3.5 per cent of all infections, while 83 per cent are in the age group 15 to 49 years (NACO 2010–2011: 5). Six states with high HIV prevalence account for over two-thirds of the HIV burden of the country. India has identified 195 priority districts across the country based on HIV prevalence rates over a three-year period with an aim to strengthen focused programmatic interventions in these districts.

The primary drivers of the HIV epidemic in India are unprotected paid sex/commercial sex work, unprotected anal sex between men and IDUs (Joint United Nations Program on HIV/AIDS (UNAIDS), National AIDS Control Organisation, Ministry of Health and Family Welfare (India) 2010: 11). HIV transmission is complicated by various socio-economic determinants that drive the epidemic: poverty, lack of livelihood options, rapid urbanization, labour migration, gender inequality and inadequate information and dialogue on sex. These factors also disable households and communities at risk and/or affected by HIV and AIDS and reduce their ability to cope with HIV-related stigma, illness and death. Although prevalence rates are lower in Asia compared to Africa, it is found that the socio-economic impact on households is so great that they are reduced to penury, and it is estimated that an additional six million households will be pushed into poverty by 2015 unless national responses are strengthened (Commission on AIDS in Asia 2008). According to the United Nations Development Program (UNDP 2005: 3) HIV has inflicted the 'single most reversal in human development'.

The National AIDS Control Program, which is in its fourth five-year cycle, is supported by national and international civil society organizations and NGOs under the Three Ones Initiative. What is noteworthy is that HIV prevention programmes in India for sex workers, IDUs and MSM have shown success through targeted interventions. In fact, in the initial days the Indian government was slow to wake up to the problem, formulating its first national action plan only in 1992. By then, civil society actors had already initiated several interventions, and some of them were recognized as best practice models nationally and internationally by the time the country responded.

The National AIDS programme, as of this date, is implemented across the country and a large emphasis is placed on expansion of testing and treatment services, service provisioning, saturating coverage through a process of community collectivization and bringing about an enabling environment through concerted efforts with the police and the media. There is a lot more that needs to be done with MSM, transgender and IDUs and their partners, groups where infection rates are still high. What is worrying is the narrowing of infection rates between men and women and urban–rural differences. The spread of infection in the general community, women and migrants has necessitated the involvement of key sector ministries, resulting in sector-specific responses to scale up HIV prevention work and improve capacities of HIV households to cope with the impact of HIV and AIDS (NACO 2010).

Vulnerable populations

Vulnerability of women to HIV

Women's vulnerability is amplified by their low literacy rate (55.7 per cent) as well as their oppressed status (Census 2011). As child marriages continue to be rampant in India, 50 per cent of women marry before the age of 18 years and complete their family by the age of 26 years (National Family Health Survey International Institute for Population Sciences (IIPS) and Macro International, 2007). Those who marry early are less likely to complete their education and face multiple vulnerabilities. The utilization of antenatal services of the public sector is poor; those who seek services from the public health system are largely represented by women of lower social economic status. The low rate of antenatal care implies that these women miss the opportunity to learn about the importance of testing under the prevention of mother-to-child transmission (PMTCT) of HIV programme. When antenatal mothers test positive for HIV in the private sector, they are selectively referred to public facilities (Dandona et al. 2006), a form of stigma and discrimination.

More than 90 per cent of women acquire HIV infection from their husbands or their intimate sexual partners. Transmission is not due to their own sexual behaviour, but instead occurs because they are partners of men who are in close sexual contact with a high risk group (HRG). These groups include clients of female sex workers (FSW), MSM or IDUs. The wider implication of this situation is that in almost 6 per cent of cases in 2008, the route of transmission of infection is from mother to child (Joint United Nations Program on HIV/AIDS (UNAIDS), National AIDS Control Organisation, Ministry of Health and Family Welfare (India) 2010: 11).

Studies show differences in the perceptions and behaviours of men and women towards HIV testing and treatment. Men from urban settings sought HIV testing, fearing their own risk behaviour or symptoms. On the other hand, women went for HIV testing only after their husbands were diagnosed with HIV, on the recommendation of their health care provider. In some cases, they reported mandatory testing by the service provider, mostly during the antenatal period (Solomon et al. 2006). In a gender-inequitable setting, HIV programmes that emphasize condom use, abstinence or faithfulness as key prevention strategies seem irrelevant for women who have no control over their own bodies and lives, especially when marital and interpersonal partner violence is very common. This is heightened in a patriarchal, male-dominated society where women have limited decision-making powers and control over their own sexuality or health.

The gender assessment study conducted in February 2010 by USAID/India (Caro et al. 2010) provided evidence for the poor health status of women. Women had fewer resources and were faced with unequal access to, and benefits from, the primary health care system. They suffered limited autonomy in reproductive choices and had poorer health and nutrition – the very factors that heighten risk and vulnerability to infection and accentuate problems when infected or affected by HIV/AIDS. Gender-based violence, the authors report, is also faced by MSM and transgender groups. Sarna *et al.* (2006) reported that there are no gender differentials in ART adherence between men and women. However, researchers such as Tarakeshwar *et al.* (2006) found that HIV-infected men receiving antiretroviral therapy experience greater satisfaction and optimism compared with women, who frequently report side effects, financial burden and inability to maintain continuity of care.

Women carry the dual burden of discrimination and being the caregivers of infected husbands or orphaned children. Evidence clearly shows that women go to the hospital not for their own health concerns, but for those of their children or husband. Furthermore, there are socio-cultural and structural barriers in terms of distance, poverty and negative attitudes of health providers. Mehta and Gupta's study (2006) shows that HIV-infected rural women report more frequent stigmatization; social isolation; compromised access to care including pregnancy, child-birth and post-natal care; and more limited financial reserves or support when compared to men. These are attenuated when women experience ill-health, are caregivers or have become widows.

Unmarried, non-pregnant or post-partum women have lesser access to testing facilities and care services. Rural women's health care is neglected, and their needs are not viewed as a priority. Although NACO has included gender mainstreaming in its programmes, this has not led to the expected impact, given the deeply entrenched attitudes towards women in the Indian psyche and the poor understanding and low commitment to a gendered response. Issues of women who are infected with HIV have not received due recognition within a gender neutral model of care, and the positive networks continue to grapple with how to deal with women's issues. Prevention interventions are largely limited to those most at risk. Women at risk due to their partner's risk behaviour are clubbed with mainstream mass communication messaging, thus perpetuating the belief that married women and women with steady partners are not necessarily at risk.

Vulnerability of most-at-risk groups

Sex workers

Among female sex workers, early marriage, lack of education and high mobility are major factors that increase vulnerability to HIV infection. Sex workers have limited power to negotiate, and this is aggravated by their impoverished situation and lack of access to most needed resources. Misconceptions such as the belief that sex with younger girls can cure HIV, the belief that AIDS affects only women who sell sex and the belief that 'casual sexual acts' (or *masti*) are not a risk for HIV and beliefs that people who 'look healthy' cannot be affected are widely prevalent. The programme has not been able to keep pace with the changing sex work patterns and sex trade dynamics. Brothel-based female sex work (FSW) is giving way to home-based commercial sex practices, making the hidden FSW population even more difficult to reach.

Stigmatization of sex work and HIV-positive status drives the epidemic underground. Female sex workers experience violence from pimps/brokers, clients and law enforcement authorities; additionally they also face family and community ostracism and self-stigma. Effectiveness of outreach efforts is dependent on an enabling environment, and hence in its absence it creates a barrier to deeper penetration of HIV/AIDS prevention, treatment, care and support. Specifically, it weakens the power of the sex worker to nego-tiate condom use and to seek STI treatment. It is largely reflected in poor condom usage with intimate and regular partners as against paid partners. The experience of domestic violence and intimate partner violence continues unabated, in spite of the efforts of the national programme to incorporate crisis intervention through community collectives. Stigma and discrimin-ation further aggravate the context of violence.

Men who have sex with men (MSM) and transgender

The withdrawal of Section 377,[2] mobilized through a concerted effort and advocacy by communities, professionals, government and judiciary, was a landmark judgement to decriminalize same-sex relationships. However, the environment is not totally facilitative for MSM to come out in the open when there is homophobia, and people practising same-sex behaviour con-tinue to be criminalized, discriminated against and not accepted.

The traditional targeted interventions for transgender are combined with MSM interventions. Evidence suggests that the transgender (TG) population was not effectively reached with prevention services, as the dynamics in the transmission of infection among and needs of the TG population are different from those of MSMs. The process of advocacy with the national programme to adopt a unique approach under targeted intervention for the TG population is in progress. Simultaneously during this process, the social concerns of the TG population received attention and led to the provision of voting rights, free legal aid services and an opportunity to interface with the Planning Commission in the current five-year plan process.

Recent evidence from prevention programmes indicates that the size and risk profile of MSM, TG persons and hijra (men who dress and act like women, also called the third gender: MTH) subpopulations has been underestimated. Emerging evidence reveals that sizable MSM and hijra communities are also living in many smaller cities and towns. In many loca-tions, the MTH communities have both commercial and non-commercial sexual partners, forming important links between high-risk and heterosexual networks.

Condom usage among MSM and TG persons is low, and they experience higher rates of HIV infection (The Global Fund 2011). When men operate as sex workers, they are even more difficult to reach, and condom usage is much more difficult to assure. Marginalization, homophobia and legal barriers coupled with reluctance among MTH to utilize preventive barriers make them more vulnerable and less amenable to prevention efforts. Their female partners are most vulnerable to HIV, as they are not aware of their partner's sexual orientation and risks.

Migrating populations

Migrant men, the bridge population, form the part of the chain that transmits infection to their unknowing wives and partners. Poor tribal persons and rural men who are less literate and have low technical skills are easily exploited as cheap labour in the urban areas (Patel 2002, cited in National AIDS Control Organisation 2010: 9). They move single to destinations such as Maharashtra (22 per cent), Andhra Pradesh (7.8 per cent), Gujarat (7 per cent) and Karnataka (5 per cent), the states with higher HIV prevalence (Verma *et al.* 2007, cited in National AIDS Control Organisation 2010: 9). Contractual male labourers are largely young (70 per cent between 18 and 29 years), over half are married, and a third reside away from their wives because of work. Over 30 per cent report having sex with FSWs (Saggurti *et al.* 2008), but they have poor knowledge about HIV and risk perceptions. Residential geographies of migrant male communities are characterized by a high density of alcohol and transactional sex venues and locales (Saggurti *et al.* 2010; Chakraborty 2004, cited in National AIDS Control Organisation 2010). The features of migration that lead to increased risk include participation of single males, access to money, lack of social and economic security, a peer culture of risk taking, easy access to alcohol, pleasure seeking and sexual experimentation. Hence, districts that are primarily migrant source points and had low prevalence a few years ago are showing trends of higher prevalence. The National AIDS Control Organisation identified 122 districts across 11 states (based on the 2001 Census) with high levels of out-migration (National AIDS Control Organization 2010–2011: 8). It has revised its migrant strategy to include interventions at source and transit points, an addition to previous destination-focused interventions (National AIDS Control Organisation 2010).

Work with transport workers was initiated from the first phase of the programme, comprising provision of information, linkage to clinical services to include treatment for opportunistic infections and later, the addition of ART. To address the structural barriers resulting out of the high level of mobility, to increase access to quality services and to improve follow-up, the programme strategy now includes transport associations and conglomerates in transport worker interventions. The effectiveness of this shift will only be known over time. The challenges in reaching out to bridge populations include the lack of systematic data on migrants and transport workers, reaching seasonal migrants and evolving low-cost strategies addressing heterogeneity among transport workers. Upscaling of migrant and transport worker interventions and the involvement of industries that cause migration has been minimal if not absent.

Injecting drug users

HIV prevalence continues to climb among IDUs, reflecting inadequate recognition and programming for this high-risk group (National AIDS Control Organisation 2008). Initially thought of as confined to the north-east region, there is an increasing concern about users in other parts of the country, and hence NACO has put in place interventions in pockets across the country. Recognizing the magnitude of the problem, NACO has in recent times incorporated methadone maintenance programmes (only in the north-east region of India) and has promoted needle exchange programmes.

Creating an enabling environment

In view of the complexity and sensitive issues surrounding the HIV pandemic, the interventions, both governmental and non-governmental, have aimed at creating an environment for people to protect themselves against infection and for positive people to come out with dignity and access services at all levels. The intervention model of care largely rested on community outreach workers or peers and on service providers linked to targeted interventions, the testing centres, PMTCT and ART centres. This has led to a significant demystification of interventions. The national programme to a large extent achieved scale, but the quality of interventions remained an issue.

To facilitate an enabling environment, the programme strengthened prevention through community collectivization and responding to some of the structural concerns such as violence; building linkages with systems; and advocating with media, police and judiciary for community-sensitive approaches. Nadkarni et al. (2010), in their study on HIV-sensitive social protection, reiterated the importance and effectiveness of the efforts of the government and civil society in strengthening access to social protection programmes for HIV-positive people and their families. The study revealed that the utilization of these programmes by PLWHA enabled the larger community of uninfected women and men to access welfare schemes available for below-poverty-line families.

The community-led crisis response system promoted under the targeted interventions led to the establishment of a mechanism to address the violence that most-at-risk populations face. The expansion of free legal aid to the TG population opened doors for justice and legal services. In a few places, sex workers have been trained as paralegal workers. Increasing evidence suggests that addressing human rights violations and creating an enabling environment can encourage behaviour change, a critical element in the fight against HIV. Interventions in some locations have been led by community-based organizations, giving the onus of care to them. These initial efforts by the government, NGOs and community initiatives have been promising, but there is a long way to go for communities to feel safe to come out and seek services.

Another challenge is how to undertake effective behavioural HIV prevention activities among people who are already positive. People who are unaware of their sero-status are very likely to transmit infections to a high proportion of unsuspecting partners. Evidence from all countries shows that individuals reduce risk behaviours and take precautions to protect their partners once they know their sero-status. With increased partner follow-up, the World Bank study on stigma and discrimination in South Asia (Stang, et al. 2010) reported that it would be possible to reach, identify and refer a large number of people or persons living with HIV/AIDS (PLWHA) for services.

The practices and locations of most-at-risk populations are constantly changing, and successful targeted interventions must evolve constantly to respond to the rapidly shifting patterns and environment. Response to stigma and discrimination is oblivious to the multi-layered structural dynamics, systemic factors and the cyclic nature of violence. Referral mechanisms for counselling are absent, and structural interventions have not received adequate attention as required.

Putting in place a management system and technical approach within a national programme is what made the programme work. A multidisciplinary technical team at NACO which also included social workers facilitated the process of shaping the programme. Dr Sujatha Rao, former Director General of NACO and Senior Leadership Fellow at the Harvard School of Public Health, explains the importance of decision-making in leadership, system strengthening and standardization of interventions and how they brought about a result-oriented approach in the national programme.

Basic guidelines on staff recruitment led to employment of qualified social workers, psychologists or human development specialists as counsellors at service points and counselling supervisors in the districts. This gave a boost to professionalizing the HIV services and provided opportunities to professional social workers to enter the field as HIV counsellors, and for social work institutions to partner with the national programme. The Tata Institute of Social Sciences[3] has pioneered training of counsellors since 1993, provided leadership to the UNAIDS-sponsored Technical Resource Group on HIV/AIDS Counselling and provided impetus for capacity building of counsellors at centres for higher learning through the Global Fund Round 7 project SAKSHAM since 2008.

The Indian HIV programme has so far depended on international funding. The global economic recession has forced the government to look for internal resources to maintain and expand upon what was built in the National AIDS Control Plan (NACP) III. Mainstreaming of HIV seems to be the pathway forward, for instance, through the integration of RCH and HIV within the National Rural Health Mission. The biggest challenge is how to make sure that programmes for most-at-risk populations receive the same attention and sensitivity within a reproductive and child health programme primarily focusing on general communities.

Maintaining quality and attracting the right human power is going to be difficult in this new scenario. An added dimension is programming effectively to scale interventions in the northern low-prevalence states with the same momentum where general health care has not been adequately reached. The challenge for HIV prevention now is to sustain the momentum for effective, complex combination efforts over the long term (Piot *et al.* 2008). Furthermore, it is important that the underlying socio-economic determinants of the epidemic and stigma and discrimination towards people engaging in high-risk behaviours (often the most marginalized in society) as well as PLHA have to be addressed for a sustained and effective response (The World Bank 2006).

Social work's response

The social work profession aims to achieve people-centred development within a human rights framework, ensuring equality and justice as the goals of social work. The International Association of Schools of Social Work (IASSW) and the International Federation of Social Workers' (IFSW) statements of ethical principles are clear that 'as a way of upholding human rights and social justice, we should not contribute to inhumane treatment of people' (section 5.2; IASSW and IFSW 2012). Social work educators and practitioners have played a very active role in the field of HIV/AIDS since the recognition of AIDS as a pandemic in India.

The social work profession is well positioned to intervene at micro, meso and macro levels; it is pertinent to state that HIV is acknowledged as a developmental and not merely a health issue. The social work profession in the health sector in India has made its mark since the first introduction of medical and psychiatric social work as a specialization in schools of social work in 1948. Health social work practice through hospitals and child guidance clinics was established well before the start of social work education in the country. Community health in social work education and practice developed based on public health perspectives. This has helped the social work profession to position itself within HIV/AIDS interventions and led to the growth of social work education.

The NACP IV provides a unique opportunity for the social work profession. The focus on improving the quality of the programmes through evidence-based interventions provides a plethora of avenues for social work professionals. This includes research, demonstration and the upscaling of innovative approaches that address barriers and bottlenecks in behaviour change. Social workers play a major role in counselling, family interventions, group counselling, peer-led approaches and training for early detection, referrals and structural responses. However, these have to be strongly supported by the changing realities, with the epidemic having crossed 28 years in the country bringing in challenges for palliative care, services for people living with HIV (PLHIV), day care and rehabilitation services.

Policy initiatives

With the origins of community organization and the UN recognition of health as a right in 1946, social workers have also worked towards community mobilization, advocacy and social action to influence development of policy and programmes at the national level for HIV/AIDS prevention, support and care interventions. The major policy shift that was initiated by professional social work educators from the Tata Institute of Social Sciences (TISS) (Mumbai, India) was the recognition of HIV/AIDS counselling as an essential part of the national programme. Professional social work was also responsible for the development of the AIDS policy draft and has been in the forefront for advocating for the AIDS law.

Working with the public health care system

The Continuum of Care and Support Project was designed as an intervention grounded on creating an enabling environment that espouses a humane policy and reducing stigma and discrimination in the treatment of PLHIV in the public hospital. Medical social workers in public hospitals were trained as preventive counsellors with skills for pre-test and post-test counselling including nutrition and health counselling. Developing close links with communities to support PLHIV to work towards reducing discriminative behaviour, it created a conducive treatment environment in the hospitals. Social work professionals undertook the strengths, weaknesses, opportunities and threats (SWOT) analysis of the service delivery system and prioritized issues and challenges to develop strategies to humanize care and reduce stigma and discrimination at public hospitals. The experiment of the project resulted in a network for people living with HIV/AIDS (PLHA) and provided lessons for an integrated approach for the national programme. The Population Council in collaboration with NACO eventually drew lessons from this project to lay down policy guidelines for HIV services at public hospitals.

Capacity building in counselling

The NACO-UNAIDS Technical Resource Group on Counselling, anchored by TISS, set the minimum standards for counselling, which became an integral part of NACP II. Over the years, professional social workers as counsellors are seen at all levels of services – prevention, treatment, care and support – within the public health care model. These concerted efforts contributed to quality counselling through the consolidation and review of training models. Today HIV/AIDS counselling has been recognized even by the Global Fund for AIDS, Tuberculosis and Malaria, which is funding capacity enhancement in counselling through the Round 7 project SAKSHAM. Through 38 institutions of higher learning across the length and breadth of the country, the initiative demonstrates the competencies of professional social work educators in a multidisciplinary team to build capacity at a macro level using an interface of social work and management skills that includes financial, programmatic, knowledge, monitoring and evaluation linked to a strong management information system. The project also illustrates the capacity of professional social workers to demonstrate leadership, largely drawn from the philosophy and values of social work, that espouses democratic participation of all stakeholders in the project.

Several professional social workers are working with the government system, at NACO and in the State AIDS Societies, as NGO consultants and full-time staff. They assist in developing local and national policies and in making operational the national polices. They participate in the selection, support of capacity enhancement, mentoring and monitoring of NGOs implementing HIV programmes. Several have started their own NGOs or are leading national and international organizations working in the field of HIV. What has led to the acceptance of social workers within the HIV programme are their multifarious skills to work at different levels, and within a variety of contexts: with individuals, groups, families and communities; through welfare, developmental, human rights and structural interventions; at the micro, meso and macro levels. However, with the newer challenges brought in by privatization, liberalization and globalization, social workers need to enhance their competencies in several ways.

The way forward

There are new and unexplored terrains to be addressed by social work professionals in HIV work. They need training to deal with HIV and sexuality issues among sexual minorities, victims of wars and riots, victims of disasters, and populations displaced as political refugees or populations of skewed development. Social work education and practice in India has remained largely static except in a few select institutions, and the profession would benefit from renewed thinking and positioning in the context of emerging themes and realities.

Need for specialized skills training

ART adherence counselling focuses on how to reduce loss to follow-up and drop-outs and is critical to prevent drug resistance. Preparing for disclosure of results and dealing with the impact on the clients remains a great challenge. Partner notification is still a grey area and needs more study and development of effective practice. Social work associations and educational institutions would need to offer refresher courses, continuing education and tailor-made upgrading of skills based on emerging needs. The mental health of HIV-positive people and of the most-at-risk populations is one of the most neglected issues for intervention. Social workers require specialist skills to be able to deal with emotional distress consequent to HIV.

Development of analytical and social action skills

While understanding HIV is important from a biomedical framework, especially when working on issues of adherence to ART, pre-test and post-test and disclosure issues, social workers have to develop analytical skills to understand HIV as a developmental and human rights issue. Access to affordable ARTs and essential medicines has been under threat in the wake of global developments in the patents regime. Without an understanding of the international politics behind this scenario, social work action would fall short. If social work is to make any difference in policies negatively impacting people infected with HIV, joining the Access to Medicine Campaign would be inevitable. Social workers would need to radically shift their perspectives from a care and rehabilitation approach to a more anti-oppressive, justice and equity-oriented approach and become sensitive to the structural dynamics of the oppression of the most at-risk groups that perpetuate and sustain the infection dynamics.

Feminist lens for work with women

Women's needs within the HIV programme are confined to preventing parent-to-child transmission. Approaching women's issues (whether HIV infected or affected) through a feminist lens would provide a very radical shift in action. Social workers, who view the programme from a functionalist framework where the women are left to fend for themselves once the medicated baby is proved negative, often miss out on the nuances of structural barriers that pregnant women and mothers, especially lactating mothers, face in caring for their children. One needs to go beyond the ART scenario and look at how women's issues rest on power dynamics, and strategize ways to address structural concerns and equity within the HIV programmes.

Reducing stigma and discrimination against most-at-risk populations

Marginalized and discriminated populations, which include sex workers, street youth, sexual minorities, drug users and so on, face barriers at service points, as medical personnel and care givers fear HIV transmission despite the availability of prophylactic medicines. NGO interventions and persistent visits by social workers, counsellors and peers to the public health care facilities seem to be partially successful. Constant alertness by social workers and counsellors has forced health systems to recognize the right to health access of the marginalized, resulting in some change in attitudes among health providers. This has been recently documented by Michielsen (2012) in his study on transformative social protection, where he found that rag-picker women affiliated to NGOs, wearing uniforms and possessing identity cards, had a better opportunity to be treated with respect compared to women connected to a non-HIV civil society organization. Sadly, there are several examples where the women infected or at risk are mistreated (Nadkarni et al. 2010). An unresolved concern has been the lack of privacy and the time constraints the counsellor faces that make communication and counselling procedural and mechanistic.

Social workers have to be constantly alert to maltreatment or negligence of HIV-positive people as well as the most-at-risk populations and play more proactive roles in addressing these concerns. With the expansion of Integrated Counselling and Testing Centres and link ART centres at private hospitals and sub-district levels, the social worker's role in counselling and providing information to the clients brings in newer challenges. They need to strategize on how they will ensure the quality of counselling in the newer contexts.

Innovating teaching pedagogies

To build in sensitivities and favourable attitudes, social work education needs to re-examine curricula to create learning and teaching pedagogies that would make students self-reflective and question their own patriarchal and moralistic attitudes towards the marginalized communities. This involves a long-term process with constant refreshers and workshops tailored to the sharing of positive and negative experiences.

Training of peer educators and PLHA networks

Efforts to date have led to success through the formation of positive people's groups that promote a sense of identity, security and the universalization of concerns. Recognizing the potential, NACO made efforts to train PLHIV and high risk groups to build competencies in programme planning, monitoring and leading interventions. Challenges have emerged in professionalizing community-led interventions. Professional social work institutions, along with management institutions, can contribute to a workable model for development wherein communities can own and lead programmes effectively.

Addressing work-related structural and systemic issues

The status of social work counsellors within the health care system is a major concern. They are vested with administrative and managerial responsibility with low salaries, high accountability and less power, and this impinges on the delivery of counselling. In these circumstances, the question is: how do we get counsellors to maintain their motivation and bring about better work and human resource policies within the national programme? Building evidence on how social work counselling and related interventions are adding value through the prevention of spread, reduction of new infections and increasing adherence to ART can help professional social workers to negotiate for better working conditions.

Social work research

Social work professionals can lead social work research. Building competence and confidence in using newer research tools and techniques in intervention studies is essential. Through research, social workers can bring into focus critical elements that need attention. Several areas where social work research can contribute are gender and social inequities, the buffering effect of social protection on risk reduction and service utilization, the impact of stigma and discrimination strategies on access to services among sexual minorities, the effectiveness of innovative sexual health interventions for adolescents, and so on. Social work teaching institutions, through international and local knowledge sharing and competence development, can support evidence generation and evidence-led interventions.

Conclusion

Social work professionals have demonstrated their contribution in the field of HIV/AIDS since the establishment of the national programme in India in 1992. They have participated as members of multidisciplinary teams in analyses of the social determinants of HIV at various levels. They have also demonstrated social interventions at all these levels. They have demonstrated success at prevention and meeting the special needs of PLHIV, as well as broad-basing HIV interventions through mainstreaming, demystification and capacity enhancement. They are working on issues beyond HIV, such as violence and sexual abuse, and integrating HIV interventions with reproductive health.

There is a lot more to do through the profession. There is a need to consolidate experiences and learning from interventions at each stage of the disease, at different points of service uptake, and for influencing national policy and programmes. There is a need to document the indigenous practices evolved over time in prevention, care and counselling, and integrate them into the curricula in schools of social work.

The bio-medical-social framework for practice does not address structural issues of poverty, gender inequality, stigma and discrimination, and cultural norms which drive the epidemic. It is here that professional social work can build upon the work done in the arena of HIV to evolve a framework on anti-oppressive or structural practice. Playing a watchdog role vis-à-vis the national programme and policy is much needed.

Notes

1 One lakh equals 100,000.
2 Chapter XVI, Section 377 of the Indian Penal Code, a piece of legislation introduced during British rule of India, criminalizes sexual activity 'against the order of nature'. The section read as follows: 'Unnatural offences: Whoever voluntarily has carnal intercourse against the order of nature with any man, woman or animal, shall be punished with imprisonment for life, or with imprisonment of either description for term which may extend to ten years, and shall also be liable to fine.' In an effort to decriminalize same-sex behaviour among consenting adults, the High Court of Delhi, on 2 July 2009, in a historic judgement, withdrew Section 377. Section 377, however, continues to apply in the case of sex involving minors and coercive sex. The law has not been amended due to appeals filed against the Delhi judgement in the Supreme Court of India (Pukaar 2012).
3 The Tata Institute of Social Sciences carried out these activities through the Cell for AIDS Research, Action and Training (CARAT) located within the Department of Medical and Psychiatric Social Work (current Centre for Health and Mental Health within the School of Social Work).

References

Caro, D., Greene, M.E., Pangare, V. and Goswami, R. (2010) *Gender Assessment USAID/India*. United States Agency for International Development. Available at: http://reliefweb.int/sites/reliefweb.int/files/resources/F70481C8D924D1D4492 57722000683B3-Full_Report.pdf (accessed 25 January 2012).

Census of India (2011) Population Enumeration Data (Final Population). Available at www.censusindia.gov.in/2011census/population_enumeration.html accessed 25 April 2015).

Chakraborty (2004) cited in National AIDS Control Organization (2010) Policy, Strategy and Operational Plan: HIV Intervention for Migrants, New Delhi, India: Department of AIDS Control, Ministry of Health and Family Welfare, Government of India.

Commission on AIDS in Asia (2008) Redefining AIDS in Asia Crafting an Effective Response. Report of the Commission on AIDS in Asia. Presented to Mr. Ban Ki-moon, UN Secretary General, on 26 March 2008. Oxford University Press, New Delhi. Available at http://data.unaids.org/pub/Report/2008/20080326_report_commission_aids_en.pdf (accessed 25 April 2015).

Dandona, L., Lakshmi, V., Kumar, G.A. and Dandona, R. (2006) 'Is the HIV burden in India being overestimated?', BMC Public Health, 6: 308.

The Global Fund (2011) Addressing Sex Work, MSM and Transgender People in the Context of the HIV Epidemic (July 2011), Global Fund Information Note. Available at: www.msmgf.org/files/msmgf//documents/R11_SOGI_InfoNote_en.pdf (accessed 26 January 2015).

International Association of Schools of Social Work (IASSW) and International Federation of Social Work (IFSW) (2012, March 3) Statement-of-ethical-principles, International Federation of Social Work. Available at: http://ifsw.org/policies/statement-of-ethical-principles/ (accessed 26 January 2015).

International Institute for Population Sciences (IIPS) and Macro International (2007) National Family Health Survey, 2005–06 (NFHS-3). Mumbai: IIPS.

Joint United Nations Program on HIV/AIDS UNAIDS (2009) 2008 UNAIDS Annual Report: Towards Universal Access. Geneva: Joint United Nations Programme on HIV/AIDS (UNAIDS). Available at: www.unaids.org/sites/default/files/media_asset/jc1736_2008_annual_report_en_1.pdf (accessed 25 January 2015).

Joint United Nations Program on HIV/AIDS (UNAIDS), National AIDS Control Organisation, Ministry of Health and Family Welfare (India) (2010) India UNGASS Country Progress Report 2010. Geneva: Joint United Nations Program on HIV/AIDS (UNAIDS). Available at: www.unaids.org/sites/default/files/en/dataanalysis/knowyourresponse/countryprogressreports/2010countries/india_2010_country_progress_report_en.pdf (accessed 25 January 2015).

Mehta, A.K. and Gupta, S. (2006) 'The impact of HIV/AIDS on women care-givers in situations of poverty: policy issues', CPRC-IIPA Working Paper No. 31. Manchester and New Delhi: Chronic Poverty Research Centre (CPRC) and Indian Institute of Public Administration (IIPA). Available at: http://r4d.dfid.gov.uk/Output/173556/Default.aspx (accessed 28 August 2013).

Michielsen J. (2012), Transformative Social Protection in Health in India: empowering the poor to claim quality health care through community health insurance, Antwerp: UA, Faculty Political and Social Sciences, Department of Sociology, PhD Dissertation.

Michielsen, J., John, D., Sardeshpande, N. and Meulemans, H. (2011) 'Improving access to quality care for female slum dwellers in urban Maharashtra, India: researching the need for transformative social protection in health', Social Theory and Health, 9(4): 376–92.

Moses, S., Blanchard, J.F., Kang, H., Emmanuel, F., Paul, S.R., Becker, M.L., Wilson, D. and Claeson, M. (2006) AIDS in South Asia: Understanding and Responding to a Heterogeneous Epidemic. Washington, DC: The World Bank. Available at: http://siteresources.worldbank.org/SOUTHASIAEXT/Resources/Publications/448813-1155152122224/southasia_aids.pdf (accessed 28 August 2013).

Nadkarni, V., Goel, S. and Pongurlekar, S. (2010) HIV Sensitive Social Protection: A Four State Utilisation Study. New Delhi: UNDP. Available at:

www.undp.org/content/dam/india/docs/hiv_sensitive_social_protection_a_four_ state_utilisation_study.pdf (accessed 28 August 2013).

National AIDS Control Organisation (NACO) (2010) *Policy, Strategy and Operational Plan: HIV Intervention for Migrants*. New Delhi: Department of AIDS Control, Ministry of Health and Family Welfare, Government of India.

National AIDS Control Organisation (NACO) (2010–2011) *Annual Report 2010–2011*. New Delhi: Department of AIDS Control, Ministry of Health and Family Welfare, Government of India. Available at: www.naco.gov.in/upload/REPORTS/ NACO%20Annual%20Report%202010–11.pdf (accessed 26 January 2015).

National Institute of Health and Family Welfare & National AIDS Control Organisation (NACO) Ministry of Health & Family Welfare (2011) *Annual HIV Sentinel Surveillance Country Report 2008–09*. National AIDS Control Organisation. Available at: http://naco.gov.in/upload/Surveillance/Reports%20 &%20Publication/HIV%20Sentinel%20Surveillance%20India%20Country%20 Report,%202008–09.pdf (accessed 26 January 2015).

National Institute of Medical Statistics and National AIDS Control Organisation (2012) *Technical Report India HIV Estimates-2012*. Department of AIDS Control, Ministry of Health and Family Welfare, Government of India. Available at: www.naco.gov.in/ upload/Surveillance/Reports%20&%20Publication/Technical%20Report%20-%20 India%20HIV%20Estimates%202012.pdf (accessed 25 January 2015).

Piot, P., Bartos, M., Larson, H., Zewdie, D. and Mane P. (2008) 'Coming to terms with complexity: a call to action for HIV prevention', *The Lancet*, 372: 845–59.

Pukaar, The Journal of Naz Foundation International. April 2012, London: NFI.

Rao, K.S. (2012) *Decision Making: Voices from the Field*. Uploaded by Harvard University: Woman in Leadership. Available at: www.youtube.com/ watch?v=WY9uA6xowT8 (accessed 16 May 2012).

Saggurti, N., Mahapatra, B., Swain, S.N., *et al.* (2010) *Migration and HIV in Districts with High Out-Migration in India*. Population Council, Draft not for circulation. UNDP and NACO, New Delhi, India cited in NACO 2010.

Saggurti, N., Verma, R.K., Jain, A.K., Rama Rao, S., Kumar, K.A., Subbiah, A. and Bharat, S. (2008) 'HIV risk behaviors among contracted and non-contracted male migrant workers in India: potential role of labor contractors and contractual systems in HIV prevention', *AIDS*, 22(Suppl 5): S127–36.

Samuel, N.M., Srijayanth, P., Dharamarajan, S. Bethel, J., Van Hook, H., Jacob, M., Junankar, V., Chamberlin, J., Collins, D. and Read, J.S. (2007) 'Acceptance of HIV-1 education and voluntary counseling/testing by and seroprevalence of HIV-1 among pregnant women in rural south India', *Indian Journal of Medical Research*, 125(1): 49–64.

Sarna, A., Gupta, I., Pujari, S., Sengar, A.K., Garg, R. and Weiss, E. (2006) *Examining Adherence and Sexual Behavior among Patients on Antiretroviral Therapy in India*. Horizons Final Report. Washington, DC: Population Council. Available at: www.popcouncil.org/pdfs/horizons/indiaart.pdf (accessed 28 August 2013).

Solomon, S., Kouyoumdjian, F.G., Cecelia, A.J., *et al.* (2006) 'Why are people getting tested? Self-reported reasons for seeking voluntary counseling and testing at a clinic in Chennai, India', *AIDS and Behavior*, 10(4): 415–20.

Stangl, A., Corr, D., Laura, B., Echhaus, T., Claeson, M. and Nyblade L. (2010). Tackling HIV-Related Stigma and Discrimination in South Asia. © 2010 The International Bank for Reconstruction and Development, The World Bank,

Washington. Available at: http://siteresources.worldbank.org/SOUTHASIAEXT/
Resources/223546-1192413140459/4281804-1231540815570/5730961-
1235157216166/5849907-1279637337320/Tackling_HIV_Stigma_July_2010.
pdf (accessed 11 May 2015).

Tarakeshwar, N., Krishnan, A.K., Johnson, S., *et al.* (2006) 'Living with HIV infection: perceptions of patients with access to care at a nongovernmental organization in Chennai, India', *Culture Health and Sexuality*, 8(5): 407–21.

United Nations Development Program (UNDP) (2005) Human Development Report 2005. International cooperation at a crossroads: Aid, trade and security in an unequal world. New York. Available at: http://hdr.undp.org/sites/default/files/reports/266/hdr05_complete.pdf (accessed 25 January 2015).

United States Agency for International Development/India (2010) *Gender Assessment*. New Delhi: United States Agency for International Development.

Verma (2007) cited in National AIDS Control Organization (2010) Policy, Strategy and Operational Plan: HIV Intervention for Migrants, New Delhi, India: Department of AIDS Control, Ministry of Health and Family Welfare, Government of India.

World Bank (2006) *World Development Report 2006: Equity and Development*. Washington, DC: The World Bank and Oxford University Press. Available at: www-wds.worldbank.org/servlet/WDSContentServer/WDSP/IB/2005/09/20/000112742_20050920110826/Rendered/PDF/322040World0Development0Report02006.pdf (accessed 26 January 2015).

Part IV

Toward the next generation

Developments in social work education

George Palattiyil, Dina Sidhva and Mono Chakrabarti

In the world of the twenty-first century, the social work profession has undergone rapid changes to withstand the challenges of globalisation (Alphonse *et al.*, 2008; Dominelli, 2010) and the widening gap between rich and poor (Annan, 2001). In no other aspect of social work is this change more visible than in social work education. In the UK, for example, social work education has undergone significant changes in the recent past, as a result of a general understanding that social work needs to raise its standards to respond to the emerging challenges of the twenty-first century. Around the same time, there have been several high profile abuse cases of children and adults, where social work became the subject of criticism by the media. Serious case reviews and other enquiries set up by successive governments to investigate such cases highlighted the importance of developing a workforce that is capable of dealing with the demands of the profession. With a view to addressing these issues, and to raise standards of practice, several steps have been taken at the policy level to standardise social work education and practice. Some of these include creating regulatory authorities in all parts of the UK with the power to approve and regulate the standards that underpin social work education; registration of social workers; creating a care commission to inspect and regulate the quality and standards of care; and developing a code of practice, to name a few.

More globally, too, social work has seen several trends in the education of new social work professionals. Much in the same way as medical and clinical education (Hoagwood *et al.*, 2001), social work is also emerging as a profession relying critically on the best available evidence to guide practice decisions (Webb, 2001; Witkin and Harrison, 2001; Glasby and Beresford, 2006). Similarly, practice wisdom and partnership with service users and carers (Beresford, 2007) are increasingly becoming a feature of social work education in the West. There is a renewed emphasis on using indigenous knowledge and First Nations expertise in social work education to train social workers who can understand and meet the needs of aboriginal people, particularly in Canada (Sinclair, 2004). A major facet of social work education in many developing countries is to equip students with the knowledge and skills to respond to structural problems such as heightened inequality, poverty, existing and emerging pandemics and natural disasters. In India, for example, many schools of social work prepare students with the knowledge and skills to respond to public health emergencies and natural disasters and make practice expeditions to the affected areas to not only engage in providing emotional and psychosocial support but also to help with rehabilitation work including building houses and roads and participate in other community and social development activities (Palattiyil and Sidhva, 2012).

Prompted by the global demand for social workers, several schools of social work in different parts of the world have also begun offering international placements, exchange programmes (Lalayants *et al.*, 2014) and twinning of social work degree programmes with overseas social work schools, with the aim of orienting students to global social work practice issues. Another interesting and perhaps a more serious development is the ever-increasing encroachment of the field of social work by other allied disciplines, such as international development, offering practice placements in social work based non-governmental organisations.

One of the latest developments in, and perhaps a real challenge for, social work education globally is the imperative for incorporating the Global Agenda for Social Work and Social Development into the social work curriculum. The Global Agenda inspires social work educators and practitioners to strengthen the international profile of social work and social development and to make a stronger contribution to policy development (Jones and Truell, 2012). The Agenda identified four fields for action by global institutions, local communities and the three organizations representing social work globally: promoting social and economic equalities, promoting the dignity and worth of peoples, working towards environmental sustainability, and strengthening human relationships (IASSW *et al.*, 2014). If social workers worldwide need to learn more about the global forces affecting societies in various stages of economic development (Hare, 2004), and if the aspirations articulated in the Global Agenda have to be achieved, it is vitally important that a concerted effort is made across the world of social work education to include the Global Agenda as a key element in the social work curriculum, such that social work can carve out a vision that rests on the core values of human rights, social justice, equality and sustainability.

Part IV examines some of these emerging trends in the education of new social work professionals and articulates the challenges facing social work in the twenty-first century.

Chapter 12 draws primarily on literature from the United Kingdom to provide a critical overview of service user and carer involvement in social work education. Chapter 13 describes and analyses the main challenges and issues affecting the process of the development of social work as a new profession in post-Soviet Russia. One of the major challenges in social work development in China is the lack of social work educators and professionals with adequate practice experience and skills. Chapter 14 describes the practice project that grew out of the response to the Sichuan earthquake. Social work can serve as a framework for social work practice in the field of disaster preparedness, response and recovery around the globe. Chapter 15 outlines a proposal for a Social Work Charter for Unexpected Disasters, based upon a needs assessment conducted by participant observers in the aftermath of the Bam, Iran earthquake. Chapter 16 examines policy and practice developments since 2000 aimed at bringing Scotland's social work practice closer in line with international standards and international research on effective approaches in the field of youth justice. Social work and the community services sector in Australia have undergone profound systemic change over the past two decades, resulting in an altered social mandate and function and a restructuring of the institutional structures and arrangements used to deliver services to marginalized and socially excluded groups and individuals. Chapter 17 examines the impact of these changes on social work practice in Australia.

References

Alphonse, M., George, P. and Moffat, K. (2008) Redefining social work standards in the context of globalisation: Lessons from India, *International Social Work*, 51(2), 145–58.

Annan, K. (2001) *We the Children: Meeting the Promises of the World Summit for Children*. New York: United Nations.

Beresford, P. (2007) The role of service user research in generating knowledge-based health and social care: From conflict to contribution, *Evidence and Policy*, 3(3), 329–41.

Dominelli, L. (2010) *Social Work in a Globalizing World*. Cambridge: Polity Press.

Glasby, J. and Beresford, P. (2006) Who knows best? Evidence-based practice and the service user contribution, *Critical Social Policy*, 26(1), 268–84.

Hare, I. (2004) Defining social work for the 21st century: The International Federation of Social Workers' revised definition of social work, *International Social Work*, 47(3), 407–24.

Hoagwood, K., Burns, B., Kiser, L., Ringeisen, H. and Schoenwald, S. (2001) Evidence based practice in child and adolescent mental health services, *Psychiatric Services*, 52(9), 1179–89.

International Association of Schools of Social Work, International Council on Social Welfare and International Federation of Social Workers (2014) Global agenda for social work and social development: First report, *International Social Work*, 57(S4), 3–16.

Jones, D. and Truell, R. (2012) The global agenda for social work and social development: A place to link together and be effective in a globalised world, *International Social Work*, 55(4), 544–72.

Lalayants, M., Doel, M. and Kachkachishvili, I. (2014) Pedagogy of international social work: A comparative study in the USA, UK, and Georgia, *European Journal of Social Work*, 17(4), 455–74.

Palattiyil, G. and Sidhva, D. (2012) Guest editorial – social work in India, *Practice: Social Work in Action*, 24(2), 75–8.

Sinclair, R. (2004) Aboriginal social work education in Canada: Decolonizing pedagogy for the seventh generation, *First Peoples Child & Family Review*, 1(1), 49–61.

Webb, S.A. (2001) Some considerations on the validity of evidence-based practice in social work, *British Journal of Social Work*, 31, 57–79.

Witkin, S. and Harrison, W. (2001) Whose evidence and for what purpose? *Editorial, Social Work*, 46(4), 293–6.

Chapter 12

Involving service users and carers in social work education

A consideration of the UK and global perspectives

Gillian MacIntyre and Pearse McCusker

Service user and carer participation has become a global phenomenon that has a high priority within many government policy initiatives (Webb 2008). This participation needs to be considered within a context of political and social change. Societies are operating within a context of globalization, migration and social exclusion, with significant financial and resource constraints. Within the UK context, the involvement of service users and carers in all aspects of social work education, from development and planning to delivery, selection and assessment of students, has become relatively commonplace. These developments have emerged partly from guidance published by governments across all four jurisdictions in relation to the requirements for social work education as set out by the Department of Health (DH; 2002), Scottish Executive (2003) and the Northern Ireland Office (2003). Under the Care Standards Act (2000), the DH issued the Requirements for Social Work Training (DH 2002) followed by the National Occupational Standards for Social Work (DH 2002) and the Quality Assurance Agency subject benchmark statement for social work (DH 2000), all of which placed central importance on service user and carer involvement in the development and delivery of social work training. Leven (2004) described the initiative as follows:

> An ambitious agenda in which the type of knowledge that service users and carers can impart is identified as a strong lever for improving social care ... [it] recognizes that service users and carers are themselves experts in what would make for more control, choice and better quality in their everyday lives and in existing services.
>
> (Leven 2004: 8)

In order to support these developments and in recognition of their significance, higher education institutions in England were allocated a small grant of around £6,000 for three years in order to develop the necessary infrastructure required to support service user and carer participation (Leven 2004).

User-led organizations such as Shaping Our Lives in England (Beresford *et al.* 2006) and Scottish Voices in Scotland (SIESWE 2004) played a crucial role in taking these developments forward. Similar requirements and developments took place across the other jurisdictions of the United Kingdom. For example, the Framework for Social Work Education in Scotland stated that institutions of higher education must set out 'policies and procedures ... [that] must include effective and appropriate ways of meeting the requirements of key stakeholders in social services ... key stakeholders include people who use services, carers and employers' (Scottish Executive 2003: 15). Similarly in Northern Ireland, the Northern Ireland Care Council stated: 'The engagement of service users and carers in training is essential for students to reach an understanding of both the quality and nature of services required and the way in which they must be delivered' (Harbison, cited in Duffy 2006: 5).

At an international level, the International Federation of Social Workers has developed a European Framework for Quality Assurance of Social Professions and has identified service user and carer involvement in the running and development of services as being essential (Anghel and Ramon 2009).

The origins of service user and carer involvement

In order to assess progress in relation to service user and carer involvement, it is important to first consider its origins. According to Barnes and Walker (1996), there are two clear philosophical principles that underpin service user and carer involvement, these being consumerism and empowerment. If the philosophy of empowerment is considered first, this can be traced largely to developments associated with the disability movement, where lessons learned from the civil rights movement in the United States resulted in an increased demand by disabled people for greater control and the right to make decisions about their own lives (Glasby and Littlechild 2009). This is perhaps best encapsulated by the Independent Living Movement, which has campaigned for greater independence, choice and control for people with disabilities (Means *et al.* 2008). Such user-led organizations have sought to develop a new understanding of disability, underpinned by the social model of disability, with an emphasis on economic, environmental and cultural barriers (Barnes and Mercer 2003). Such rights are now arguably underpinned by human rights legislation such as the Human Rights Act 1998, which incorporated the European Convention on Human Rights and the Disability Discrimination Act, 1995 and the Equalities Act, 2010.

The second philosophical principle underpinning service user and carer involvement is that of consumerism. In the 1980s the Conservative government in the United Kingdom began to apply market principles to health and social care services. This involved a shift in focus, with service users being regarded as consumers, and was characterized by greater choice, flexibility and efficiency (Means *et al.* 2008). This need for efficiency and effectiveness is felt keenly across all developed countries, particularly in areas where public funding and finances play a role (Evers 2003). The idea is that more efficient and effective services are more likely to occur if they more closely relate to the expressed views and wishes of service users and carers (Bowl 1996). This shift in ideology afforded a much greater role for service users and carers in a consultancy capacity, and there was an increased expectation that service providers should consult with service users and carers as the customers of their services (Glasby and Littlechild 2009). This led to an increased focus on collaborative working and co-production, with service users and carers being increasingly viewed as active partners in their care. While this can be viewed in a positive light, the move towards a consumerist notion of service user and carer involvement has also attracted criticism that the primary motivation can be regarded as reducing costs, with service user and carer participation being viewed as a means to 'reduce operations and maintenance costs' by government agencies (Carey 2009: 184). Ferguson (2007) refers to service user and carer involvement in the form of personalization as a type of 'privatization by the back door', where risk is privatized and becomes an individual concern rather than a responsibility of the state.

Bound up in this is the perceived threat to the social work profession usefully highlighted by Manthorpe *et al.* (2009) who suggest that developments in relation to individual budgets for service users have led social workers to become increasingly uncertain about their role. Also, and perhaps somewhat ironically, this new system of consumerism is located within the old system of welfare paternalism, where people are defined in the terms of service providers as service users (Croft and Beresford 1989), thus creating an in-built power imbalance where the potential for change is reduced.

Webb, writing in an Australian context, helpfully theorizes service user and carer involvement in terms of 'degrees of participation in relation to the demand by government directives to nurture it' (Webb 2008: 273). In other words, he suggests that the approach taken by different governments to service user and carer involvement will depend on their initial motivations for this involvement. He identifies a number of models that can be used in order to assess the type or level of participation. The 'direct democratic model', for example, assumes a direct ciphering of views and does not acknowledge or explore issues of power. The model suggests that service users' and professionals' views are treated with equal regard with neither holding primacy over the other. This view does not appear to acknowledge the power imbalances inherent in this field. The economic model involves the inclusion of organizations with the finances and resources to support service user and carer involvement, such as the National Society for the Prevention of Cruelty to Children (NSPCC) or MIND, a national mental health organization. Webb suggests that they 'combine money with expertise and research that has the ear of government' (Webb 2008: 274). Such organizations often adopt a campaigning function on behalf of their members and are afforded a level of independence (although this is increasingly questionable); however, service user and carer empowerment and increasing the range of participants is not the primary focus. A social model of participation, on the other hand, has the inclusion of service users and carers at its centre. However, this model views participation or involvement as an end in itself and does not look to measure or evaluate outcomes. The ideological model, meanwhile, highlights the views and beliefs of service users and carers and is aimed at shaping or changing policy or services (Webb 2008).

These models (or variations of these) often co-exist, for example, a more traditional welfarist approach might exist alongside a consumerist or rights-based approach (Evers 2003). The different models will likely result in service users and carers being viewed in different ways – for example as citizens with entitlements, as consumers to be consulted or as vulnerable individuals to be protected (Evers 2003). Perhaps what each of these models has in common is the extent to which power is transferred from the state or from organizations to individual service users and carers.

The range of models indicated might also relate to some extent to the notion of a hierarchy of participation. Drawing on the work of Arnstein (1969) in terms of her ladder of participation, theorists have developed various hierarchies of participation that include, for example, the levels of *no involvement, passive involvement, token involvement* and *collaboration and partnership* (Stickley 2006). At the highest level of the hierarchy, involvement will encompass an equal relationship between service users and professionals, with decisions being made jointly, different forms of knowledge being valued equally and power being shared.

By considering the origins of user and carer involvement and the different models of involvement outlined above, it is possible to begin to review some examples of user and carer involvement, considering some of the benefits, before moving on to identify a number of key challenges that remain.

The impact of service user and carer involvement in the UK context

Service user and carer involvement in British institutions of higher education occurs at a number of levels, from the development and planning of courses to direct contact with students in the delivery of teaching, recruitment and selection, and assessment. These different types of involvement can be linked to the hierarchy of participation outlined above. A plethora of material has been published in recent times that illustrates some of the work that has been carried out in partnership with service users and carers. Anghel and Ramon (2009) for example, have discussed involvement that has focused on personal testimony and a model that views service users and carers as consultants and co-trainers. The power of hearing about service user experiences directly from them is well documented, the reason for which Baldwin and Sadd (2006: 351) encapsulated succinctly: 'It was easy enough for a social work lecturer to say the words, [but] it is the medium (service user voice) that conveys the message.'

Allain *et al.* (2006) described user and carer involvement in one institution of higher education from the perspective of a range of key stakeholders, including service users, carers, tutors and students. This piece suggested the transformative potential of service user and carer involvement, describing how service users have grown in confidence since participating in the programme (Allain *et al.* 2006). Such work is well developed, with numerous examples of service user and carer involvement in both the development and particularly in the delivery of direct teaching. Less well developed appears to be service user involvement in selection and in assessment processes (Barnes *et al.* 2000), although this differs across institutions of higher education. A survey of service user and carer involvement in Scottish institutions of higher education reported by Ager *et al.* in 2005 suggested that, in relation to teaching, overall involvement was limited to occasional classes. In relation to assessment, only a small proportion of service users and carers had been directly involved in giving feedback, suggesting that further developmental work is needed here. Similar findings were reported in a Social Care Institute for Excellence (SCIE) review of service user and carer involvement published in 2011. The report was developed by service users and carers in order to provide evidence to support the view that service user and carer involvement is of central importance to social work education. The report identified a range of benefits, although it was argued that involvement needed to move beyond 'sharing personal stories' in teaching (SCIE 2011).

The SCIE report is indicative of the widespread agreement as to the benefits of service user and carer involvement; however, as Robinson and Webber (2013) have pointed out, there is very little empirical evidence that evaluates the impact of service user and carer involvement on practice. As a result, a growing body of studies has begun to question and critically analyse the impact of service user and carer involvement. The weight of the current evidence base appears to lie with self-reported evidence from service users, carers, students and staff, which suggests that service user and carer involvement is highly valued by those involved. For example, Anghel and Ramon (2009) reported findings from an evaluation of user and carer involvement indicating students felt that input from service users and carers changed their perspectives, suggesting that involvement made an impact at a personal level. There are also reported benefits for service users and carers in terms of their own personal and skills development (Barnes *et al.* 2000). Likewise, Humphries (2005) reported positive feedback from both service user organizations and students, while recognizing the limitations of such involvement. She argued that a project where students worked alongside service users and carers to consider different experiences of discrimination was 'a step towards good practice [in] mainstreaming the involvement of service users in social work education, rather than a step towards radical transformation' (Humphries 2005: 802).

This raises the question as to what radical transformation might look like. Referring back to Webb's models of involvement (2008), one might hypothesize that radical transformation may involve privileging the knowledge of service users and carers over other forms of knowledge. It would certainly involve a significant shift in the balance of power. Despite the advances made in terms of user and carer involvement, professionals continue to exercise considerable power over the lives of service users and carers (Barnes and Mercer 2003). This is clear even from the language adopted by each profession, which often serves to exclude users and carers, given that they are unlikely to be privy to the professional knowledge base it is informed by (Barnes and Mercer 2003; Carey 2009; Cowden and Singh 2007). This relates closely to the arguments made by Carey (2009) in his critical commentary on service user and carer participation. He questions the way in which service user and carer involvement is organized as well as 'the overall philosophy of an apparently vibrant counter-culture' (Carey 2009: 181). He argues that as service users and carers become increasingly involved, both individually and organizationally, in official government and professional agendas, they become part of that agenda, thus inadvertently promoting inequality between themselves and those service users and carers who are not involved. In other words the message that service users and carers bring becomes lost within those of the organization; hence the ability to promote change is greatly reduced. A slightly different but related point was raised by Felton and Stickley (2004), who have suggested that the closer a service user becomes to the educational structures, the more distant they are assumed to have become from their own experiences. Speaking specifically about those who use mental health services, they draw on the work of Szasz (1960), who discusses stereotypical perceptions of those experiencing mental ill health as irrational, irresponsible and dangerous. As service users who are involved with delivering education challenge these perceptions there is then an assumption that they are not typically representative of the group. Rather than challenging the stereotype, in some cases they are dismissed as being unrepresentative. Hence they find themselves in a no-win situation. This suggests an element of exclusivity within the service user and carer movement, with the accounts of some service user and carer groups being privileged over those of others. Evidence suggests that members of black and minority ethnic groups, for example, remain under-represented (Yeung and Ng 2011).

The problem with service user and carer involvement

Service users and carers find themselves with a dilemma: to become part of the 'establishment' and risk losing their independence, or to maintain their independence and have their voices further marginalized. Indeed some organizations have not felt that it was within their best interests to pursue traditional forms of involvement. Mad Pride, a movement of people who use mental health services, for example, did not pursue involvement, adopting a more archaic approach in terms of campaigning (Stickley 2006). They have actively sought to reclaim terms such as 'mad', 'nutter' and 'psycho' from misuse. Indeed, Tew (2005) has suggested that ideas of citizenship and rationality have been used somewhat cynically to 'regulate political dissidence and to legitimate forms of discrimination and injustice' (Tew 2005: 85).

Those organizations that wish to promote service user and carer involvement also face a number of challenges in order to promote meaningful rather than tokenistic participation. This involves first identifying what meaningful involvement might look like. Webber and Robinson (2012), in a study examining stakeholder views, found no agreed definition of meaningful involvement, with definitions ranging from adding value to the course to empowerment of service users and carers; however, these findings relate primarily to the perceived purpose of involvement.

Meaningful involvement is likely to incorporate a number of practical measures that have been well documented elsewhere and can be considered good practice when working with service users and carers (see, for example, Beresford 2007; Carr 2004; Duffy 2006; Leven 2004; SCIE 2009). Although meaningful involvement might be considered a difficult objective to fully achieve, it is by no means impossible (Tyler 2006). Such practical steps include, for example, providing service users and carers with adequate training and support prior to their involvement, as well as adequate guidance in terms of what is expected, preferably arriving at an agreement around expectations in partnership. Brown and Young (2008) identify the benefits of providing training to service users in order to develop capacity, as well as the need for ongoing support for service users and carers. Meaningful involvement also involves not stretching service user and carers' knowledge and expertise simply to fit in with the existing structure of a module or programme (Humphries 2005). There should also be the opportunity for adequate debriefing after involvement, for students and service users, as well as the provision of timely and constructive feedback. This support has to be balanced, however, with not making assumptions about service users' perceived vulnerabilities. As Taylor (1997: 178) argues: 'Whereas it is appropriate to consider issues of safety for all guest presenters, to single [service] users out as a particularly vulnerable group is discriminatory.' Indeed, institutions of higher education are not free from discrimination or stereotypes, and certain groups of service users in particular (such as those with mental health issues) may be viewed as unreliable or incapable of contributing (Bassett et al. 2006).

Barnes and Mercer (2003) report that from the perspectives of service users and carers, a number of constraints have been identified. These range from too little time for meaningful discussion, to having little access to senior staff within organizations. Institutions of higher education are essentially hierarchical institutions, with a built-in pecking order (Bassett *et al.* 2006). The notion of expertise is significant here, and in some quarters resistance in terms of letting go of the role of expert might be apparent (Bassett *et al.* 2006). Indeed, drawing on the work of Carr (2004), it is possible to hypothesize that many of the barriers to meaningful participation relate essentially to power differentials: 'Exclusionary structures, institutional practices and professional attitudes can affect the extent to which service users can influence change ... power sharing can be difficult within established mainstream structures' (Carr 2004: 267).

There are a number of particular cultural barriers that relate to stigma. When considering the Chinese community, for example, there are those who wish to respect their 'family secret', for example (Yeung and Ng 2011). Many traditional Chinese families are reluctant to involve outsiders and may continue to retain traditional beliefs and thinking (Yeung and Ng 2011). There are also practical considerations such as language barriers that need to be taken into consideration.

Until this point, the assumption has been that greater levels of participation are something that service users and carers seek. This does not consider the experiences of a great many service users who do not use services on a voluntary basis. Such service users, for example, those who use children and families social work services, criminal justice service users and those subject to compulsory measures under mental health legislation, may not necessarily wish for greater levels of engagement with social work in any form (Smith *et al.* 2012), making the prospect of creating meaningful service user and carer involvement all the more challenging. Smith *et al.* (2012), drawing on evidence from a knowledge exchange project carried out in collaboration with social work practitioners, emphasize the importance of building trusting relationships as a starting point for meaningful engagement with involuntary clients. In addition, taking time to communicate with and provide information to service users and their families was thought to be vital. This can be considered good practice in promoting service user involvement amongst all service user groups.

Alongside these considerations, the importance of adequate remuneration for service users and carers has been well documented. The challenges of achieving this have also been considered (see, for example, Branfield 2009). Barriers in processing payments or even making payments at all as a result of unnecessary bureaucracy within institutions of higher education can leave service users feeling devalued (Bassett *et al.* 2006). However, overcoming these barriers is crucial if accusations of tokenism are to be avoided.

Addressing these issues will require further investment of resources (SCIE 2011). In a time of financial constraint this is likely to be challenging. In

Scotland, for example, monies provided to institutions of higher education by the Scottish Government via the Scottish Social Services Council to support the development of service user and carer involvement in Scottish institutions of higher education have ceased to be available. Thus it appears that the commitment to service user and carer involvement at a policy level is not always backed up by ongoing financial support.

What do we need to learn? Lessons from a global context

The current financial constraints faced by developed countries mean that sustaining current levels of service user and carer involvement, let alone developing these advances further, will prove to be particularly challenging. It is helpful to look to other countries in order to consider what lessons, if any, might be learned in terms of involving service users and carers. In South Africa, for example, it appears that service user and carer involvement has been limited during the 20 years of democracy. In relation to mental health, for example, a study of four African countries (South Africa, Ghana, Uganda and Zambia) found that, with the exception of Zambia, service users were not consulted widely during policy development, despite the requirements of the World Health Organization report (2001) which recommended that mental health service users and their families be included as critical stakeholders in decision-making and review processes that inform the development of laws, policies and services (Cooper *et al.* 2011).

It appears that service user and carer involvement in the developing world is by no means standard practice. However, when it does occur, developing countries make use of strategies for social action aimed at reducing stigma and supporting social inclusion, and perhaps developed countries might learn from this. User-led advocacy has begun to develop across African countries, although these developments are in their early stages: 'The challenge is for governments and NGOs to partner with user support groups, advocacy bodies and self-help initiatives to expand and strengthen these initiatives throughout Africa' (Cooper *et al.* 2011: 319).

Within developing or low-income countries, community-based organizations have a central role to play in working with professionals to promote effective partnership working with previously excluded or marginalized people (Herrman 2010). It is essential for professionals to take time to develop a trusting relationship with service users, as work from a Chinese context suggests (Yeung and Ng 2011). Cross-cultural studies of service user and carer involvement have identified the importance of involving someone in a position of trust in order to engage with hard-to-reach communities. Identifying these key insiders, such as community leaders, at an early stage can promote a greater level of engagement with those who have not traditionally been involved (Bowes and Sim 2006; Yeung and Ng 2011). Similarly, with reference to involving service users and carers with differing experiences of sectarianism in Northern Ireland, Coulter *et al.* (2013: 11) stress the importance of creating an environment of trust or safety in the classroom that encourages students to leave their comfort zones and enter a 'process of open and critical enquiry'.

In many ways the barriers faced in terms of progressing service user and carer involvement are the same across developed and developing countries. The struggle, for example, to define what counts as knowledge is as keenly felt in South Africa as it is in the United Kingdom. For example, Sithole (2011: 89) argues that in South Africa knowledge production is both racialized and gendered, reflecting power positions in the West. He argues: 'Indigenous knowledge from Africa is seen as embarrassing to articulate ... yet most western knowledge that ended up being scientific has its origins in indigenous theories.' Similar arguments can be made as to the primacy held by professional knowledge as opposed to service user knowledge.

In times of financial constraint, in this area as in all areas of social work, the pressure to demonstrate outcomes is ever greater (Miller 2012). Robinson and Webber identify a number of outcome-focused models of user and carer involvement within the literature characterized by the need to evidence change or improvement. However, little systematic evaluation of the impact of such models has been carried out, making it difficult to assess their success or otherwise (Robinson and Webber 2013). This suggests a need for further research that focuses on specifically measuring the impact of involvement.

Conclusions

It is clear from this discussion that service user and carer involvement in social work education is a complex activity that can take many different forms, which arise from a range of philosophical standpoints and are influenced by local and national political, economic and cultural factors. As such, when seeking to develop or improve service user and carer involvement within a particular institution of higher education, a key imperative from the research evidence would appear to be ensuring that the aims and objectives are clarified at the outset. This would require the relevant stakeholders, including academics, service users, carers and students, to stipulate what it is they hope to achieve and, importantly, what the limitations of the involvement would be. In others words, aiming for a degree of power and control that is likely unattainable, regardless of how laudable the aim might be is likely to result in demotivation and disengagement. Indeed, Cowden and Singh (2007: 5) suggest that it is perhaps more realistic for service user and carer perspectives to be 'neither privileged or subjected but to be situated in a process of creative critical dialogue'. Allied to defining the aims and objectives of involvement underpinned by a particular model or philosophy is the need to establish the funding source that would support it, both directly in relation to payments to service users and carers, and indirectly for those costs associated with lecturing and administrative staff time.

With the model of involvement and financial arrangements established, the current research base, particularly in the United Kingdom, provides a rich source of information on how service user and carer involvement can be facilitated. This is particularly the case for involvement in direct teaching, although the evidence for other activities, including assessment and selection, is increasing. For example, paying adequate attention to ensuring that service users and carers have been able to prepare sufficiently and matching service user and carer input to specific course aims and intended learning outcomes is essential, in order to avoid the activities being tokenistic.

Despite the numerous challenges outlined in this chapter and across the literature, the growing evidence base suggests that service user and carer involvement may have significant transformative pedagogic potential. The self-reported nature of much of the research findings to date from students, service users and carers should not invalidate this message. Rather, the consistency with which it is made calls for new research designed to evaluate the impact on students' knowledge and behaviours as they move from educational institutions into practice. This will be essential in order to safeguard funding streams in addition to making the argument for increased levels of involvement, both of which appear at risk in the current economic climate.

A number of questions remain, and perhaps further research might address these questions. How meaningful involvement is defined and measured, for example, continues to be a conundrum for those working in this field. Likewise, the contested nature of what constitutes knowledge needs to be explored in order for a shared understanding to be achieved. It was hoped that drawing on literature from other countries and cultures might shed some light on these questions. What was discovered, however, was a fledgling service user and carer movement facing, to a greater or lesser extent, a range of similar challenges to those that have been highlighted in the UK context.

The global economic crisis raises doubts around how service user and carer involvement can be sustained at its current level, let alone being further developed, and building a robust evidence base is imperative in order to make this case in a climate of competing demands. However, providing the evidence base to show what works in relation to service user and carer involvement must be viewed positively, as it is only when this evidence is made widely available that some of the more cynical or tokenistic ways of involving service users and carers can finally be laid to rest.

References

Ager, W., Dow, J. and Gee, M. (2005) 'Grassroots networks: a model for promoting the influence of service users and carers in social work education', *Social Work Education*, 24(4): 467–76.

Allain, L., Cosis Brown, H., Danso, C., Dillon, J., Finnegan, P., Gadhoke, S., Shamash, M., and Whittaker, F. (2006) 'User and carer involvement in social work education – a university case study: manipulation or control?', *Social Work Education*, 25(4): 403–13.

Anghel, R. and Ramon, S. (2009) 'Service users and carers' involvement in social work education: Lessons from an English case study', *European Journal of Social Work*, 12(2): 185–99.

Arnstein, Sherry R. (1969) 'A ladder of citizen participation', *JAIP*, 35(4): 216–24.

Baldwin, M. and Sadd, J. (2006) 'Allies with attitude! Service users, academics and social service agency staff learning how to share power in running social work education courses', *Social Work Education*, 25(4): 348–59.

Barnes, C. and Mercer, G. (2003) *Research Review on User Involvement in Promoting Change and Enhancing the Quality of Social 'Care' Services for Disabled People*, Leeds: Centre for Disability Studies, University of Leeds.

Barnes, D., Carpenter, J. and Bailey, D. (2000) 'Partnerships with service users in interprofessional education for community health: A case study', *Journal of Interprofessional Care*, 14(2): 189–200.

Barnes, M. and Walker, A. (1996) 'Consumerism versus empowerment: A principled approach to the involvement of older service users', *Policy & Politics*, 24(4): 375–93.

Bassett, T., Campbell, P. and Anderson, J. (2006) 'Service user/survivor involvement in mental health training and education: Overcoming the barriers', *Social Work Education*, 25(4): 393–402.

Beresford, P. (2007) 'User involvement, research and health inequalities: Developing new directions', *Health and Social Care in the Community*, 15(4): 306–12.

Beresford, P., Branfield, F., Taylor, J., Brennan, M., Sartori, A., Lalani, M. and Wise, G. (2006) 'Working together for better social work education', *Social Work Education*, 25(4): 326–31.

Bowes, A. and Sim, D. (2006) 'Advocacy for black and minority ethnic communities: Understandings and expectations', *British Journal of Social Work*, 36(7): 1209–25.

Bowl, R. (1996) 'Legislating for user involvement in the United Kingdom: Mental health services and the NHS and Community Care Act 1990', *International Journal of Social Psychiatry*, 42: 165–80.

Branfield, F. (2009) *Developing User Involvement in Social Work Education*, SCIE Workforce Development Report No. 29, London: SCIE.

Brown, K. and Young, N. (2008) 'Building capacity for service user and carer involvement in social work education', *Social Work Education*, 27(1): 84–96.

Carey, M. (2009) 'Happy shopper? The problem with service user and carer participation', *British Journal of Social Work*, 39(1): 179–88.

Carr, S. (2004) *Has Service User and Carer Participation Made a Difference to Social Care Services?* SCIE Position Paper No. 3, London: SCIE.

Cooper, S., Bhana, A., Drew, N., Faydi, A., Fisher, A., Kakuma, R., Kleintjes, S., Lund, K., Ofori-Atta, A., Skeen, S. and the MHAPP Research Consortium (2011) 'Recommendations for improving mental health systems in Africa: Lessons from Ghana, Uganda, South Africa and Zambia', in K. Kondlo and C. Ejiogu (eds) *Africa in Focus: Governance in the 21st Century*, Cape Town: HSRC Press.

Coulter, S., Campbell, J., Duffy, J. and Reilly, I. (2013) 'Enabling social work students to deal with the consequences of political conflict: Engaging with victim/survivor service users and a "pedagogy of discomfort"', *Social Work Education*, 32(4): 439–52.

Cowden, S. and Singh, G. (2007) 'The "user": friend, foe or fetish?: A critical exploration of user involvement in health and social care', *Critical Social Policy*, 27(1): 5–23.

Croft, S. and Beresford, P. (1989) 'User involvement, citizenship and social policy', *Critical Social Policy*, 9(26): 5–18.

Department of Health (2000) *A Quality Strategy for Social Care*, London: Department of Health.

Department of Health (2002) *Requirements for Social Work Training*, London: Department of Health.

Duffy, J. (2006) *Participating and Learning: Citizen Involvement in Social Work Education in the Northern Ireland Context, a Good Practice Guide*, Belfast: University of Ulster.

Evers, A. (2003) '*Current strands in debating user involvement in social services: Discussion paper for the group of specialists on user involvement in social services*', Council of Europe.

Felton, A. and Stickley, T. (2004) 'Pedagogy, power and service user involvement', *Journal of Psychiatry and Mental Health Nursing*, 11(1): 89–98.

Ferguson, I. (2007) 'Increasing user choice or privatizing risk? The antinomies of personalisation', *British Journal of Social Work*, 37(3): 387–403.

Glasby, J. and Littlechild, R. (2009) *Direct Payments and Personal Budgets: Putting Personalisation into Practice*, Bristol: Policy Press.

Great Britain (1998) *Human Rights Act 1998: Elizabeth ll. Chapter 42*, London: The Stationery Office.

Herrman, H. (2010) 'WPA Project on partnerships for best practices in working with service users and carers', *World Psychiatry*, 9(2): 127–8.

Humphries, C. (2005) 'Service user involvement in social work education: A case example', *Social Work Education*, 24(7): 797–803.

Leven, E. (2004) *Involving Service Users and Carers in Social Work Education*, SCIE Guide No. 4, London: SCIE.

Manthorpe, J. (2000) 'Developing carers' contribution to social work training', *Social Work Education Journal*, 19(1): 19–27.

Manthorpe, J., Jacobs, S., Rapaport, J., Challis, D., Netten, A., Glendinning, C., Stevens, M., Wilberforce, M., Knapp, M. and Harris, J. (2009) 'Training for change: Early days of Individual Budgets and the implications for social work and care management practice: A qualitative study of the views of trainers', *British Journal of Social Work*, 39(7): 1291–305.

Means, R., Richard, S. and Smith, R. (2008) *Community Care: Policy and Practice* (4th edn), Basingstoke: Palgrave Macmillan.

Miller, A. (2012) *Individual Outcomes: Getting Back to What Matters*, Edinburgh: Dunedin Academic Press.

Northern Ireland Office (2003) *Northern Ireland Framework Specification for the Degree in Social Work*, Northern Ireland: Department of Health, Social Services and Public Safety.

Robinson, K. and Webber, M. (2013) 'Models and effectiveness of service user and carer involvement in social work education: A literature review', *British Journal of Social Work*, 43(5): 925–44.

Scottish Executive (2003) 'The framework for social work education in Scotland'. Available at: www.gov.scot/Publications/2003/01/16202/17015 (accessed 10 February 2015).

SIESWE (2004) 'Scottish voices: Service users and carers at the heart of social work education', a conference report.

Sithole, P. (2011) 'Wrestling with intellectual hegemony: The dwarfed status of knowledge production in South Africa', in K. Kondlo and C. Ejiogu (eds) *Africa in Focus: Governance in the 21st Century*, Cape Town: HSRC Press.

Smith, M., Gallagher, M., Wosu, H., Stewart, J., Cree, V., Hunter S., Evans S., Montgomery, C., Holiday, S. and Wilkinson, H. (2012) 'Engaging with involuntary service users in social work: Findings from a knowledge exchange project', *British Journal of Social Work*, 42(8): 1460–77.

Social Care Institute for Excellence (2009) *Building User and Carer Involvement in Social Work Education*, SCIE At a Glance Report No. 19, London: SCIE.

Social Care Institute for Excellence (2011) *'We Are More Than Just Our Story': Service User and Carer Participation in Social Work Education*, SCIE Report No. 42, London: SCIE.

Stickley, T. (2006) 'Should service user involvement be consigned to history? A critical realist perspective', *Journal of Psychiatric and Mental Health Nursing*, 13(5): 570–7.

Szasz, T. (1960) 'The myth of mental illness', *American Psychologist*, 15: 113–18.

Taylor, I. (1997) *Developing Learning in Professional Education: Partnerships for Practice*, Buckingham: Open University Press.

Tew, J. (ed.) (2005) *Social Perspectives in Mental Health: Developing Social Models to Understand and Work with Mental Distress*, London: Jessica Kingsley Publishers.

Tyler, G. (2006) 'Addressing barriers to participation: Service user involvement in social work training', *Social Work Education*, 25(4): 385–92.

Webb, S. (2008) 'Modelling service user participation in social care', *Journal of Social Work*, 7(3): 269–90.

Webber, M. and Robinson, K. (2012) 'The meaningful involvement of service users and carers in advanced-level post-qualifying social work education: A qualitative study', *British Journal of Social Work*, 42(7): 1256–74.

World Health Organization (WHO) (2001) *The World Health Report 2001 – Mental Health: New Understanding, New Hope*, Geneva: WHO.

Yeung, Y. and Ng, S. (2011) 'Engaging service users and carers in health and social care education: Challenges and opportunities in the Chinese community', *Social Work Education*, 30(3): 281–98.

Chapter 13

Social work in Russia

Between the global and the local

Elena Iarskaia-Smirnova and Pavel Romanov[1]

Introduction

This chapter describes and analyses the main challenges and issues affecting the process of development of social work as a new profession in today's Russia. At the end of the Soviet Union, the engagement of Russia with the West increased, but still the tensions between Russia and the West exist, and at times these tensions become even stronger. It is of particular interest to explore the specific implications of these relationships for social work. Since social work's establishment as an occupation and training programme in the early 1990s, educators, students, administrators and practitioners have not only implemented several shifts in the national policy agenda but have also addressed various global influences and incorporated them into the local policy context. The development of social work is being shaped by different power relations. Looking at these power relations from three interrelated analytical perspectives – those of actors, institutions and discourses – we will consider the role of international cooperation in the field of social work. We shall refer to the qualitative interviews with social work practitioners and managers in three social service agencies conducted during 2011–2012 in Saratov, Russia. These services were chosen because they were a part of international projects.

We shall start with a short historical background on the policy context in the Soviet past and provide a brief introduction to current developments in the profession in post-communist Russia. Then we briefly outline some of the issues regarding global/local knowledge transfer in social work and consider the power relations that are embedded in different contexts of international collaboration. The chapter continues by addressing questions about the scope and characteristics of actors, institutions and discourses, which constitute a framework for the development of social work in Russia, taking into account global and local interrelationships. We conclude with a discussion of changes in social work within the wider context.

Historical background

Since 1917, following the demise of czarism with its relatively rudimentary social services, Russia experienced the transition to socialist principles of welfare, exemplifying the dual characteristics of universalism and employment-based provision (Standing 1996: 227). These principles underwent various major changes during the Stalinist years, the Second World War and its aftermath, as well as in the late Soviet period and of course in the more recent post-Soviet/communist period. State ideology in socialist times combined elements of conservative and social democratic value systems (using the typology of Esping Andersen (1990)), and while the early Soviet political rhetoric appealed to the values of self-government and equality, the shift was soon made towards paternalism and differential inclusion. This was reflected in changes relating to the understanding of social problems, their causes and ways of tackling them, reforming social support and service provision (Iarskaia-Smirnova 2011a).

The state and its various agents carried out this double-faced task of care and control at all levels of social life, moving gradually from tough and selective schemes of social security and insurance to the 'bright future' of a socialist welfare state. The Soviet system of social welfare shaped by the 1950s served as a model for the states of the Eastern socialist bloc (Dixon and Macarov 1992; Schilde and Schulte 2005). In the 1960s and 1970s, the Soviet government built one of the most advanced systems of social assistance in the world, in terms of equality of access as well as the volume and quality of services.

Political transformation and market reforms in the early 1990s led to the appearance of significant social distinctions and the accelerated formation of discrete social classes: a comparatively small stratum of the very rich and a rather large proportion of the poor and impoverished, living on the poverty line (Lokshin and Popkin 1999). Compared to Soviet society, the gap between the rich and the poor suddenly became extraordinary. In the 1990s and 2000s, new forms of social inequality were deepened by the differences in capabilities and lifestyles of people living in big cities and small towns, the level of education and the availability of health care and social networks. It was a time of big political changes and painful social transformations that were accompanied by dramatic changes in society (Titterton 2006). Russia, as did many other post-communist societies, experienced the serious deterioration of welfare indicators, the depths of distress, including evidence of declining life expectancy, rising morbidity, erosion of schooling, lack of social protection and mass unemployment (Standing 1998), as well as increases in poverty (Cook 2007: 3).

For the welfare states emerging in post-Soviet Russia, as in other post-socialist countries, it was not an easy task to compete with the previous welfare system (Pascall and Manning 2000). Free education, public health care and social benefits that had been a fact of life for decades in the Soviet Union have now become an object of deep nostalgia for many people, especially the elderly. However, it was evident that previous social institutions could not cope with rising social problems.

In the 1993 Constitution, Russia was declared a 'social state', and a series of new social laws were adopted. Russia became a member of the Council of Europe, a signatory to the Universal Declaration of Human Rights, and has ratified a number of other international human rights instruments as well as the European Social Charter. In order to assume its place in the Western international order, new democratic institutions had to be introduced (Huntington 1996: 94). Social work, as an element of this new institutional system that embodied liberal values of human rights, was introduced in Russia at the very beginning of the 1990s (see Iarskaia-Smirnova and Romanov 2002).

Social work in post-Socialist Russia: an overview

It is important to give a general picture of the state of social work in post-communist Russia in order to articulate the key issues and to show various areas in which social workers are engaged. Some general facts and figures will be presented in relation to the context, policy drivers and challenges facing social work in today's Russia.

The first four universities began to teach social work courses in 1991, and by 2011 the number of university programmes of social work was 175, and they covered the entire country. In addition, there were 115 university programmes in social pedagogy. Currently the number of social work university programmes is gradually decreasing, due to a falling number of applicants as well as budget cuts. All universities are involved in a process of transformation towards the Bologna system, switching to four-year BA (1992) and two-year MA (1996) levels, but many of them also continue to offer traditional five-year diploma programmes for 'specialists in social work' (1991). The system has created problems in the labour market for the graduates of such programmes. Due to the low salaries offered to qualified social workers, young university graduates are choosing other jobs for themselves.

In the early 1990s, four professional associations were created: the Association of Social Workers, the Association of Social Pedagogues and Social Workers, the Association of Social Services Employees, and the Association of Schools of Social Work. Several periodicals on social work have been established, and a Code of Ethics has been elaborated based on international examples. Since 2001, the Union of Social Pedagogues and Social Workers has been acting as the national association, with over 4,500 members in 70 regions of the Russian Federation. The Union has been active in promoting the prestige of social work and building a national community of social work practitioners, administrators and educators, but it has not been in possession of self-regulatory and licensing mandates.

Until recently, there was no special legal regulation of professional social work practice in Russia. In the Law on Bases of Social Services (1995), the term *social service workers* is used. During the 1990s, a wide network of social services was established under the responsibility of the Ministry of Labour and Social Development (recently the Ministry of Labour and Social Protection). This social services network has been expanding rapidly during the last 20 years. The workforce of social services workers provides care in many different settings, which, according to the Social Service Federal Law (1995), includes home care, social assistance for families and children, social rehabilitation services for children and youngsters under 18; helping children who are left without parents; shelters for children and adolescents; psychological-pedagogical help to the population; hot-line services; night stay hostels; day care for lonely elderly people; residential social services (nursing homes for elderly and disabled people, psycho-neurological nursing homes, nursing homes for children with mental retardation, nursing homes for children with disabilities); and elderly care. Residential care established in state-owned institutions and other state-based social care services are also found in Russia. Outreach work with delinquent youth, drug addicts and homeless people is conducted mainly by non-governmental organizations (NGOs), including religious organizations, which are active in big cities (see Romanov and Kononenko (2014) for an account of social work in the parishes of the Orthodox Church).

The term *social worker* is defined in a draft of a new Law on Social Services (under consideration in 2011–2013) as a specialist with professional education relevant to the job functions, who works in any kind of organization that performs social services. The new law formulates the rights, responsibilities and guarantees of a social worker. In spring 2013, the ethical code became an issue of governmental concern. New legislation is being elaborated concerning the ethical code of practitioners working in social services.

In the 2000s, the monopolized position of public social services persists in Russia. At the same time, the idea of neo-managerialism has entered the social services sector, which means that the central government intends to make relationships between the citizens and the state more efficient and effective. It also opens possibilities for NGOs to compete with municipal services for budget finances. This process is, however, limited by a lack of standards in social services, a weak knowledge base concerning the methods of working with clients and standard regulation in this field, and a lack of skills in project management and evaluation among many public organizations and NGOs. The concept and skills of empowerment, an important component of social work education, is not yet recognized by practitioners and administrators in Russia. In order to mobilize the resources of local communities to help vulnerable groups fully realize their social citizenship, social workers need to collaborate with non-governmental services, including women's organizations, trade unions and human rights organizations. By contrast, NGOs, which have grown out of the service users' associations and grassroots movements, have developed a strong emancipatory view in their work. The number of such organizations is rather limited and unstable due to the economic and political situation in Russia, where the involvement of foreign donors is not encouraged, while national funds to support non-governmental activities are scarce (Iarskaia-Smirnova 2011b).

Global/local relations in international projects in social work

Social work has a broad international dimension (Cox and Pawar 2006; Payne and Askeland 2008) that includes research, professional training visits and exchanges, field placements, practical work and supervision, administration and policy-making activities. Globalization leads to changes that challenge social work practice and education (Payne and Askeland 2008: 2). The international viewpoint proposes that there is one social work with its local variations, and therefore a global standard for social work education should be accepted (Sewpaul and Jones 2005). Such a 'grand narrative' of social work is questioned by other viewpoints that warn about the risks of considering Western models as universal ideals (Gray 2005; Webb 2003) and suggest the existence of alternative forms of social work with different cultural roots (Payne and Askeland 2008: 5).

International projects in social work have been considered as knowledge transfer (Healy 2008; Trygged and Eriksson 2009). Direct transfer and application of professionally specific concepts is hardly possible, and a number of authors are concerned about whether it is appropriate and genuinely helpful to support these developments by introducing new models, from a variety of European and transatlantic countries in particular, to Eastern Europe and Russia (Breslauer 1995; Bridge 2000; Montague *et al.* 2008; Penn 2007; Ramon 1996; Simpson 2009; Williams 2003). Such criticisms are not unique to Russia/Eastern Europe of course, but in each region there are peculiar contextual characteristics of such developments.

Lyons (2006: 377) warns about different expectations of the role of the state and of the family that should be taken into account while conducting studies of international and global processes in social work. Doel and Penn (2007) admit that cross-national projects possess not only a technical side of knowledge transfer but also a socio-political dimension.

Global and international institutions and processes impact on national policies and practice in the social welfare field (Lyons 2006: 377) that result in globalization of social work training and practice. However, the processes of globalization are very complex and diverse; they can be linked to importing and authentication (Walton and El Nasr 1988; Yunong and Xiong 2008), as well as 'regionalization, triadization, international localization, and cross-borderization' (Jessop 2009: 151). Indigenization is considered as a modification of the foreign social work discourse by adapting it to the political context and socio-cultural patterns in the receiving country (Walton and El Nasr 1988). This process involves power relations between different agents and agencies trying to produce or reproduce social order through institutional process in order to secure their interests (Yan and Cheung 2006: 63–4).

Analysis of power relations in such policy processes can be conducted around three interlocking perspectives: those of actors, institutions and discourses (Jones 2009; Sumner and Jones 2008). The long-term effects of the changes induced by global policy and local actions within international collaborative projects have been related to such factors as legal, political and administrative, technical and cultural feasibilities (Cooper and Vargas 2004; Trygged 2009). Legal, fiscal and technical 'rules of the game' constitute institutional mechanisms for selective appropriation of the foreign social work model. Societal values and ethical concepts shared by the occupational group are framing discourses of thought, meanings and actions, generated by different institutions (Yan and Cheung 2006).

Actors

Looking at the development of social work from this perspective, we see as its driving force interest groups possessing differential allocations of resources that are competing over their own definitions and formulation of rules and regulation (Jones 2009). Professional development of social work in Russia has been affected by the local and global interests of government, the market and civil society. The local context can be seen as configured by the national civil society and universities, and mostly by the welfare state that operates within national borders but is subject to worldwide economic challenges as well as 'globalized social policy – accompanied by international organizations' (Deacon et al. 1997: 53).

The 'professional project' (Larson 1977) of social work began to develop in Russia simultaneously as a new occupation and university programme. This profession was imported into Russia from the West through the efforts of universities, individual scholars and social work practitioners, who became involved in the various forms of collaboration, knowledge exchange, academic mobility and the establishment of joint degree programmes. A new occupation and educational programme has been viewed by its advocates as a crucial component of modern social justice and the welfare state. Local academics have been actively engaged in such cooperation.

Social work trainers from the universities and social service agencies have been supported by public and private, national and international donors. The mission was to adopt the best practice, which would catalyse positive changes to be based on principles of human rights and social justice.

Russian governmental agencies and social service administrators played an important role in inviting the foreign experts into the local practice field.

Russian NGOs and universities have been actively involved in international projects, and this experience was converted into influential power resources, both material and symbolic. Speaking of material resources, various projects related to the development of social work and ranging from €10,000 to €1,000,000 have been implemented during the last 20 years by the universities, governmental agencies and third sector organizations. International projects differed by size and tasks, but those implemented in social work practice usually allocated less money for mobility from Russia to the West than projects focusing on the development of higher education (see analysis of international projects in social work education: Iarskaia-Smirnova 2011b).

Symbolically, the power resource was increased through acquiring new knowledge, skills and social capital due to participation in such projects. For the practice-oriented projects, usually no foreign language training was provided, and short-term study visits were arranged for officials and experts from federal and regional ministries and administration of services, accompanied by their interpreters. Selected staff from the agencies also visited foreign countries to familiarize themselves with social welfare systems, to observe social work practice and to participate in training in theory and methods of social work (see analysis of Swedish-Russian collaboration: Trygged and Eriksson 2009; UK-Russian collaboration: Doel and Penn 2007).

Usually, the small-scale grants limited the influence of foreign donors by the selection of a project proposal written by the local organizations to be supported. In other cases, through a series of training sessions, knowledge, skills and values have been transferred from global into local contexts. Some of the projects aimed to develop the competence of the practitioners within one or several agencies, while others were intended to induce structural changes of the system, for example, to develop a new approach to the treatment of juvenile offenders.

Since the 1990s a wide network of social services has been built under the jurisdiction of the Ministry of Labour and Social Development (currently Ministry of Health Care and Social Development). This system has been expanding rapidly during the last 20 years. According to the Social Service Federal Law (1995), 'the system of social service agencies includes organisations under the control of both Federal and regional authorities, in addition to municipal systems which involve municipal organisations of social services. Social service can also be provided by organisations and citizens representing different sectors of the economy'. By now, there are about 6,000 public agencies with more than 500,000 employees who provide services for the elderly, people with disabilities, and families with children, along with a few non-governmental services.

There is still no common definition of the term *social worker* among service administrators and practitioners (Trygged 2009: 214), although it has been possible to undertake higher education in social work for more than 20 years (for a more detailed discussion on the recent development of social work education in Russia, see, for example, Iarskaia-Smirnova 2011a; Penn 2007). Lack of national consensus about what constitutes the professional core of social work practice (Trygged 2009: 214) was obvious not only in Russia but in Eastern Europe, too, where the profession has been re-established since the 1980s and has become a 'growth area with funding from a variety of sources to help promote East-West partnerships' (Doel and Penn 2007: 367).

It seems that the array of resources for disseminating global social work experience, values and knowledge is decreasing at present. Availability of local resources for training and retraining is hardly better. This is going on under policy reform. As one administrator at a centre for work with families noted, 'After the restructuring of the social service system in the region, several agencies have been merged, specialists were cut down and we've lost the teams'. This is an impact of neo-liberal social policy, which should combine a focus on the needs of the individual customer with a focus on effectiveness. In Russia, only the second element has been undertaken, and this has led to a reduction in the numbers of well-qualified staff, the merging of agencies, and a decrease in the of costs of professional social work intervention.

An important structural effect of international projects in a number of regions has been connected with the development of cooperation between universities, social service agencies and local authorities. This effect was emphasized by our informants, social work practitioners and administrators who took part in European projects as well as training projects focused on the development of social service practice. Within the framework of project implementation, some university departments or faculties managed to substantially influence social policy and the ways of tackling social problems in the region. For instance, participation in an IREX[2] sponsored project enabled the head of the social work department at Perm University and her colleagues to elaborate and apply a new approach to coping with the problem of child abandonment.

Much attention has been paid to adopting new technologies and standards and their application to work practice at a local level. Training events sometimes involved local university teachers, but more often they involved specialists from abroad and from Moscow and St. Petersburg. These events were arranged in short-term thematic seminars and practice training workshops as well as big conferences. After some years of implementation of the adopted technique, it might not be recognized as having an imported or foreign origin, especially by the new workers who learned about new methods from their colleagues in the service.

Institutions

This perspective highlights the context that shapes formal and informal 'rules of the game', legal rules and cultural norms. Knowledge and ideas can be accepted and institutionalized or 'refracted, altered and translated to fit prevailing institutions, or certain types of knowledge may be excluded entirely' (Jones 2009: 5).

Due to foreign influence, the rules have been subject to change, but mostly the process of change occurs within individual organizations. For example, in a rehabilitation centre for children with disabilities, international projects resulted in the acquisition of new skills and knowledge by the staff, as well as the development of new services and approaches to management. As one social work specialist commented, 'After these training courses, individual rehabilitation programs have been elaborated for children. The council was set up that engaged all specialists working with a child'.

Some informants see the development of inter-agency cooperation and the introduction of the institute of supervision as important institutional changes. One administrator at a centre for family services commented, 'We were firstly those who were supervised and then we have got the diploma of trainers and supervisors ourselves. It was very important because social workers here did not know about such instruments earlier'.

In this example, an innovation emerges as a local action derived from the global context, but it can be institutionalized in the region and even throughout the country. The story of an idea turning into action may soon be forgotten if the idea does not receive institutional support. The legal, financial and administrative feasibility of such changes may be increased by building a consensus, or changes may be fought for in an uneasy struggle. Trygged and Eriksson (2009) compared two large international efforts to build a new social work model in Russia and concluded that it was easier to make a change by building something new than to make changes within an existing establishment.

Discourse

This perspective 'sees knowledge and power as intertwined, with considerable power held in concepts and ideas seen as relevant for policy, and exerted through interactive processes of communication and policy formulation' (Jones 2009: 5). Popular media and textbooks are important components of a context in which clients understand their personal life situation in respect to the existing system of support, and social workers create their own understanding of social problems (see analysis of Russian textbooks on social policy and social work: Iarskaia-Smirnova and Romanov 2008). In their interactions with each other and with the institutions of the social welfare system, the process of knowledge production occurs.

Doel and Penn (2007: 347) admit, 'Western visits are often interpreted as inspections, and ... this perception inhibits transparency'. However, when the collaboration is sustained, the outcomes go beyond the acquired new knowledge and skills. New understanding has led to the reconceptualization of both imported and native values. The limits and borders have been shifted towards critical reflection on existing practices and concepts. In our interviews, this reflection was spoken of in terms of a reconsidered notion of the term *norm*. One social work specialist at the rehabilitation centre for children with disabilities commented, 'From the project we also learned how to form self-service skills in children with cerebral palsy. In our literature, that we used previously, everything was directed to working with "normal" children'. Similarly, a specialist at a service centre for women, families and children commented, 'They [the clients] are special people. Now I understand why social workers here are mad at them. The whole system of work here is like they were a "norm", with overestimated demands'.

Some social service organizations have developed a reflexive, holistic approach in working with clients and have become exemplary resource centres for others in terms of their developed competences and the humanist philosophy of social work. They conduct supervision and training courses for their colleagues from other agencies.

An idea can become institutionalized, but what if it does not earn legitimacy within the wider socio-political and cultural context? A project may be perceived differently by politicians and the general public. One example is presented by a case of social work in the courts, as an element of the juvenile justice system developed in Russia during the last 12 years. Juvenile courts were first introduced in Russia more than 100 years ago, but they functioned only until 1918. During Soviet times, there was no juvenile justice, and the policy on punishment of youngsters was rather strict (see McAuley and MacDonald 2007). In 1990, Russia signed the UN Convention on Children's Rights, and in 1996 it joined the European Council. These political actions required reform of the treatment of young offenders. Juvenile justice was reintroduced into Russia in 1999 under a French-Russian project designed to change the system towards a preventive approach. In a few years, 20 Russian regions set up juvenile courts as an experiment, with the support of the UNDP, UNICEF and foreign agencies and foundations (e.g. agencies from France and Sweden) and with the involvement of the Supreme Court of the Russian Federation. A number of social workers, judges, probation officers, policemen, administrators and specialists in a youth colony and regional public officials were trained in the new treatment methods to be used. Social workers were trained to establish an environment to rehabilitate, support and help the child. Teaching materials and recommendations have been prepared and conferences have been held in order to disseminate the new models. A strong emphasis was made on changing the attitudes among staff towards young offenders, who should be seen as individuals within their social contexts, and on involving their families and social networks in treatment (Trygged 2009; Trygged and Eriksson 2009). A special Act of the Supreme Court has emphasized the security of interests and rights of juveniles in conflict with law as well as prevention of repeated crimes. As a result, the proportion of repeated crime has significantly decreased among the juveniles, as well as the number of young people in custody facilities intended for adults. Manuals for preventive work and follow-up among young offenders have been prepared and applied in practice. In several regions, this experiment was conducted with the active support of the regional administration, and the results were positively evaluated.

Some progress and reforms were thus possible. As a result of the project, cooperation between judges and social workers has been strengthened, and more young offenders have been treated in open care before or instead of going to trial (Trygged and Eriksson 2009). However, in some regions, training of social workers has occurred irregularly, only as on-the-job training in the workplace, through coaching by more experienced social workers.

Such a switch in approach implied a change of attitude from punishment to social treatment. However, gaps in the legislative and normative base, insufficient training and a lack of consent among the key stakeholders of this process have formed a background for the lack of legal and administrative feasibility of adopting this innovation properly and rooting it in local institutions.

In the second half of the 2000s, negative public opinion towards juvenile justice was shaped by a moral panic. The mass media accelerated this moral panic using contradictory claims: on the one hand, juveniles, including homeless children, were represented as a threat to society; on the other hand, it was stressed that punishment should be softened or even replaced by rehabilitation work.

Introducing such surveillance techniques as providing child protection officers at schools and monitoring children for drug usage were debated by the public as a Western idea of state control over private life. At the same time, children and adolescents were depicted as insecure victims who should be protected from careless parents, paedophiles, drugs, etc. These claims were formulated by the conservative media, nationalist groups and the Church, but sometimes they were also initiated or supported by representatives of the government. The child protection agencies in these discourses were referred to by the term *juvenile services*. Thus, the term 'juvenile' assumed a negative connotation, which in turn led to a discrediting of the concept of juvenile justice.[3]

In popular protests, various arguments were presented, and juvenile justice was depicted as a Western idea and a threat against families. Moral panic increased. An analytic report on child poverty in Russia recently published by UNICEF (2012) has received harsh criticism by the opponents of the new system. This report is referred to in blogs and mass media as a 'new weapon of the adepts of juvenile justice' (Karpov 2012). The critics claim that the focus on children and their economic status undermines the important role of family and the spiritual component of socialization: 'An approach to children as some market acquisition is unseemly. It means that economic indicators are for a person more important than love and the wish to continue one's own kin on the earth' (Karpov 2012).

Juvenile justice still functions in several Russian regions, for instance, in Rostov-on-Don, St. Petersburg and Perm. Social work still exists in courts in these regions, but it is arranged in different ways. In some cases it is carried out by assistants of the judges. In other regions, social workers' positions have been moved from the courts to social work agencies, or their positions have been cut down. Some of the judges who were trained during the project have left the courts, and social workers have found their position to be weakened in several regions. Some members of the public, social services, ombudsmen and NGOs support juvenile justice, but the national legislation reform on juvenile justice has been blocked due to the intense popular unrest and stigmatization of the idea itself. According to some authors (L'vovski 2010), anti-Western attitudes are used as a base for political consolidation.

Conclusions

Globalization impacts social policy by the lowering of social and labour standards, privatization of public services (Deacon 2000; Yeates 2002), creation of global health and welfare markets and growing reliance on voluntary and informal provision, as well as an increase in the technocratic rationale of social work (Dominelli and Hoogvelt 1996). One of the themes of globalization is a strong neo-liberal trend in policy reforms that tend to 'erode social citizenship and weaken, if not repudiate, an earlier commitment to a social minimum as of right' (Mishra 1999: 51). Globalizing strategies impact on national and local policies, but they are also being regulated or opposed (Yeates 2002), and their logic is reconceptualized by various agents in a number of spheres.

The analysis shows the imported techniques of working with clients as well as how social work discourse is modified in local context (see Romanov and Kononenko 2014). Various agents contribute to the constitution of knowledge and the value base of the profession. Among these agents can be social service administrators, social work practitioners, service users, educators and scholars, policy-makers and mass media. The state has the main jurisdiction over the new profession and provides it with financial and symbolic capital. However, by setting up inadequate wage policies for social workers, the state has reinforced the societal assumption that social work is cheap women's labour, as well as the lack of professionalization, as university graduates avoid careers in social services.

Foreign and local governmental and non-state actors, universities, social services, individual educators, administrators and practitioners compete and create coalitions in order to maximize their own symbolic and material capital, to gain the right to formulate the rules of the game. They contribute to different definitions of social work, trying to modify or sustain the existing social arrangements through institutional mechanisms that selectively appropriate foreign models of social work in frames of societal and professional values.

Post-socialist social work is developing in a context where global and local forces intersect, paternalistic and liberal values compete and socialist and pre-socialist legacies meet neo-liberal policies and form a new complex agenda for the development of the profession (Romanov and Kononenko 2014: 443). Through international projects, social work practice and education become part of global/local policy processes constituted by power relations on different levels. These processes are never unidirectional. Global and international actors make efforts to influence local social policies and social work practices by establishing new rules and promoting new discourses, which interact with national and local agents, institutions and cultures. The effects of such global/local interactions in social work are conditioned by legal, political, administrative, technical and cultural feasibilities. When innovations are arriving without support in the local institutional, cultural and political environment, they are at risk of slipping through the cracks. The decisions of political actors can support changes proposed by international collaboration as well as induce conflicts between different interest groups, thus hindering the process of direct adaptation of a non-native model.

Not all innovations can be sustainable. Some social service administrators and the local authorities can have somewhat more flexibility to implement changes on their own. Administration of a service or inter-agency cooperation can stop or catalyse the change, while personnel turnover and replacement of administrators minimize its longevity and continuity. The scope and longevity of changes may be supported by the personal commitment of a high official on the federal level. However, if the project aims to promote structural changes on a wide scale, strict regulations on the national level may obstruct the reform completely.

On the societal level, however, lack of legitimacy of an imported idea may discredit the whole reform, even though it lies within the global agenda of human rights, which itself appears to be a highly contested area. Gray and Webb (2007) raise the issue of the dangers of applying liberal Eurocentric ideals, such as individual freedom, human rights and political empowerment, in non-Western, non-democratic contexts. But some alarming trends can arise from localization, too. 'Localisation is a two-edged sword; it can provide a positive community development experience, or it can strengthen the forces of exclusion, prejudice and oppression' (Ife 2000: 3).

An important component of social work education, which is not yet recognized by Russian practitioners and administrators, is the concept of empowerment. In order to mobilize the resources of local communities to help vulnerable groups fully realize their social citizenship, social workers need to collaborate with non-governmental organizations, including women's organizations, trade unions and human rights organizations.

It is worthwhile to pay more attention to retraining programmes and to raise the level of skills of staff who already work for social service agencies, because the vast majority of staff in those agencies do not get basic training in the field. Education is called upon to contribute to the development of such reflexive professionals who would be able to recognize inequality at individual and institutional levels, in direct contacts with clients or on a structural level during organizational, social and political interaction, and come up with innovative means of tackling these problems.

The importance of improving such training increases due to the intensive growth of social services and the demand for well qualified personnel. There is a growing need for appropriate professional literature as well as for the popularization of civil society and social work values by the mass media. An effective mechanism for the independent evaluation of social services is also needed, to make it possible to target educational and fundraising activities. It is important for the government, national and international foundations, and the professional and academic community to focus more on critical issues in social work, both locally and globally.

Acknowledgements

This chapter consists of findings that emerged from projects implemented with the support of the Russian Foundation for Humanities, grant No. 14-03-00778 and the Basic Research Programme of the National Research University Higher School of Economics for 2015. The chapter was co-authored, and finalized by Elena Iarskaia-Smirnova.

Notes

1 Pavel Romanov sadly passed away before the book could be completed. This chapter was completed by his co-author, colleague, research partner and wife, Elena Iarskaia-Smirnova.
2 International Research and Exchange Board – a United States-based non-profit organization committed to international education in academic research, professional training and technical assistance.
3 Power abuse by child protection officials who are responsible for excessive termination of parental rights has received a crucially negative public reaction. In particular, according to Article 121 of the Family Code (the amendment of 2009), children will be taken into custody when the activity or inactivity of parents threatens children's life and health or hinders their normal upbringing and development. The fuzzy words *normal upbringing* provide a legal foundation to take children into custody merely on the basis of poverty. There are clearly risks

involved in this legislation: authorities from child protection services, housing services and the police have the power to decide whether the conditions in the family comply with the arbitrarily defined standards in the code.

References

Breslauer, G.W. (1995) 'Aid to Russia: what difference can western policy make', in G.W. Lapidus (ed.) *The New Russia: Troubled Transformation*, Boulder: Westview Press.

Bridge, G. (2000) 'Reflections on the process of developing social work in Eastern Europe', *Social Work in Europe*, 7(1): 31–9.

Cook, L.J. (2007) *Postcommunist Welfare States: Reform Politics in Russia and Eastern Europe*, Ithaca, NY: Cornell University Press.

Cooper, P. and Vargas, C.M. (2004) *Implementing Sustainable Development: From Global Policy to Local Action*, Lanham: Rowman & Littlefield.

Cox, D. and Pawar, M. (eds) (2006) *International Social Work: Issues, Strategies, and Programs*, Thousand Oaks: Sage.

Deacon, B. (2000) *Globalization and Social Policy: The Threat to Equitable Welfare*, Occasional Paper 5, Geneva: United Nations Research Institute for Social Development.

Deacon, B., Hulse, M. and Stubbs, P. (1997) *Global Social Policy: International Organizations and the Future of Welfare*, Thousand Oaks: Sage.

Dixon, J. and Macarov, D. (eds) (1992) *Social Welfare in Socialist Countries*, London: Routledge.

Doel, M. and Penn, J. (2007) 'Technical assistance, neo-colonialism or mutual trade? The experience of an Anglo/Ukrainian/Russian social work practice learning project', *European Journal of Social Work*, 10(3): 367–81.

Dominelli, L. and Hoogvelt, A. (1996) 'Globalization and the technocratization of social work', *Critical Social Policy*, 16(47): 45–62.

Gray, M. (2005) 'Dilemmas of international social work: paradoxical processes in indigenisation, imperialism and universalism', *International Journal of Social Welfare*, 14(2): 230–7.

Gray, M. and Webb, S.A. (2007) 'Global double standards in social work – a critical review', *SW & S News Magazine*, 8 March 2007. Online. Available at: www.socmag.net/?p=56 (accessed 14 October 2013).

Healy, L. (2008) *International Social Work: Professional Action in an Interdependent World*, 2nd edn, Oxford: Oxford University Press.

Huntington, S.P. (1996) *The Clash of Civilizations*, New York: Touchstone Books.

Iarskaia-Smirnova, E. (2011a) *Gender and Class in Russian Welfare Policy: Soviet Legacies and Contemporary Challenges*, Goteborg: University of Goteborg, Ineko.

Iarskaia-Smirnova, E. (2011b) 'Professional ideologies in Russian social work: challenges from inside and outside', in S. Stanley (ed.) *Social Work Education in Countries of the East: Issues and Challenges*, Hauppauge: Nova Science Publishers.

Iarskaia-Smirnova, E. and Romanov, P. (2008) 'Gendering social work in Russia: towards anti-discriminatory practices', *Equal Opportunities*, 7(1): 64–76.

Ife, J. (2000) *Local and Global Practice: Relocating Social Work as a Human Rights Profession in the New Global Order*, Eileen Younghusband Memorial Lecture, IFSW/IASSW Biennial Conference, Montreal, 31 July 2000. Online. Available at:

http://info.humanrights.curtin.edu.au/local/docs/LocalGlobalPractice.pdf (accessed 14 October 2013).

Jessop, B. (2009) 'The spatiotemporal dynamics of globalizing capital and their impact on state power and democracy', in H. Rosa and W. E. Scheuerman (eds) *High-Speed Society: Social Acceleration, Power and Modernity*, University Park: The Pennsylvania State University Press.

Jones, H. (2009) *Policy-Making as Discourse: A Review of Recent Knowledge-to-Policy Literature*, Joint IKM Emergent–ODI Working Paper No. 5. Online. Available at: http://wiki.ikmemergent.net/files/090911-ikm-working-pa per-5-policy-making-as-discourse.pdf (accessed 14 October 2013).

Karpov, A. (2012) 'Analiz polozhenia detei – novoe oruzhie juvenalshchikov' [Analysis of the position of children is a new weapon of the adepts of juvenile justice], 16 February 2012. Online. Available at: http://ruskline.ru/monitoring_smi/2012/02/16/analiz_polozheniya_detej_novoe_oruzhie_yuvenalwikov/ (accessed 14 October 2013).

Larson, M.S. (1977) *The Rise of Professionalism: A Sociological Analysis*, Berkeley: University of California Press.

Lokshin, M. and Popkin, B. (1999) 'Emerging underclass in Russia: poverty and income dynamics 1992–1996', *Journal of Economic Development and Cultural Change*, 47(4): 829–37.

L'vovski, S. (2010) 'Pod znakov juvenal'noi justitsii', *Pro et Contra*, January–April 2010: 20–41.

Lyons, K. (2006) 'Globalization and social work: international and local implications', *British Journal of Social Work*, 36: 365–80.

McAuley, M. and MacDonald, I.K. (2007) 'Russia and youth crime: a comparative study of attitudes and their implications', *British Journal of Criminology*, 47: 2–22.

Mishra, R. (1999) *Globalization and the Welfare State*, Cheltenham: Edward Elgar.

Montague, J., Morgan, J. and Sommerville, A. (2008) 'Travelling on an East-West social work journey: issues in trans-national collaborative working', in P. Salustowicz (ed.) *Social Policy and Social Work: From an International Development Perspective*, European Perspectives on Social Development Series, Berlin: LIT Verlag.

Pascall, G. and Manning, N. (2000) 'Gender and social policy: comparing welfare states in Central and Eastern Europe and the former Soviet Union', *Journal of European Social Policy*, 10(3): 240–66.

Payne, M. and Askeland, G.A. (2008) *Globalization and International Social Work: Postmodern Change and Challenge*, Hampshire: Ashgate.

Penn, J. (2007) 'The development of social work education in Russia since 1995', *European Journal of Social Work*, 10(4): 513–27.

Ramon, S. (1996) 'West-East European social work educational initiatives: continuing dilemmas', *Social Work in Europe*, 3(2): 52–4.

Romanov, P.V. and Kononenko, R.V. (2014) 'Globalization processes in Russian social work', *International Social Work*, 57(5): 435–46.

Schilde, K. and Schulte, D. (eds) (2005) *Need and Care – Glimpses into the Beginnings of Eastern Europe's Professional Welfare*, Leverkusen: Barbara Budrich Publishers.

Sewpaul, V. and Jones, D. (2005) 'Global standards for the education and training of the social work profession', *International Journal of Social Welfare*, 14(3): 218–30.

Simpson, G. (2009) 'Global and local issues in the training of "overseas" social workers', *Social Work Education*, 28(6): 655–67.

Standing, G. (1996) 'Social protection in Central and Eastern Europe: a tale of slipping anchors and torn safety nets', in G. Esping-Andersen (ed.) *Welfare States in Transition: National Adaptations in Global Economies*, London: Sage.

Standing, G. (1998) 'Societal impoverishment: the challenge for Russian social policy', *Journal of European Social Policy*, 8(1): 23–42.

Sumner, A. and Jones, N. (2008) 'The politics of poverty policy: are pro-poor policy processes expert-led or citizen-led?', *International Development Planning Review*, 30(4): 359–76.

Titterton, M. (2006) 'Social policy in a cold climate: health and social welfare in Russia', *Social Policy and Administration*, 40(1): 88–103.

Trygged, S. (2009) 'Social work with vulnerable families and children in 11 Russian regions', *European Journal of Social Work*, 12(2): 201–20.

Trygged, S. and Eriksson, B. (2009) 'Implementing Swedish models of social work in a Russian context', *Social Work and Society*, 7(2). Online. Available at: www.socwork.net/sws/article/view/78/337 (accessed 14 October 2013).

UNICEF (2012) *Analiz polozhenia detei v Rossiiskoi Federatsii: na puti k obshchestvu ravnykh vozmozhnostei* [Analysis of the position of children in the Russian Federation: on the way towards a society of equal opportunities]. Moscow: UNICEF, Independent Insitute of Social Policy. Online. Available at: www.budget-solution.ru/uploads/materials/inkl_doc.pdf (accessed 22 January 2015).

Walton, R.G. and El Nasr, A.M.M. (1988) 'The indigenization and authentization of social work in Egypt', *Community Development Journal*, 23(3): 148–55.

Webb, S. (2003) 'Local orders and global chaos in social work', *European Journal of Social Work*, 6(2): 191–204.

Williams, J. (2003) 'Is inclusion of an international perspective relevant or feasible in social work education?', *Social Work in Europe*, 10(2): 31–6.

Yan, M.C. and Cheung, K.W. (2006) 'The politics of indigenization: a case study of development of social work in China', *Journal of Sociology and Social Welfare*, 33(2): 63–83.

Yeates, N. (2002) 'Globalization and social policy: from global neoliberal hegemony to global political pluralism', *Global Social Policy*, 2(1): 69–91.

Yunong, H. and Zhang, X. (2008) 'A reflection on the indigenization discourse in social work', *International Social Work*, 51(5): 611–22.

Chapter 14

Indigenous social work in China

Wai-Fong Ting and Eric Blyth

Introduction

China is the world's second largest economy and the world's largest exporter (Central Intelligence Agency 2011), exercising significant global political and economic weight – an influence emphasized in the aftermath of the 2008 global financial crisis that brought a number of developed economies close to implosion. This notable accomplishment has been realized in little more than three decades following the introduction of the socialist market economy in 1978. China has a World Bank classification as an 'upper middle income' country (per capita gross national income of US$3,976 to $12,275; World Bank 2012). However, this masks massive variation, as evidenced by China's GINI Index of 41.5 as of 2007 (Central Intelligence Agency 2011), and in particular, disparities between the country's more prosperous urban dwellers and those who live in the countryside. Even though the workforce needs of China's developing industry have seen the internal migration of more than 200 million workers and their dependents from the rural hinterlands to the coastal and south eastern industrial zones, more than half of the total 1.3 billion population still live in rural areas. Here the principal means of livelihood remains subsistence farming, with agriculture comprising 38.1 per cent of the country's labour force (Central Intelligence Agency 2011). According to 2007 data, the annual income of 21.5 million of China's rural population fell below the official 'absolute poverty' level (approximately US$90 per annum), and an additional 35.5 million had annual incomes below the official 'low income' level (approximately US$125 per annum; Central Intelligence Agency 2011).

Social work in China

Social work as an academic discipline in the form that would be recognized today was introduced in China in 1917, notably in Shanghai and Beijing, as a sub-branch of sociology. Social work was largely confined to a small number of large cities, but at the founding of the People's Republic of China in 1949, it was proscribed along with other 'capitalist' academic disciplines. The state assumed responsibility for the welfare of its citizens, principally through work units and a range of government agencies (Li and Yeung 1989). Social work did not reappear in China until the mid-1980s during the post-Maoist era of 'reform and openness', although it did so in piecemeal fashion, once again located in regional pockets – notably Shanghai, Beijing, Shenzhen, Guangzhou and other large cities. A national programme for social work development was noticeably absent.

The development of China's 'socialist market economy' – with a fair measure of neoliberal underpinnings – inevitably resulted in massive upheavals to Chinese society. The urban work unit system changed dramatically; some ceased to operate completely and others scaled down the services they provided for their workers. New economic enterprises without either the experience of, or the motivation for, providing welfare services began to emerge. Formerly comprehensive state welfare provision became less comprehensive (Chow 1990). The period also witnessed the beginning of mass internal migration from the countryside to China's new industrial heartlands; rapid mass urbanization bringing with it a raft of new social problems such as poverty, unemployment, family breakup, crime, street children, HIV/AIDS, prostitution, corruption, ethnic tensions, environmental pollution, drug addiction and gambling, and increasing disparities between rich and poor. In short, while the sources of personal support declined, the need for them increased. At the same time, the government was acutely aware that in a period of rapid and massive social transition, threats to its authority might easily emerge, the rapid dismantling of the Soviet empire providing a salient reminder of such a prospect. An overwhelming priority for the central authorities therefore was to oversee China's fast-paced modernization and alleviate ensuing social problems in order to minimize social unrest and maintain the 'harmonious' society. Social work's moment had arrived in China; it offered the government a means by which stability could be fostered: a means to help others 'help themselves, alleviate social tensions and promote social justice' rather than advocate for 'the downtrodden' (Sigley 2011: 107).

In 2007 the government announced an ambitious plan to train two million social workers by 2015 and three million by 2020 (People's Republic of China Government 2010). Three major issues faced the government in realizing these aspirations. The first is the 'numbers challenge'. While Chinese social work educators and practitioners celebrated the arrival of the 'spring of social work' in China, much doubt was cast on how to build from scratch such a large workforce of skilled social work practitioners in the absence of competent experienced practitioners or researchers to impart the necessary expertise. If this huge force of two million social workers were to arrive in China by 2015, there would be 149 social workers per 100,000 persons, which is 48 more than in the United States (Ting and Zhang 2012: 204).

This 'numbers challenge' is immense and encourages speculation that this may represent yet another misguided 'great leap forward' in China (Ting and Zhang 2012: 203). Related to this is the challenge of quality in social work education and continuous professional development. Within 23 years after its re-instatement, the growth of social work education in China has been phenomenal. Within the last decade the number of undergraduate social work programmes jumped from 28 to 270, and MSW programmes from zero to 72 (Liu *et al.* 2012; Ting and Zhang 2012). This represents close to 50 per cent of the total number of Council on Social Work Education (CSWE) accredited social work programmes in the United States (CSWE 2013), a country where the roots of social work and social work education go back more than a century. It is again no small challenge to find a sufficient number of competent educators to teach in these programmes. Despite this, the Chinese Association of Social Work Education (CASWE), since its inauguration in 2001, has contributed to uplift and safeguard the quality of social work education programmes in China. Recently, it has completed an important task in developing national standards for assessing social work programmes. Its efforts also extend to organizing annual programme meetings and encouraging the publication of references and literature in the local context (Ting and Zhang 2012).

A second challenge for the government as well as for the profession is that social work as a profession has little social recognition. This has to do with the half-century of tradition in communist China in which grassroots party cadres dictated every aspect of citizens' non-material life, including getting party consent to get married and conceive children; accessing education and recreational services, resolving interpersonal and familial conflicts, etc. This was a culture of 'party cares' in which there was no role for social work. Despite the intention of both central and provincial governments to create more social work posts, without a culture of social work, few people know what social workers do or how they could be employed. Ironically, therefore, social work graduates in China do not find it easy to gain suitable employment (Chinese People's Political Consultative Conference 2005). A recent study of frontline social workers revealed that the lack of public or societal recognition has sabotaged the development of a core professional identity among newly graduated social workers (Liu *et al.* 2012). Furthermore, many of those who had been able to find employment in the social work field were considering quitting the profession due to various occupational and societal hurdles preventing them from developing a long-term commitment to the profession (Liu *et al.* 2012).

One of the hurdles deemed most difficult to overcome is the inherent contradiction between a regime that emphasizes undivided allegiance to the political and administrative leadership and a profession that values human rights, equality and social justice. Many social workers, especially those who had been exposed to and attracted to these 'Western' values, found it hard to work in these social and organizational environments. Many social workers felt powerless and helpless to change the structural factors that were the causes of their clients' predicaments (Liu *et al.* 2012). While China has been reaping material dividends in the globalized economy, this has largely been paid for by the migrant workforce, many of whose working conditions are Dickensian (BBC News 2010; Chan and Ngai 2012; Ngai and Smith 2007).

The toughest question to answer has been what sort of social work is best suited to the Chinese context. Whilst there is a general desire to 'learn from the West', as a socialist country, China remains suspicious of the political ideology of Western capitalism. Consequently, what has been sought from Western social work is not its underpinning ideology, but merely its instrumental functions in cushioning the effects of social mishap. To a large extent, Chinese national and provincial governments and academic institutions have looked to Hong Kong for assistance in the process of capacity-building in social work education, resulting in several joint programmes (Chow 2008). Collaboration with Hong Kong partners has suited China's specific needs well. However, because Hong Kong is a former British colony, social work in Hong Kong has been much influenced by both British and American social work concepts and ideologies. Nonetheless, Hong Kong scholars have increasingly challenged the necessary transferability of these ideologies to countries with different history, culture, values and politics, and has begun to offer alternative models of indigenous social work theory and practice (Chau 1995; Chow 2008; 朱[Chu] 1999; Kwong 1996; Lam 1996; Law and Gu 2008; 李[Li] 1999; Ngan 1993; Tsang 1997; Xu and Zhang 2005; 葉[Yip] 2001, 2004; Yuen and Sung-Chan 2002; Yuen and Wang 2008). Significantly also, Hong Kong returned to Chinese sovereignty in 1997. However, since the culture of mainland China, the problems to be addressed and the context in which social work needed to operate were markedly different in many respects from those pertaining in Hong Kong, the nascent Chinese model of social work emphasized integrated social and economic development and capacity-building rather than individualized clinical practice, which played a largely secondary role (Yuen and Wang 2002).

When the Wenchuan earthquake struck, China's social work profession was unprepared and untested, and social workers were no more ready to deal with large-scale disaster relief than anyone else. However, as a consequence of the Chinese government's unprecedented willingness to open up the relief effort to the rest of the world, a 'shop window' was offered to social work to demonstrate what it could offer the Chinese community in its hour of need.

The 5.12 Wenchuan earthquake

At 2:28 p.m. on 12 May 2008, a major earthquake measuring magnitude 8.0 struck Wenchuan County in Sichuan Province, in the southwest of China.

The scale of destruction caused by the earthquake, also referred to as the 5.12 Wenchuan earthquake, was so extensive that precise enumeration of casualties has proved elusive. However, data provided by the State Council Press Office have cited 69,227 deaths, 17,923 missing and 374,643 injured (Sina.com 2004). Millions of homes and other buildings were destroyed or rendered unsafe for human use, resulting in the evacuation of 15 million people from their homes (ReliefWeb 2008a). More than 46 million people were known to have been affected, primarily in Sichuan itself, and in the neighbouring provinces of Gansu and Shaanxi (ReliefWeb 2008b).

Particularly hard hit were schools, with Jiang et al. (2008) claiming that 13,616 educational institutions were partially damaged or destroyed. Suspicions that the apparent increased susceptibility of schools to earthquake damage and the high number of school-aged casualties may have resulted from construction faults earned these structures the derisive tag of 'tofu-dregs' (Lantier 2008) and generated demands from both activists and grieving parents for a government investigation into possible corruption involving builders and government officials (Bristow 2008; Wong 2008).

Sichuan is a largely rural, impoverished province that well exemplified the disparities between China's affluent urbanites and the rural poor. The already limited services and infrastructure – roads, communications, power supply, water and sanitation facilities – were also badly damaged by the earthquake. Post-earthquake landslides due to after-shocks impeded efforts to implement rescue and recovery in the most severely affected areas, poorer rural villages located in difficult-to-access terrain.

Indigenous post-disaster social work in Wenchuan

The 5.12 earthquake generated a massive relief effort. It was estimated that over three million frontline volunteers, another ten million volunteers providing support services, and hundreds of NGOs participated in the post-disaster relief work (Ministry of Civil Affairs 2009). Although social workers took part in the initial relief effort, the real challenges for social work emerged during the post-disaster discovery phase occurring about six months after the earthquake. However, existing evidence-based practice models for recovery intervention that had been developed in response to disasters occurring in the West were not compatible with the geographical, cultural, social and economic context in which social workers found themselves (Iravani and Ghojavand 2005; Puig and Glynn 2003). Survivors were particularly resistant to offers of personal therapy, so much so that a derisive saying gained great popularity, to be 'mindful of fire, theft, and psychotherapy' (Sim 2009), and some local residents affixed notices to their doors stating 'psychological counsellors do not enter' (Sigley 2011). While the prior absence of a social work culture in China meant that no one knew what to expect of social workers, it also provided social workers with a unique opportunity to create and define their role within communities that had lost possessions, homes, livelihoods and family members, were critical of government relief efforts, lacked 'hope and vision for the future' and in which '[t]here was a real sense of hopelessness and despair' (Xu Yongxiang cited in Sigley 2011: 111). Thus social workers perceived the need to help build a sense of community spirit and repair the strained relations between the survivors and the government (Sigley 2011). Teams of social workers from across China participated in the post-disaster social reconstruction, demonstrating that social work could 'become Chinese' and not be reliant on Western imports (Xu Yongxiang, cited in Sigley 2011). Below we provide an account of one such reconstruction project that was led by the first author and which illustrates characteristic features of indigenized post-disaster social work practice.

A three-year, asset-based community reconstruction programme (Kretzmann and McKnight 1993), running from February 2009 to January 2012 and funded by the Zeshan Foundation, was set up in partnership with two rural communities in Sichuan: Xingxiu and Qingping. The project located in Qingping Town subsequently became known as 'Experiencing Rural Qingping'. The project team comprised two Hong Kong colleagues of the first author, and a local team of one supervisor and four social workers. In early June 2008, the municipal and county government set up a Qingping Town 'cabin community' providing temporary accommodation for 6,000 survivors 32 kilometres away from their destroyed villages. In February 2009, the five local team members took up residence in cabins in Qingping Town made available by the local authorities and opened the Qingping Town Social Work Station. Prior to the earthquake, Qingping had comprised 2,027 households, 6,240 villagers and a transient population of 6,000 workers in the phosphorous mine. Two hundred and forty-seven villagers were killed by the earthquake, and 74 sustained serious injuries. It was estimated that another 120 visitors/workers died and 1,000 were injured. The livelihoods of all surviving villagers were seriously affected. Prior to the earthquake, approximately 55 per cent of the population had been economically active, engaged primarily in mining, transportation, tourism, forestry, poultry and animal husbandry. Mining was the predominant industry in Qingping; however, the phosphorus mine which the villagers owned collectively was completely destroyed, thus preventing former miners from returning to work there. There was a knock-on effect for the employment of other villagers, such as self-employed van or truck drivers, who had previously been engaged in transporting minerals and mine workers. Prior to the earthquake, tourism had been a thriving industry, since Qingping had been a popular mountain retreat for vacationing residents of Chengdu (Sichuan's capital city, with a population in excess of 14 million inhabitants). However, many of the area's restaurants and guest houses offering bed and breakfast were also destroyed. Many of these establishments had outstanding development loans. The earthquake thus destroyed the homes and livelihoods of villagers engaged in tourism as well as their means of repaying their loans on properties that no longer existed.

In the first three months of the project, door-to-door visiting by team members enabled both pre- and post-earthquake household profiles to be developed and solicited villagers' views/visions for the post-disaster recovery. The resultant community profile identified four priorities for action: (1) home reconstruction; (2) livelihood renewal; (3) restoration of historical and cultural heritage; and (4) concerns for youth development (although this latter project was never developed because of the inability to secure the necessary funding).

Home reconstruction

Repairing damaged and rebuilding destroyed homes was a priority recognized by the government and survivors alike. An integral ingredient of the reconstruction programme devised by the State Council had been to pair earthquake-stricken areas with a specific province/city in more affluent and unaffected regions in China to coordinate post-disaster reconstruction support. Jiangyin City, located in Jiangsu Province on China's Pacific coast, and its wealthiest province, was responsible for repairing and building roads, houses, schools, clinics, government offices, etc. By the end of August 2009, the Jiangyin Assisted Reconstruction Unit had completed more than 200 new homes. However, there were major problems with the new homes related to affordability for villagers, their design and location. Government subsidies for the purchase of new homes covered, at most, two-thirds of the cost, and so villagers had to obtain a loan from local banks to pay the outstanding balance. Some survivors – including those with outstanding bank loans, retirees, and those seriously injured in the earthquake who were economically inactive – were ineligible for bank loans that they could not repay. Furthermore, despite the good intentions of Jiangsu Province, the design of the new homes suited east coast towns rather than the needs of mountain villagers living in an earthquake zone. In addition, villagers were reluctant to invest in new homes because of fears of a further earthquake (fears that were tragically realized barely two years after the 5.12 earthquake – see below) and concerns that the site of the new homes was at high risk of flooding by a so-called 'quake lake' (one of many lakes created in the region by the earthquake). The project team identified households that were least able to help themselves to re-build their damaged houses and established a mutual-aid programme for the building of light, steel-framed earthquake-resistant houses under which participants agreed to help build each other's homes in exchange for financial assistance. However, funding limitations meant that only three households, each comprising impoverished farmers with varying disabilities, were able to participate in this scheme.

Livelihood renewal

The 5.12 earthquake demolished much of the villagers' means of earning a living through mining, agriculture and tourism. The project team focused its efforts to re-build economic activity at both individual and enterprise/community levels. Following discussions within the community, two livelihood mutual-aid groups whose efforts complemented each other were established with associated micro-financing to promote business start-up and ensure cash flow: one for eco-(organic) farming and one for eco-tourism. The eco-farming project encouraged both the rearing of livestock and cultivation of local wild vegetables. Eco-farming augmented the eco-tourism project and a market for surplus produce was promoted by means of a Fair Trade shop and liaison with other local NGOs to develop a niche market. The eco-tourism project has enabled visitors to experience and participate in rural life, including engagement with eco-farming, such as feeding animals and harvesting vegetables, as well as learning traditional dances and songs, touring sites associated with the earthquake and mudslide disasters and listening to disaster-related stories.

Restoration of historical and cultural heritage

Despite the damage wreaked by the earthquake, Qingping's rich historical and cultural heritage was not destroyed. During initial data gathering, the project team became aware of a sense of 'uselessness' among the economically inactive members of the community, primarily elderly villagers, who were physically incapable of contributing to the reconstruction effort. On the other hand, elderly villagers were effectively the custodians of the community's history and traditions. In addition to their knowledge, they also had the time to contribute to its reconstruction. The project team realized that conscious articulation of the community's cultural and historical heritage could help counter the prevalent sentiment of loss and despair, enable community seniors to make an active contribution to the restoration effort and augment the eco-tourism industry. Thus an oral history project was initiated in which seniors' stories about local architecture, marriage customs, local folk songs and dances, religious practices, local cuisine, etc. were collected. Volunteers, including local youth, were engaged in recording and writing up these stories, acting as translators where the villager did not speak Putonghua, to produce a local history book, which also included pictures provided by the villagers. These 'story tellers' have also regularly participated in community-wide gatherings in which these stories are told and circulated and have contributed to the cultural programme associated with the eco-tourism project. Other villagers have also contributed to the preservation and dissemination of local cultural activities, such as a group of women who wished to promote traditional dancing for which they needed resources such as a rehearsal venue, music tapes/videos, a sound system and costumes. They were able to provide for what they needed except for costumes. The project arranged a micro-loan so that the women's costumes could be tailor-made.

The Ginkgo Cultural Festival provides another example of the importance of collective community endeavours to overcome the effects of the earthquake. Over the past two decades, thousands of ginkgo trees had been planted in the area in support of the government's policy of promoting reforestation. Since ginkgo is widely promoted as a health food, an annual Ginkgo Cultural Festival had been held for several years. This festival had been very successful, attracting more than 50,000 tourists each year, thus boosting the local tourism industry. Because of the severe damage to the main road providing access to the area and the local government's focus on repairs and reconstruction, it decided not to re-establish the festival even after the villagers returned home. However, the villagers and the project team thought that the festival had significant meaning to local people and the failure to reinstate it would reinforce their sense of helplessness. The project team collaborated with the community, and in April 2010 the festival was held, albeit on a smaller scale compared to previous years, although it was widely regarded as a success.

Reference has previously been made to villagers' fears of further earthquakes and in the early hours of 13 August 2010, following exceptionally heavy rain, Qingping experienced a large scale landslide, a second disaster to hit the community, whose damage was comparable to that of the 5.12 earthquake. Although there were fewer human casualties (nine deaths and four injuries), the only road to the city was damaged, most local roads, five bridges, 603 houses, the newly built schools, water station and the county government offices were either completely flooded or sustained various degrees of damage (although the three new homes built with the support of the project were unaffected, possibly owing to their location). Two supervisors from the Qingping social work station and several volunteers from Hong Kong and Sichuan, together with other Qingping villagers, had to be rescued by PLA helicopter, thus highlighting the privations and dangers experienced by social workers serving the community. Following the landslide, large areas of housing and farming in Qingping were covered by mud and other debris. More than 400 households were forced to resettle again (even though many homes had been completed only a few months before the landslide). The mining industry, which had gradually recovered following the earthquake, was completely closed following the landslide. The new initiatives in eco-farming and eco-tourism were also set back. Many villagers suffered further economic and psychological distress, since their only financial assets remaining after the earthquake had been used to build their new homes, which had now also been destroyed. By the summer of 2011, all of the homes of villagers participating in the eco-tourism project had been rebuilt and started taking visitors again.

Villagers' resentment against the government escalated after the landslide, as resistance to the government's refusal to allow the villagers to relocate to a safer location intensified. Villagers blocked roads to prevent clear-up operations and renovation, petitioned the government to buy back their 'Jiangyin' homes so that they could move to a safer area and asked for greater transparency in distributing disaster subsidies and compensation. It should be noted that in rural China, such acts of civil disobedience were previously unheard of.

Reflections on the project

Since its inception, the project upheld important core values that are aligned with the social transformative framework that advocates development of a broad range of assets (Pieterse 2010). When contemplating a viable model for redevelopment, the prime concern of the project had been to ensure villagers' ownership of the development project rather than imposing a plan from outside. This approach may be contrasted with the government tendency to impose solutions, which created a sense of dependency on the part of survivors and ultimately generated resistance. The policy of the government governing disaster management is characterized as 'the party leads' (dang wei ling dao), 'government executes' (zheng fu fu ze), 'society supports' (she hui xie tong) and 'individuals participate' (gong zhong can yu) (Jiang 2008; State Council 2008; Sun 2004).

While the project acknowledged villagers' needs for economic well-being, discussion with them revealed a much wider concept of human, social and cultural capital and provided a framework for collaborative work. As discussed at length elsewhere (Ting and Chen 2012), the importance of resurrecting these various 'capitals' in an integrative approach for post-disaster (re)development is underscored; for example, the need to bring 'social' back to development by mobilizing 'poor people's capacity for cooperation and social organization on the basis of norms of reciprocity and a culture of social solidarity' (Ting and Chen 2012; Veltmeyer 2011: 124).

This discussion is of particular relevance in the context of China, where the dominance of the central government in many aspects of people's lives has inevitably crowded out civil society initiatives. This project thus advocated an alternative model of development that fostered equal participation among villagers. It resembles the Social Economy Charter's (European Union 2004) emphasis on 'voluntary and open membership' and the 'partnership, sustainability and democratization' that is depicted in Pieterse's social transformation model (2010). Moreover, the project also accentuated the significance of local ownership in which members will take charge of the project direction. This again is echoed in the European Union's Social Economy Charter (2004) and Wright's (2010) social economy model that underscores the importance of democratic control by membership. The project approach reiterated that the development focus should not be on economic/financial sustainability alone, but that environmental, social and cultural sustainability are equally imperative, if not more so. While the government and mass media depicted survivors as helpless and in desperate need of help, the project, focusing on the utilization of their personal, social, cultural and natural assets, reassured them that they were indeed survivors whose survival experiences told a lot about their own strength. It is thus apparent that financial outcomes alone cannot capture the comprehensive gain and development made by the villagers. Respect for local culture, as illustrated by the eco-tourism project inviting visitors to experience the rural way of living, was another prominent theme of this project and illustrated that an endogenous model of modernization can ensure the sustainability of indigenous culture.

The objective of the community economy project 'Experiencing Rural Qingping' was to help Qingping villagers to rebuild their livelihoods. However, in addition to securing improvements to their livelihoods, participating villagers were able to (re)build their social capital, resurrect their cultural capital and further develop their human capital. Moreover, this project fostered urban–rural connections and understanding as a means to redress the 'city-developed-superior and rural-undeveloped-inferior' discourse that has been so prevalent globally and in China. This effort has resulted in urban visitors beginning to appraise the uniqueness and beauty of rural life, which in turn restored the rural villagers' pride in their hometown, their knowledge and skills in rural living and their identity. This is particularly important in the midst of the irreversible outflow of the rural population to urban cities, resulting in fewer people engaged in farming (the major source of food production), a trend that, if continued, will have a deleterious impact, not only on rural residents.

Since its operation, the post-disaster redevelopment project has employed over ten locally trained frontline social workers and offered training opportunities to two doctoral students and more than 20 Chinese undergraduate social work students. As discussed above, one of the major challenges in social work development in China is the lack of social work educators and professionals with adequate practice experience and skills. One way to address this challenge is to develop practicum sites based on practice projects like the current one in Qingping (Ting and Zhang 2012). These experiences enable the further development of indigenous social work through theorization of practice. As the development of social work and social work education is interwoven in China, this project therefore contributes to the enrichment of social work curriculum and field education, especially in the area of post-disaster community-based social work intervention in China.

References

BBC News (2010) 'Foxconn suicides: "Workers feel quite lonely"', BBC News Asia-Pacific, 28 May 2010. Online. Available at: www.bbc.co.uk/news/10182824 (accessed 28 April 2013).

Bristow, M. (2008) 'China reins in quake school fury', BBC News, 3 June 2008. Online. Available at: http://news.bbc.co.uk/2/hi/asia-pacific/7434054.stm (accessed 28 April 2013).

Central Intelligence Agency (2011) *CIA World Factbook: China*. Online. Available at: www.cia.gov/library/publications/the-world-factbook/geos/ch.html (accessed 28 April 2013).

Chan, J. and Ngai, P. (2012) 'Global capital, the state and Chinese workers: The Foxconn experience', *Modern China*, 38: 383–410.

Chau, K. (1995) 'Social work practice in a Chinese society: Reflections and challenges', *Hong Kong Journal of Social Work*, 29(2): 1–9.

Chinese People's Political Consultative Conference (2005) *Issue of Employment Problem of Social Work Graduates*. Online. Available at: www.douban.com/group/topic/1004365/ (accessed 18 January 2015).

Chow, N.W.S. (1990) 'Social welfare in China', in D. Elliott, N.S. Mayadas and T.D. Watts (eds) *The World of Social Welfare: Social Welfare and Services in an International Context*, Springfield: Charles C. Thomas Publisher.

Chow, N.W.S. (2008) 'Social work in Hong Kong – Western practice in a Chinese context', *China Journal of Social Work*, 1(1): 23–35.

Council on Social Work Education (CSWE) (2013) *Accreditation*. Online. Available at: www.cswe.org/Accreditation.aspx (accessed 15 October 2013).

朱偉志[Chu, W.C.] (1999) 〈香港社會工作本土化藍圖再檢視〉載於何潔雲、阮曾媛琪主編,《邁向新世紀: 社會工作理論與實踐新趨勢》, (414–440), 新澤西: 八方文化企業公司。

Chu, W.C. (1999) 'Re-visit the blueprint of indigenous social work', in K.W. Ho and W.K. Yuen-Tsang (eds) *Social Work Theory and Practice in the New Millennium*, New Jersey: Bafen Corporation.

European Union (2004) *Social Economy Charter*.

Iravani, M.R. and Ghojavand, K. (2005) 'Social work skills in working with survivors of earthquake: A social work intervention – Iran', *Social Work & Society*, 3(2): 265–72.

Jiang, J. (2008) 'A review on disaster relief and reduction policies of China since the reform and opening up', *Social Science of Beijing*, 5: 61–5.

Jiang, L., Wang, J. and Liu, L. (2008) *People's Republic of China: Providing Emergency response to Wenchuan Earthquake* (Technical assistance consultant's report). Beijing: Ministry of Civil Affairs, People's Republic of China, and Asian Development Bank.

Kretzmann, J. and McKnight, J. (1993) *Building Communities from the Inside Out: A Path Toward Finding and Mobilizing a Community's Assets*, Evanston: The Asset-Based Community Development Institute, Institute for Policy Research, Northwestern University.

Kwong, W.M. (1996) 'Local knowledge, indigenous practice: Linking the cultural, the personal and the professional in social work practice', *Hong Kong Journal of Social Work*, 30(1): 22–30.

Lam, C.W. (1996) 'Indigenization of social work values in Hong Kong: A brief review', *Hong Kong Journal of Social Work*, 30(1): 10–21.

Lantier, A. (2008) 'Rising death toll, popular anger in China quake', World Socialist Web Site, 21 May 2008. International Committee of the Fourth International (ICFI). Online. Available at: www.wsws.org/articles/2008/may2008/quak-m21.shtml (accessed 28 April 2013).

Law, K.C. and Gu, J.X. (2008) 'Social work education in mainland China: Development and issues', *Asian Social Work and Policy Review*, 2: 1–12.

李潔文[Li K.M.], (1999) 〈社會工作文化問題初探: 從社會科學本土化到社會工作文化反〉載於何潔雲、阮曾媛琪主編, 《邁向新世紀: 社會工作理論與實踐新趨勢》, (391–413), 新澤西: 八方文化企業公司。

Li, K.M. (1999) 'Exploring cultural issues of social work: From indigenization of social sciences to reflection of culture of social work', in K.W. Ho and W.K. Yuen-Tsang (eds) *Social Work Theory and Practice in the New Millennium*, New Jersey: Bafen Corporation.

Li, E. and Yeung, W.T. (1989) 'China's social welfare in the 1980s', in J.Y.S. Cheng (ed.) *China: Modernization in the 1980s*, Hong Kong: The Chinese University Press.

Liu, Y., Lam, C.M. and Yan, M.C. (2012) 'A challenged professional identity: The struggles of new social workers in China', *China Journal of Social Work*, 5(3): 189–200.

Ministry of Civil Affairs (2009) *He Daofeng: Ideal in the Secular Evolution of Mud*, 5 November 2009. Online. Available at: http://cszh.mca.gov.cn/article/gyzx/200911/20091100041447.shtml (accessed 16 October 2013).

Ngai, P. and Smith, C. (2007) 'Putting transnational labour process in its place: The dormitory labour regime in post-socialist China', *Work, Employment and Society*, 21: 27–45.

Ngan, R. (1993) 'Cultural imperialism: Western social work theories for Chinese practice and the mission of social work in Hong Kong', *Hong Kong Journal of Social Work*, 28(2): 47–55.

People's Republic of China Government (2010) Online. Available at: www.gov.cn/jrzg/2010-06/06/content_1621777.htm (accessed 18 January 2015).

Pieterse, J.N. (2010). *Development Theory: Deconstruction/Reconstruction* (2nd edn), London: SAGE Publications.

Puig, M.E. and Glynn J.B. (2003) 'Disaster responders: A cross-cultural approach to recovery and relief work', *Journal of Social Service Research*, 30(2): 55–66.

ReliefWeb (2008a) 'China: HK gov't proposes 2 bln HKD in support of Sichuan reconstruction', ReliefWeb, 16 July 2008. Online. Available at: http://reliefweb.int/node/273542 (accessed 28 April 2013).

ReliefWeb (2008b) 'China: focus – the Sichuan earthquake', ReliefWeb, 30 June 2008. Online. Available at: http://reliefweb.int/node/271942 (accessed 28 April 2013).

Sigley, G. (2011) 'Social policy and social work in contemporary China: An interview with Xu Yongxiang', *China Journal of Social Work*, 4(2): 103–13.

Sim, T. (2009) 'Crossing the river stone by stone: Developing an expanded school mental health network in post-quake Sichuan', *China Journal of Social Work*, 2(3): 165–77.

Sina.com (2004) Online. Available at: http://news.sina.com.cn/c/2008–09-25/183514 499939s.shtml (accessed 24 February 2012).

State Council (2008) *The Notice of Print and Distribution of the Overall Planning of Post-Wenchuan Earthquake Recovery by State Council*. Online. Available at: www.gov.cn/zwgk/2008-09/23/content_1103686.htm (accessed 16 October 2009).

孙绍聘 (2004) 中国救灾制度研究, 北京: 商务印书馆。[Sun, S. (2004) *A Study of the Chinese System of Disaster Relief*. Beijing: Commercial Press].

Ting, W.F. and Chen, H. (2012) 'The alternative model of development: The practice of community economy in disaster-stricken Sichuan', *China Journal of Social Work*, 5(1): 3–24.

Ting, W.F. and Zhang, H.Y. (2012) 'Flourishing in the spring? Social work, social work education and field education in China', *China Journal of Social Work*, 5(3): 201–22.

Tsang, N.M. (1997) 'Examining the cultural dimension of social work practice: The experience of teaching students on a social work course in Hong Kong', *International Social Work*, 40: 133–44.

Veltmeyer, H. (ed.) (2011) *The Critical Development Studies Handbook: Tools for Change*, New York: Pluto Press.

Wong, E. (2008) 'A Chinese school, shored up by its principal, survived where others fell', *New York Times*, 15 June 2008. Online. Available at: www.nytimes.com/2008/06/15/world/asia/15iht-quake.1.13714011.html?pagewanted=1 (accessed 28 April 2013).

World Bank (2012) *China*. Online. Available at: http://data.worldbank.org/country/china (accessed 28 April 2013).

Wright, E.O. (2010) *Envisioning Real Utopias*, London: Verso.

Xu, Y.X. and Zhang, X.L. (2005) 'The reconstruction of the role of Chinese government in relation to social welfare [Zhongguo zhengfu zai shehui fuli zhong de jiaose chongjian]', *Zhongguo Shehui Kexue*, No. 5.

葉錦成 (2001) 香港社會工作本土化的沈思(一): 本土化的回顧與前瞻, 香港社會工作學報 8, 51–78. [Yip, K.S. (2001) Contemplation of Hong Kong Social Work Localization: Retrospect and Prospect, Hong Kong Journal of Social Work, 8: 51–78.]

Yip, K.S. (2001) 'Reflection of the indigenisation of social work (1): Review and forward looking of indigenisation', *Hong Kong Journal of Social Work*: 51–78.

Yip, K.S. (2004) 'A Chinese cultural critique of the global qualifying standards for social work education', *Social Work Education*, 23(5): 597–612.

Yuen, A.T. and Sung-Chan, P.P.L. (2002) 'Capacity building through networking: Integrating professional knowledge with indigenous practice', in N.T. Tan and I. Dodds (eds) *Social Work around the World II*, Berne: International Federation of Social Workers.

Yuen, A.T. and Wang, S.B. (2002) 'Tensions confronting the development of social work education in China: Challenges and opportunities', *International Social Work*, 45(3): 375–88.

Yuen, A.T. and Wang, S.B. (2008) 'Revitalization of social work in China: The significance of human agency in institutional transformation and structural change', *China Journal of Social Work*, 1(1): 5–22.

Chapter 15

A social work charter for unexpected disasters

Lessons from the Bam, Iran earthquake

Edward Kruk and Habib Aghabakhshi

Introduction

Human social life is situated at the interface of the natural and human worlds. Contrary to human-made calamities, natural disasters do not implicate human beings, although they sometimes create human disasters. These types of events produce critical situations where conventional methods of intervention have limited utility at best, and can exacerbate the tragedy at worst – a tragic natural disaster has taken place, response time is short, and a lack of familiarity and preparedness may lead to ineffective and even harmful decisions being made in the course of disaster relief work.

Among natural happenings and casualties, an earthquake is characterized by its unpredictability as well its destructive after-effects as its primary features; these are often combined with the lack of preparation for disaster relief efforts. The earthquake immediately causes human calamities which leave direct, indirect and secondary destructive impacts on people, their habitat and society; such situations require the immediate intervention of social workers trained in individual, family, group and community work, and in crisis intervention. The involvement of social workers is critical in both the rescue and recovery stages of the disaster, particularly in regard to identifying and linking the victims' needs with resources (Chou 2003). In addition, social work educators can play a critical role in training in disaster aid, although such training is rarely included in current university social work curricula.

The aim of this chapter is to outline the main lessons of the Bam, Iran earthquake of 2003, the largest earthquake in the region in over 2,000 years (Aghabakhshi and Gregor 2007), and to offer a framework for social work intervention in disaster response around the globe, in the form of a Social Work Charter for Unexpected Disasters. It is based on reports on the stated needs of Bam earthquake survivors as recorded by 40 social work participant observers from the Social Welfare and Rehabilitation Sciences University in Tehran, particularly during the first days of the Bam earthquake. It details social group mutual aid efforts among earthquake survivors after the disaster and procedures adopted by human service organizations in the difficult aftermath of the earthquake. A situation of massive human calamity resulted from the Bam event, mostly the result of a lacuna of organized aid plans and crisis management inadequacies.

In this disaster, in spite of emergency measures imposed by government officials as part of a national strategy of earthquake relief, the efforts of government welfare agencies and international aid organizations largely failed to address the stated needs of the earthquake survivors. An atmosphere of distrust emerged, as a result of deficiencies in crisis management, lack of organized programmes by aid organizations, unequal and disrespectful distribution of goods and food, discrimination among survivors in the provision of initial emergency requirements, and other factors. The immigration of neighbouring groups facing poverty exhausted food supplies and took aid attention away from the earthquake survivors. Most importantly, essential human needs in the aftermath of the earthquake were not sufficiently addressed. As detailed by Aghabakhshi and Gregor (2007), Javadian (2007) and Doostgharian (2009), the survivors became rapidly disenfranchised from the relief efforts, and social capital – social networks and connections, and the norms of reciprocity and trustworthiness that arise from them (Coleman 1988; Mathbor 2007) – diminished significantly. This was the end result of feelings of betrayed trust that emerged among survivors, a consequence of unmet needs and the poorly coordinated efforts of government social welfare agencies, as well as lack of coordination between government and international aid organizations.

In preventing human disasters, the best method is to impede their occurrence, but in the case of an earthquake, which cannot be controlled, disaster preparedness is the crucial first step, aimed towards the prevention of additional crises after the disaster. Disaster preparedness includes both public education measures and the establishment of a disaster aid headquarters, responsible for the coordination of aid facilities and resources, including aid organizations. Such specialized planning and the equipping of interveners trained in disaster relief, on the alert for unpreventable yet predictable natural disasters, is critical (Banerjee and Gillespie 1994). The second step is the rescue stage immediately following the occurrence of the disaster; it entails facing the disaster promptly and addressing the circumstances of the crisis. During this stage, addressing the critical situation and preventing the expansion of damage are of paramount importance. The third step is the recovery stage, which focuses on crisis reduction as well as the resulting impacts. In this stage damages should be compensated for quickly in an effort towards crisis reduction. Finally, the fourth step is the stabilization stage, focused on the normalization of the situation so that normal life comes back to the area (Banerjee and Gillespie 1994; Chou 2003; Dodds and Nuehring 1996; Drabek 1986; Dufka 1988; Seroka et al. 1986; Zakour 1996).

Although social workers have long been involved in disaster relief work (Zakour 1996), this has not been the focus of much social work theory and research (Yanay and Benjamin 2005), and disaster intervention is most often not a component of professional social work education (Dodds and Nuehring 1996). The majority of social workers thus have at best limited training in disaster aid and relief.

The Bam earthquake: methodology

Iran lies in an earthquake zone. It sits on a number of seismic fault lines and has had more than 20 major earthquakes, with a magnitude above 6 on the Richter scale, in the past century. Iran is located on the Himalaya-Alp earthquake belt, where the Eurasian and Arabian tectonic plates meet, and is always expecting earthquakes (Goudarzi 2004). On Friday morning, 26 December 2003, at 5:30 a.m., Bam was violently shaken by an earthquake registering 6.8 on the Richter scale; afterwards few buildings remained. The earthquake levelled the city, which had a population of 120,000, killing 32,000 people. Since that time an additional 11,000 have died, bringing the toll to 43,000 dead. Eighty per cent of the city's remaining population of 88,000, a total of 75,000 people, were left homeless by the earthquake. Thirty thousand were injured, with 4,000 remaining permanently disabled. An estimated 2,500 orphan survivors were left without parents. Property damage was estimated in excess of the amount of US$1 billion (Aghabakhshi and Gregor 2007; Ghafory-Ashtiany and Eshghi 2005).

Despite consecutive stirrings of the earth at night and after midnight, those who slept did not take the warnings seriously and the institute responsible for transmitting disaster warning messages did not warn residents of Bam of the impending earthquake, even though there were small quivers indicating the activation of the earth in that area. The morning immediately after the disaster, people of the neighbouring city of Kerman, three hours away, rushed to find their neighbouring compatriots in serious trouble, before government authorities arrived, and transported the injured to Kerman facilities using their automobiles, vans and even trash trucks.

In Iran as elsewhere, in addition to government agencies responsible for disaster response, the United Nations, through its various bodies, such as the UN High Commission for Refugees, and civil society organizations such as the International Federation of the Red Cross and Red Crescent Societies, are key agencies through which humanitarian aid in disaster situations is delivered, particularly in the immediate aftermath of a disaster event. In this context, their activities focus on providing food, water, shelter and medical supplies on a non-discriminatory basis. Social workers become involved in the aid process via these public and private agencies, assessing need, coordinating and delivering goods and services, assisting in family reunification, supporting individuals and communities in rebuilding their lives and developing resilience and capacity to minimize risks for future disasters (Dominelli 2007).

In the immediate aftermath of the Bam tragedy, aid organizations seemed confused and acted without evident preparation. Disorganization and diffuseness in aid and the lack of coherent predetermined techniques and programmes made the distribution of goods and transportation of the injured difficult.

The almost-immediate presence of physicians from the neighbouring city of Kerman on the morning of the disaster was remarkable. But lack of security and organization in the region resulted in serious problems among survivors. Donated goods were insufficient, and looting occurred.

On the day of the earthquake, the School of Social Work of the Social Welfare and Rehabilitation Sciences University temporarily suspended its educational operations and volunteered faculty and students for the relief effort, under the supervision of the School's director, Dr Mostafa Eghlima. On the morning of the following day, a bus carrying 40 social work students of the School arrived and set up tents in Bam's Farmandari Square. They came to face the catastrophe, devoting themselves to the disaster relief, rescue and recovery effort. They worked in an unaffected and sympathetic manner, out of the glare of publicity. In the rescue stage, they accompanied victims waiting for family members to be rescued from collapsed buildings, digging out corpses from the debris, arranging for funerals, searching for shelters and transportation between the shelters and the wreckage, collecting and distributing food and supplies to the victims. Support to the injured and the families of the dead, collection of disaster information, seeking out vulnerable populations, linking victims' needs with resources, and empowering other volunteers in disaster relief work rounded out their activities.

Despite the existence of many common methods of more precise quantitative measurement, the observations and interviews of the social workers, recorded in field notes, was recognized as the most appropriate data collection method during the first few days after the disaster. In keeping with the recommendations of Dodds and Nuehring (1996) on social work research in the context of natural disasters, brief notations on individual and organizational behaviours during the rescue stage proved to be an effective and efficient data collection method in the context of limited time when the social work students were engaged in disaster relief work. After the students had returned to the School of Social Work, they were able to share their field notes and undertook a grounded theory method in identifying core themes and categories from their collected data. In addition, the students were surveyed on their impressions about the needs of Bami survivors that were met and unmet, and they participated in the development of recommendations for disaster aid work by social workers, culminating in the development of a Social Work Charter for Unexpected Disasters. This charter, it is hoped, will provide a template for social work practice in the field of disaster aid and intervention across the globe.

Results: conduct of the survivors and aid organizations

The following constitute summaries of what the students recorded in the first few days of the disaster:

Supplies are minimal and tents are few. The bitterly cold Bam nights in December are intense. Many people do not have tents or blankets and await the arrival of equipped foreign tents. The survivors experience the looting and pillaging of their city during the first days and prefer to stay on the debris of their destroyed homes and ignore efforts at obtaining food in the interests of saving their property underground. Goods and food aid are taken by the poor of the neighbouring regions from trucks, thus vulgarizing the distribution of goods. Honorable Bamis and seniors do not move from their debris and do not pay attention to obtaining food and making use of aid facilities. The distribution system is so flawed that the poor from outside the region that pour into Bam in search of relief agencies are also discriminated against; according to the Deputy Minister of Health, who is present in the region, 'What is most pitiful is the trespass of human dignity and benevolence'.

After seven days, essential needs are still not identified. The condition of women and children in particular is worse, and no one is thinking of women and girls' hygienic needs. There is no sign of a field bathroom and restroom. Today, on the seventh day of the disaster, the demolished city of Bam is seeing street cleaners with sweepers in their hands who do not know whether to consider the thousands of mineral water bottles, left by pedestrians, as trash or a life-giving substance! The distribution of goods is the same; we still see heaped and castoff clothes and bread all over the city.

Non-governmental organizations, without caring about the cameras and all the publicity, are aiding more effectively. The nurses and social workers of the university, as well as volunteer professionals accompanying them, are doing their best, but a lack of proper management in critical situations has reduced our efficiency and some of the volunteers have left. International aid teams have ignored their New Year celebrations and are working in an unpretentious and organized way.

Social work interviews with some of the hurt Bamis, most of whom had injured fingertips, which they used as tools for searching for loved ones under the rubble, revealed the bitter fact that they believed they would soon be forgotten – in a matter of days. They still did not know when and how the reconstruction of demolished houses would be done; some were still in deep shock; some were searching for their loved ones or possessions in the rubble; some were clinically depressed as a result of their losses; some felt guilty about being the only family member who had survived; and some considered God as responsible for their punishment. People were very dissatisfied with the manner of distributing goods and food, as well as the behaviour of the aid organizations. The influx of the neighbouring poor, mainly refugees from Baluchistan and Afghanistan, and the hijacking of goods trucks, shocked the Bamis; it intensified the prevailing atmosphere of distrust. Rumours developed, and some whispered, 'This catastrophe was not an earthquake, but the impact of atomic weapons testing'.

From the students' field notes

As the Bami survivors are desperately looking for their missing loved ones, some social welfare and aid organizations are transferring seemingly orphaned, forlorn children to Tehran. In fact, the aid organizations have ignored the need for the participation of survivors, from local trustees and confidantes. Cooperation with local groups is virtually non-existent. They do not care about people's contributions to the relief effort and underestimate the potential strengths of the survivors. Admittedly, there is a feeble connection between the real needs of the survivors, people's participation in relief work, and the issue of aid. Bami survivors, who have experienced plunder, prefer to look after their underground properties in their own debris and do not move to other places; whereas the aid organizations tend to settle them in camps far from their houses, as this is more expedient.

The people are truly claiming, based on the manner of distributing goods and food, that the aid organizations provide most of the goods and food for the poor refugees who have rushed to the city. This is because the organizations do not use the help of local persons to identify who is from Bam and who is not. The combination of the neighbouring refugees with the hurt people of Bam is seriously straining the aid organizations.

As men and women survivors are wandering about aimlessly enriching the mourning culture, the social welfare organizations do not make use of their energy and adaptability with the existing situation in providing and distributing goods and food, and instead they themselves do the distribution inappropriately. These governmental welfare organizations' power in attempting to force normalization of the situation also causes more disorganization and inefficiency in their activities.

A marked decrease in the efficacy of the relief work becomes evident when social welfare organizations use their administrative staff instead of volunteer professionals, and when they are not up to the task, return them in despair. The administrative staff, bearing the false belief that the people who are hurt are weak and cannot make their own decisions, make decisions for them and against their interests and well-being; such actions will cause negative reactions in the near future.

Iranian non-governmental organizations present in the Bam region focused on identifying the essential needs and requirements of the survivors, and their relief efforts were more effective as a result. However, they tended to distribute goods directly, and not under the supervision of and in coordination with governmental and public aid organizations. Inequitable distribution of goods thus added to the general sense of distrust and despair at the community level.

To the social work student participant observers, it was clear that the Bam survivors constituted the best resource for understanding the core needs of those hurt in the earthquake, but this resource was not utilized.

Some organizations, particularly the military forces, do not consider the stated wishes of the local people, including even those in convalescent homes.

Lack of coordination in the activities of social welfare organizations resulted in the performance of aid activities in a haphazard manner. Also, in some parts of Bam, different aid organizations formulated vastly different visions and interpretations of needs, services and facilities, often arguing with each other in this regard. This caused further pessimism among the most vulnerable and hurt survivors and made them even more resolute in staying put on their own debris. Some aid organizations hide their supplies and consider other organizations as a competition instead of being part of an aiding team.

The unintended negative consequences of some aid organizations' interventions were evident in the decision to remove the elderly and children from the region, ignoring the fact that extended family and relatives might still have been alive, and that social network supports still existed in the region. The survivors tended to seek out their own families in obtaining social support, and in case that was not possible, they looked for relatives to obtain social supports within their family network. The responsibility of aid organizations to strengthen social networks to support family members and relatives was largely ignored.

On the other hand, foreign aiding teams tirelessly aided survivors in organized teams from dawn to dusk:

The seventh day after the disaster was concurrent with Western New Year celebrations; when the team members were told, 'Instead of celebrating the New Year, you are among the injured and hurt people', they replied, with full satisfaction, 'there is no joy better that helping others ...'. And how well they have realized the meaning of, 'Humans are parts of one single body'.

When the students returned to the School of Social Work, they shared their field notes and impressions. The following data were obtained from the student participant observers:

- Forty out of 40 stated that the primary need of the Bam earthquake survivors was respect for the inherent dignity and the innate strengths and capacities of the survivors. Some referred to this as the need for 'honour'.
- Forty out of 40 indicated that the primary need of the Bam earthquake survivors for respect for their inherent dignity and strengths

was not addressed by aid organizations, as solutions were imposed in a 'top-down' manner, much to the detriment of the survivors. This included a lack of knowledge of who were and who were not genuine survivors, and the ignoring of native, local knowledge in the relief effort.

- Thirty-nine out of 40 students indicated that aid organizations made no use of survivors' participation in the relief effort.
- Thirty-nine out of 40 students identified that survivors' basic health needs were not met by the aid organizations. Access to essential primary healthcare was lacking, and the rebuilding of sanitation systems, establishment of temporary health clinics (and rebuilding of damaged ones), and training health care workers was impeded by a lack of overall coordination of the relief effort.
- Thirty-nine out of 40 students expressed that survivors' shelter needs were not adequately addressed in the relief effort.

Proposal for a Social Work Charter for Unexpected Disasters

The Bam earthquake disaster is not the last natural disaster that Iran will face. It did provide an opportunity, however, to identify how a lack of disaster relief preparedness can lead to the emergence of a human-made calamity more traumatic than the natural disaster itself. This has implications for social work disaster relief work around the globe. As an essential part of such preparedness, aid groups should organize and make transparent their activities, resources and services at each stage of the disaster relief effort. Inter-organization cooperation in relief efforts is otherwise not possible. The establishment of local disaster aid management committees, responsible for the coordination of aid facilities and resources, including aid organizations, is an essential preventative step, in which capable and qualified aid organization managers are able to plan and make effective decisions.

The human calamity following the Bam disaster, observed by the social work participant observers, provided the impetus for the development of a Social Work Charter for Unexpected Disasters which, it is hoped, will provide a template for disaster preparedness and relief efforts globally.

Our proposal for a Social Work Charter for Unexpected Disasters follows the four stages of natural disaster aid, and is aimed at the prevention of human calamities following natural disasters, enhancing social capital at each stage. Social work roles and functions for each stage are delineated. These are based on the data gathered by the 40 social work student participant observers to the 2003 Bam earthquake disaster, as well as on existing literature on social workers' involvement in natural disaster aid (Banerjee and Gillespie 1994; Chou 2003; Desai 2007; Dominelli 2007; Dufka 1988; Pyles 2007; Seroka *et al.* 1986; Yanay and Benjamin 2005; Zakour 1996).

Social Work Charter for Unexpected Disasters

The Social Work Charter for Unexpected Disasters delineates the core needs of affected populations and essential interventions to address these needs, towards achieving the predetermined objective of prevention of human calamity attendant to natural disaster. The charter is divided into the four stages of (1) pre-disaster preparedness: public education measures and the coordination of aid facilities and resources, including aid organizations; (2) the rescue stage: the first days of the disaster; (3) the recovery stage: the weeks after the disaster; (4) the stabilization stage: the return to normalcy (see Table 15.1).

1. Disaster preparedness

The concept of disaster preparedness and readiness applies to a broad range of social services when circumstances overwhelm the usual means of responding to problems. Preparedness may be defined as the degree of readiness to deliver services in response to a disaster, and it involves actions taken prior to disasters to improve response efforts. There is a strong connection between preparedness and aid effectiveness of rescue, recovery and stabilization work; whatever the type of disaster, high levels of preparedness reduce deaths, injuries, property damage and financial loss (Banerjee and Gillespie 1994). Preparedness results in more effective relief response, faster recovery and lower cost (Drabek 1986).

As the Bam earthquake situation illustrates, although natural disaster cannot always be prevented, human mismanagement and exploitation that add to the disaster can be. As all communities are vulnerable to disasters, social service agencies and administrators that ignore potential disaster hazards are taking a serious risk. Banerjee and Gillespie (1994) recommend that social service agencies providing residential care, family counselling, homeless shelters, and social and economic development, as well as professional schools of social work, incorporate disaster preparedness within the scope of their activities. Knowledge of human responses to disasters, role conflict and role abandonment, previous disaster experience, and inter-organizational coordination are crucial elements of any disaster preparedness programme.

Disaster preparedness also includes public education measures as well as the establishment of local disaster aid management committees, responsible for the coordination of aid facilities and resources, including aid organizations. Such specialized planning and the equipping of efficient forces trained in disaster relief is critical. Although disaster preparedness cannot be directly assessed until response to a natural disaster occurs, it can be indirectly assessed prior to disaster occurrence through the existence of disaster plans, inter-organizational coordination, disaster-relevant training, and public education. Social workers have an important role to play in regard to each of these measures.

Table 15.1 Stages of natural disaster aid, identified needs and social work functions

Stages	Identified needs	Social work roles
1. Disaster preparedness	• Community preparedness • Preparedness/readiness of aid organizations	• Internal social welfare organization preparedness: disaster aid training • External preparedness: inter-organizational coordination; establishment of disaster aid headquarters • Public education • Professional education
2. Rescue	• Securing food • Shelter • Clothing and blankets • Gathering information on family and friends • Looking after injured • Burying the dead • Special needs of children, elders, disabled and injured	• Establishment of disaster aid headquarters • Needs assessment • Enumeration of survivors • Sharing data with aid groups • Support for individuals and families • Advocacy and linking victims' needs with resources • Locating family members • Search and rescue; organizing funerals • Setting up temporary accommodation • Collecting and distributing food and supplies • Connecting injured with non-injured survivors • Identifying vulnerable populations
3. Recovery	• Physical health problems • Mental health problems; emotional stress and trauma • Special needs of children, elders, disabled and injured • Adequate accommodation • Community disorganization • Inter-agency disorganization	• Ongoing needs assessment • Modifying disaster aid plans • Setting up prefabricated accommodation • Inter-organizational coordination • Working with and protecting vulnerable populations • Locality development • Creating work opportunities for survivors • Support to professional and volunteer aid workers
4. Stabilization	• Normalization	• Reconstruction • Rehabilitation • Public education

Police and fire departments, emergency management agencies, hospitals and organizations such as the Red Cross and Red Crescent may have legal mandates to respond to disasters. Social services agencies, on the other hand, may not have such a legal mandate but often get involved in disaster response with services of sheltering, feeding, counselling and rehabilitation. Following a disaster, the number of people requiring such services increases dramatically.

Both internal preparedness in social work organizations and external preparedness in the form of participation in the formation of disaster aid headquarters are important for social workers. Internal preparedness may include training in disaster relief and recovery work, budgeted funds for disaster aid work, keeping ready mobile equipment, supplies and communication mechanisms, and coordinated planning. External preparedness includes coordination of efforts with other organizations in the development of national and local disaster plans.

2. The rescue stage

The rescue stage immediately follows the occurrence of the disaster, facing the emergency promptly, and addressing the circumstances of the disaster. During this stage, preventing the expansion of damage, dealing with the crisis and restricting the critical situation is the focus of work. Shock and panic, dissociative behaviour and emotional numbing are frequent reactions to sudden natural disasters.

In Bam, social workers assumed the following roles in the first few days of the disaster:

- Immediate outreach and accurate assessment of the primary needs of survivors; conducting an enumeration of survivors in the region and relaying this information to aid groups and organizations.
- Direct support and provision of information to individuals and families; identifying and locating vulnerable populations of survivors and attending to their needs.
- Advocacy and linking victims' needs with resources.
- Searching for the missing and accompanying survivors and search and rescue teams; digging out corpses from under debris and supporting grieving family members; assisting in organizing funerals for the dead and supporting grieving survivors.
- Helping in the establishment of disaster aid headquarters to set up urgent temporary accommodation for children, women, elderly and the disabled in the region; arranging transportation between the temporary shelters and the wreckage.
- Collecting and distributing food and supplies to the victims.
- Identifying and locating family members and kin of child survivors; accommodating them in the region and avoiding hasty moves to other

locations, as children who were evacuated from Bam had significantly more fearful reactions and problems than those who did not leave.

- Establishing a connection among physically healthy survivors and the injured, especially for injured survivors with no family members in the region.

After the first few days, rescue efforts gradually began to shift towards recovery. Social workers then assumed the following roles:

- Assessing temporary accommodation situations and longer-term settlement needs; in particular, working to establish adequate food preparation, washing and toilet facilities and sanitation systems.
- Creating uni-gender facilities for vulnerable groups, particularly facilities for children and youth without parents or family members, where parents searching for children can be directed.
- Utilizing the strengths and capacities of physically healthy survivors instead of prolonging their mourning; enlisting their cooperation for mutual aid. Survivors possess abundant energy which can be harnessed towards a more efficient and successful rescue effort. The active involvement of survivors in organizing the rescue effort also bodes well for survivor involvement in the future reconstruction of the region.

3. The recovery stage

The recovery stage follows in the weeks after the disaster. During this stage, crisis intervention gradually shifts towards an emphasis on longer-term planning, particularly with respect to linking survivors with resources, and focusing on coordination among disaster relief groups and organizations now in the region. In Bam, social workers assumed the following roles in the weeks after the disaster:

- Reviewing disaster aid plans and making modifications where required, based on ongoing needs assessment; assessing the effectiveness of interventions in the rescue phase and relaying this information to disaster aid headquarters.
- Managing temporary shelters; helping in the construction of more appropriate accommodation, such as moving from tents to more stable prefabricated structures.
- Creating work opportunities for survivors in the recovery effort and preventing dependency; providing short-term employment for those unable to find a role in the recovery effort.
- Working with vulnerable populations, including those with no immediate relatives or family members; forming new family cores via social network intervention.

- Finding relatives of child survivors; establishing a kindergarten for young children.
- Engaging in locality development: involving the community in initial planning for the reconstructing the region, particularly in relation to housing, with the cooperation of local authorities.
- Coordinating the efforts of disaster aid social welfare organizations and finding meaningful roles for volunteers and non-governmental organizations; developing service programmes to address unmet needs.

4. Stabilization

Over the longer term, the task for social workers and other helping professionals consists mainly of rehabilitation and reconstruction, focused on the normalization of the situation so that normal life comes back to the area. Again, emphasizing the full participation in planning, decision-making and executing the reconstruction of their homes is critical to survivors' longer-term well-being and adjustment. One of the tragedies of the Bam disaster was the fact that many survivors refused the new homes built for them because they were not involved in the planning and building of these houses.

The longer-term rehabilitation of survivors is focused on tasks such as interventions for traumatic stress disorders and helping survivors identify, express and deal with difficult feelings; communicating a sense of hope in the context of hopelessness and fear that life can never again be joyful and normal; and educating the community on aspects of human response to crisis. Creative outreach is important. Public education in the form of information about longer-term stress reactions that accompany disaster recovery are critical, and they go a long way towards community acceptance of therapeutic services which effect a more rapid recovery for the disaster-affected population.

Conclusion

Social work practice in the field of natural disasters involves a complicated set of tasks and should be recognized as a vital component of social work practice and the profession. This is a major challenge for future social work practice and education. The experiences and observations of the 40 social work student participant observers in the Bam, Iran earthquake disaster made clear that social workers have important and unique contributions to make in the disaster preparedness, rescue, recovery and stabilization stages of disaster aid work. After a disaster, in the context of traumatic stress and collective suffering, the expertise of social workers in crisis intervention, ecological approaches, strengths-based practice, and promoting change in micro, mezzo and macro systems is central to the task of needs assessment, linking needs with resources, providing therapeutic interventions to survivors, supporting vulnerable populations, and coordinating the efforts of groups and organizations to provide effective responses. As a natural disaster such as earthquake induces shock and fear among victims, it is imperative that non-injured survivors be quickly mobilized towards goal-oriented rescue and recovery functions, and that recovery efforts serve to enhance social capital and improve the community's ability to address its own unmet needs. Following a disaster, survivors are preoccupied with gathering information on the whereabouts of family and friends, as well as securing food, shelter, clothing and blankets; taking part in the rescue operation, as well as looking after the injured and burying the dead, is fundamental to short- and longer-term coping. Anxiety and fear, guilt, powerlessness, loss and depression, and the increasing dependency needs of vulnerable groups such as children, elders, and the disabled and injured provide a more specific focus for social work intervention during the rescue and recovery stages. Over the longer term, crisis intervention is replaced by stabilization efforts focused on rehabilitation and reconstruction.

It is in the area of disaster preparedness, however, that social workers can perhaps make their most important contribution. The findings presented here underscore the need for preparedness in the form of disaster plans, both within social welfare and aid organizations and externally in the form of local disaster aid management committees of which social workers are a part. Adequate preparedness reduces the disruption following natural disasters, and can prevent the 'second (human) disaster' that all too frequently follows a natural disaster. Massive natural disasters with heavy human casualties occur in all parts of the world; exactly one year after Bam, the Southeast Asian tsunami struck, and nine months later, Hurricane Katrina destroyed the city of New Orleans and surrounding areas. With global population growth, disadvantaged populations are increasing in areas vulnerable to disaster. Social work agencies and social welfare organizations which are currently on the periphery of disaster preparedness networks can and should get involved in preparation efforts, and both social work administrators and educators need to be involved in disaster preparedness planning and education in regard to assessment and intervention in disaster aid work, and contributing to inter-organizational coordination for disaster response. In addition, contributing to public education campaigns and disseminating information related to disaster aid and rescue, and implementing disaster rehearsal, is an important social work role in the preparedness stage.

Finally, descriptive and empirical studies on human responses to disaster, as well as research on the effectiveness of assessment protocols and intervention strategies, are needed to meet the acute and long-term needs of disaster victims. It is hoped that this study and accompanying charter, although from a distant land, will spearhead the development of this field of practice in the global context.

References

Aghabakhshi, H. and Gregor, C. (2007) 'Learning the lessons of Bam: the role of social capital', *International Social Work*, 50(3): 347–56.

Banerjee, M.M. and Gillespie, D.F. (1994) 'Linking disaster preparedness and organizational response effectiveness', *Journal of Community Practice*, 1(3): 129–42.

Chou, Y. (2003) 'Social workers' involvement in Taiwan's 1999 earthquake disaster aid: implications for social work education', *Social Work and Society*, 1(1). Online. Available at: www.socwork.net/sws/article/view/251 (accessed 21 October 2013).

Coleman, J. (1988) 'Social capital in the creation of human capital', *American Journal of Sociology*, 94: S95–S120.

Desai, A. (2007) 'Disaster and social work responses', in L. Dominelli (ed.), *Revitalising Communities in a Globalising World*, Aldershot: Ashgate.

Dodds, S. and Nuehring, E. (1996) 'A primer for social work research on disaster', *Journal of Social Service Research*, 22(1/2): 27–56.

Dominelli, L. (ed.) (2007) *Revitalising Communities in a Globalising World*, Aldershot: Ashgate.

Doostgharin, T. (2009) 'Children affected by earthquakes and their immediate emotional needs', *International Social Work*, 52(1): 96–106.

Drabek, T.E. (1986) *Human System Responses to Disaster: An Inventory of Sociological Findings*, New York: Spinger-Verlag.

Dufka, C.L. (1988) 'The Mexico City earthquake disaster', *Social Casework*, 69(3): 162–70.

Ghafory-Ashtiany, M. and Eshghi, S. (2005) 'Bam earthquake of 05:26:26 of 26 December 2003, Ms 6.5', *Proceedings of the International Symposium on Earthquake Engineering Commemorating Tenth Anniversary of the 1995 Kobe Earthquake* (ISEE Kobe 2005), E-23–E26.

Goudarzi, M. (2004) 'The biggest quakes of Iran and the world', *Journal of Culture and Research*, 13(10): 55–67.

Javadian, R. (2007) 'Social work responses to earthquake disasters: a social work intervention in Bam, Iran', *International Social Work*, 50(3): 334–46.

Mathbor, G.M. (2007) 'Enhancement of community preparedness for natural disasters: the role of social work in building social capital for sustainable disaster relief and management', *International Social Work*, 50(3): 357–69.

Pyles, L. (2007) 'Community organising for post-disaster development: locating social work', *International Social Work*, 50(3): 321–33.

Seroka, C.M., Knapp, C., Knight, S., Siemon, C.R. and Starbuck, S. (1986) 'A comprehensive program for postdisaster counseling', *Social Casework*, 67(1): 37–44.

Yanay, U. and Benjamin, S. (2005) 'The role of social workers in natural disasters: the Jerusalem experience', *International Social Work*, 48(3): 263–76.

Zakour, M.J. (1996) 'Disaster research in social work', *Journal of Social Service Research*, 22(1): 7–25.

The changing face of social work in youth justice in Scotland

Bill Whyte

Introduction

Scotland's Children's Hearing system has, for over 40 years, attempted to deal with young people who offend as part of its integrated social work services to children and families. In many respects the approach is consistent with the requirements of the United Nations Convention on the Rights of the Child (UNCRC) (G.A. Res 44/25, 1989) and its associated guidance, which focus on well-being as a paramount consideration, extra-judicial solutions and socio-educational rather than punitive interventions. However international standards and European rules have highlighted challenges to all jurisdictions in establishing 'child-centred' policy and practice for dealing with young people within and outside criminal processes, particularly those under the age of 18 years involved in serious and violent offending.

Approaches to dealing with children and young people who break the law vary much more widely across jurisdictions than the equivalent justice systems for adults. In addition to cultural and institutional differences, youth systems vary in their structures and age jurisdiction as well as in the underlying normative and value assumptions underpinning policy and practice.

Many Western countries pursued youth crime policies during much of the twentieth century that eroded the distinction between the young person in need and the delinquent youth. In the early twenty-first century, welfare-oriented approaches were often superseded by punitive law-and-order ideologies driven by politicians under pressure to be seen as tough on crime. The predominance of 'punishment' as a cultural response, for example, has often meant that the public framing of provision for responding to youth crime has been dominated by a language of punishment, without consideration of how best to respond to the characteristics and circumstances of the young people in ways that are likely to result in positive change. As a consequence, less consideration is also given to the well-being and safety of the community as a whole (Brown, 1998).

Justice and welfare – children first?

The combination of two concepts, special responses to children and young people and equal rights under the law, create tension in practice on how best to reconcile the competing claims of the law, judicial process and punishment, with the need to consider the best interests and the rights of the child or young person while effectively reducing offending.

Systems dealing with young people who offend are often differentiated along the broad dimensions of 'justice' and 'welfare'. As with all ideal types, models are seldom found in a pure form. All countries remain uncomfortable with a rigid distinction between youth justice and child welfare/protection, and in practice most combine elements of the different approaches. Legislation tends to maintain a separation between systems dealing with the care and protection of children and young people (child welfare) and responses to offending by children and young people (youth justice). With respect to young people in their teens who offend, the second half of the twentieth century saw a swing away from welfare approaches to systems associated more with access to due process, particularly in English-speaking jurisdictions directed by principles of proportionality and accountability, and towards greater recognition of the place of victims. Nonetheless all countries allow for varying degrees of overlap and convergence between child welfare and youth justice systems, with the age of transition (from shared responsibility to individual criminal responsibility) to the youth justice system ranging from 8 to 15 years. The philosophy of child protection continues to hold sway in mainland European countries up to the mid-teens. However, because the peak age for offending is typically in the mid- to late-teens, the majority of young people who offend, notwithstanding diversionary measures, are commonly dealt with by courts with a justice and criminal orientation.

Scotland's children's legislation reaches to the age of 18, yet many, if not most young people involved in crime are 'criminalized' in some way long before that age, despite the evidence suggesting that early criminalization is one of the best predictors of sustained criminality (McAra and McVie, 2007). These circumstances present day-to-day challenges for practitioners concerned with effectiveness, values, rights and ethical practice. They must contend with variable definitions and statutes on what constitutes 'a child' and 'a youth' and demarcations between those who are and are not deemed 'fully criminally responsible', or between those considered best dealt with in criminal proceedings and those not.

In a criminal justice paradigm, no adult need accept any shared responsibility for a young person's action, despite the intentions of children's legislation and UNCRC principles. Indeed criminalization can be seen to absolve adults and service providers from accountability for 'failure'. In this regard all UK jurisdictions stand accused by the UN Committee on the Rights of the Child (UNComRC) of poor child-centred approaches to youth crime; of high levels of criminalization and detention of young people, many with public care backgrounds. It is only in recent years that political views in Scotland have begun again to embrace the idea that a low age of criminal responsibility (eight in Scotland) is symbolic of a lack of shared adult responsibility for young people's behaviour.

Youth justice in a global context: international standards

The near universal ratification of the UNCRC has placed importance on establishing a 'level playing field' for all children through progressive universal provision and early social intervention measures. In relation to youth crime, UNCRC and its associated guidance – the Beijing Rules, 1985; the Directing Principles of Riyadh, 1990; the Havana Rules, 1990; the Tokyo Rules, 1990; the Vienna Guidelines, 1997 – stress the importance of the following:

- well-being as a paramount consideration;
- an age of criminal responsibility based on maturity;
- socio-educational interventions rather than punitive ones;
- extra-judicial solutions;
- deprivation of liberty only as a last resort; and
- safeguards for the use of alternatives to custody.

Benchmarks for practice have been set by international agreements and regulations. UNCRC (G.A. Res 44/25, 1989, Article 3) requires that 'in all actions concerning children, whether undertaken by public or private social welfare institutions, courts of law, administrative authorities or legislative bodies, the best interests of the child shall be a primary consideration' (para. 1). The qualification of 'a' primary rather than 'the' primary consideration can find expression in quite different practices which invoke the public interest as overriding the interests of the child when it comes to criminal matters for relatively minor, even if persistent, offending.

The preamble to UNCRC stresses the dynamic nature of the framework and that it expects it to be continually developed on the basis of research and practice-related evidence. The international practice model recommended is one of diversion as far as possible from criminal proceedings up to the age of 18, stressing the value of early preventive intervention. UNCRC is not incorporated into law in UK jurisdictions; nonetheless international law requires that the United Kingdom should adhere to the spirit and principles of the Convention. UNCRC should represent the standard for measuring any appropriate system of youth justice, particularly as the European Convention of Human Rights (ECHR), which is incorporated in UK and Scots law, does not comment on whether there are, or should be, positive obligations on states to safeguard or promote the welfare of children and young persons. It is difficult to argue from evidence on the levels of criminalization and detention of young people under the age of 18 in all UK jurisdictions that the obligations implied by UNCRC have featured greatly as a priority.

UNComRC, which monitors the application of UNCRC, published a list of concerns and criticisms regarding the United Kingdom's performance in 1995, along with a comprehensive set of recommendations on how better to meet practice obligations and protect children's rights. In revisiting these concerns in 2002, it remained highly critical of UK practices and expressed disappointment that the majority of the recommendations from 1995 had not been acted on (Harvey, 2002).

The UK delegation argued that the low age of criminal responsibility in all UK jurisdictions allowed for early intervention while recognizing children's responsibility for their crime. It also argued that children's legislation, although providing protection and guarantees of services for children up to the age of 18, did not apply to children in detention. However signal judgments of the High Court in England, following judicial reviews instigated by the Howard League in 2002 and 2007, confirmed that English, and by extension UK, jurisdictions cannot designate young people under 18 as 'ex-children' simply by their entrance into the criminal justice system. The High Court held that the Children Act 1989 did apply to children held in custody. The judge said that the Howard League had 'performed a most useful service in bringing to the public attention matters which, on the face of it, ought to shock the conscience of every citizen' (*R* v. *Secretary of State*, 29 November 2002; Case No CO/1806/2002, para. 175).

The decision confirmed that local authorities retain a statutory duty to safeguard the welfare of children, even if they are in prison, and that this should result in more child protection investigations inside prisons and greater involvement of social services in assessing the needs of the most vulnerable children. In July 2007, in a further Court of Appeal decision in the case of J, who was 15 when she committed the offence leading to detention, three Law Lords confirmed that local authorities should provide her with the care due under s20 of the Children Act 1989 (Provision of accommodation for children); in effect that local authorities have the same duties to children who leave custody as to 'children in need'. The wording of the 1989 Act in England and Wales is almost identical in Scots law.

This judgment highlighted that 'local authorities across the country were failing to provide proper assessments and care plans for vulnerable children' entering and leaving detention, particularly 'where children are in danger of returning to precisely the same situations that led to their crimes and imprisonment in the first place' (Howard League press release, 26 July 2007). These decisions confirmed that young people involved even in serious crime do fall within the children services policy framework and are entitled to aftercare support to ensure their personal and social integration and long-term desistence from crime. However, giving practice expression to these duties is a difficult matter without multi-disciplinary protocols and shared resources among criminal justice/probation, youth justice, children's services, housing, education and employment, leisure and health-related provision; in other words a whole systems approach to youth justice.

European standards

If UK politics have ensured that practice standards have remained ambivalent towards international UNCRC benchmarks, it could be argued that this should be less so in the context of ECHR, which has been incorporated into UK law. The Commission of Human Rights (CoE, 2005) noted that the United Kingdom had not been immune to a tendency to consider human rights as excessively restricting the effective administration of justice and public protection. The report noted that it was difficult to avoid the impression that 'juvenile trouble-makers are too rapidly drawn into the criminal justice system and ... too readily placed in detention, when greater attention to alternative forms of supervision and targeted early intervention would be more effective' (CoE, 2005, para. 81). It commented that extensive programme development appeared to have made little impact on the numbers detained, noting that the United Kingdom had among the highest rates of juvenile detention in Western Europe, high rates of reconviction following the release, and an apparent lack of appropriate psychological care and inadequate educational assistance for young people. It suggested 'young adults should leave prison with something other than advanced degrees in criminality', and drew the conclusion that preventive intervention was 'minimal' (para. 94).

European Guidelines on Child-Friendly Justice (CJ-S-CH (2010) 3 E) and European Rules on Juvenile Offenders subject to Sanctions and Measures (CM/Rec 2008 11E) further strengthen the position of young people involved in offending. In particular, they stress the importance of desistence and social integration, and avoiding adult criminal proceedings, irrespective of the gravity of their crime; and that, with some exceptions for serious crimes, records should not be disclosed on reaching the age of majority.

Youth justice in Scotland: a distinct philosophy

The Social Work (Scotland) Act 1968 introduced a distinctive approach to youth justice in Scotland in 1971, which has lasted for over 40 years (Lockyer and Stone, 1998). Scottish youth courts were disbanded and replaced by lay decision-making tribunals – Children's Hearings – which deal with children at risk of abuse and neglect and children who offend within a unified welfare system.

The system is based on the philosophy of justice advocated by the Report of the Kilbrandon Committee (SHHD, 1964; Stone, 2003). It recommended an extra-judicial system of Children's Hearings and the reorganization of social work services under the umbrella of all-purpose local authority social work departments, with responsibility for child care and protection and youth justice, alongside responsibilities previously undertaken by the national probation service, which was also disbanded.

Lord Kilbrandon's report took the view that the criminal process was unsuccessful in its attempts to compromise between crime, responsibility and punishment on one hand and the welfare and interests of the young person on the other and that a new approach was needed. It viewed the criminal process as having two fundamental functions: the adjudication of the legal facts, whether or not an offence had been established beyond reasonable doubt – viewed as requiring the skills of a professional judge – and decisions concerning disposal once the facts had been established, for which criminal judges had no particular claim on expertise.

Accordingly, the Scottish system separates adjudication and disposal – the former continues to be the responsibility of criminal courts and the latter the responsibility of a welfare tribunal of trained community representatives (panel members). If the young person and their family accept the 'grounds', i.e. that the offence has been committed, at the opening of a hearing, the hearing will deal with the 'What should we do about it?' and operates as a welfare tribunal geared to acting in the best interests of the young person, assuming this to be in the best interests of the community as a whole. As a consequence a Children's Hearing has no power to determine questions of innocence or guilt. Nonetheless, the Hearing has the powers to make young people subject to 'compulsory measures' in the community with their family or with alternatives or in institutional provision, if they accept the offence ground or if it has been proven in a court.

Access to representation and legal aid is available to all young people and parents who dispute the facts of the case, deny the offence, are unable to understand the evidence against them or wish to appeal against the outcome. This is intended to safeguard legal rights and provide a check against over-enthusiastic intervention. In practice, the vast majority of children and young people brought before Hearings in Scotland accept the facts and are therefore dealt with in this welfare setting. The resulting welfare-based system has a clear commitment to the 'paramountcy principle' outlined as a foundation principle in UNCRC, up to the age of 16 and to a lesser extent to 18.

A Children's Hearing is a tribunal consisting of three trained lay panel members (at least one man and one woman), intended to be representative of the community; one of these acts as chairperson. The procedure, including the decision-making, is conducted in front of all the participants, usually in a round-table discussion. Changes to strengthen and modernize the structure and organization of the Children's Hearing system, including a new independent national body, Children's Hearings Scotland (CHS), responsible for the system, were introduced under the Children's Hearings Act (2011) in 2013. Policies renewing the emphasis on early intervention and the whole systems approach to provision are being promoted.

Children's Reporters are the gatekeepers to the system, combining the function of a child welfare official and 'prosecutor' in the child's best interests. They must consider that a young person who has offended may be in need of 'compulsory measures' to justify referral to a Hearing and have powers to require reports and assessments to assist in their judgment. Where an offence referral is made to a Hearing, the Reporter attends and provides expert legal advice but does not take part in the official deliberations in respect of disposal. Challenges under the ECHR have resulted in a review of the Reporter's role and provisions updated in the Children's Hearings Act 2011.

While not recommending a specific age of transition to criminal proceedings, the UNCRC Committee has tended to criticize jurisdictions in which the minimum age is 12 or less and has urged UK countries to raise the age of criminal responsibility (Harvey, 2002). UK countries have among the lowest ages of criminal responsibility of any of the continental European states, with Scotland as the lowest at age eight (Buist and Whyte, 2004: 59).

The issue of maturity in regard to criminal responsibility is a complex one for all jurisdictions, and few have arrived at a consensus on how best to respond to troubled and troublesome children and young people. In 2010 the Scottish Government introduced immunity from prosecution for young people under the age of 12, and while no children between eight and 12 can be prosecuted in court, the age of criminal responsibility remains age eight, allowing for this age group to be referred to a welfare Hearing because of criminal behaviour. The Children's Hearings Act 2011 re-introduced the original intention of the system that offences accepted as grounds at a Hearing would not be considered criminal convictions for any purpose in the future. The 2011 Act left scope for some categories of offences, e.g. serious sexual offences, to be 'recorded'.

The vast majority of offence referrals are diverted from formal Hearings by doing very little other than communicating with parent/carers – radical non-intervention (Schur 1973) or receiving 'advice, guidance and assistance' from local authorities under a 'voluntary agreement' as a form of early and preventive intervention consistent with the UNCRC principle of progressive universal responses.

Arrangements can be made with the agreement of parents and the young person to confiscate weapons, provide a letter of apology to the victim, or agree to make restitution with the assistance of a voluntary agency. Other restorative practices including conferencing and victim awareness programmes are available to Reporters in many local authority areas, and legislation makes provision for Reporters to give victims information on decision-making and outcomes. By diverting cases from the Children's Hearings the whole system has a crucial role in minimizing the risk of 'net-widening' which is sometimes associated with welfare-oriented systems.

While no clear theoretical exposition or any precise definitions of its founding principles were outlined at the time, the Kilbrandon proposals were based on key assumptions recognizable in current theoretical debates and in more recent international and European regulations. An integrated system for dealing with all such children was proposed because 'the true distinguishing factor … is their need for special measures of education and training, the normal up-bringing processes having, for whatever reason, fallen short' (para. 15). Early effective intervention policies and the promotion of whole systems approaches in Scotland have seen a reduction of referrals in some pilot areas of around 40 per cent (Capgemini Consulting, 2011).

The Children's Hearing system is not intended, simplistically, to separate out 'offending' and 'non-offending' children. In principle, the system is structured as a system of diversion from prosecution and early intervention intended to address the needs of the whole child in partnership with parents, where possible, not simply or exclusively focusing on offending. It is, nonetheless, one of the explicit objectives of the system to try to help young people stop offending through decision-making in a setting which, by its informality and allocation of time, would ensure, as far as practically possible, effective participation by the young person and adults in resolving problems and deciding on future action (Lockyer and Stone, 1998).

Consequently key principles of the system stress the importance, where possible, of working in partnership with parents and family networks to find coordinated community-based solutions directed by social educational principles (Smith and Whyte, 2008) rather than relying on formal criminalization and its associated risks. Young people who offend are to be viewed not simply as offenders but as young people first, whose upbringing has been unsatisfactory and where the responsibility for their offending behaviour should be a shared one between the young person, the family, the community and the state, and where possible resolutions are sought without recourse to formal proceedings.

Theories of victimology, though undeveloped at the time, are nonetheless implicit in the assumptions that young people are often themselves victims of their upbringing and circumstances as well as 'villains' or perpetrators of crime (Anderson et al., 1994). It was never argued by Kilbrandon that social adversity caused or fully explained offending. It drew on developments in the social sciences at the time, which suggested that social and emotional deprivation associated with disorganized neighbourhoods, family disruption, separation and poor parenting would have a major impact on the subsequent behaviour of the young. The importance of positive schooling and the crucial role of parental supervision in preventing delinquency were strongly emphasized.

Scots law places a statutory duty on local authorities to 'promote social welfare' (Social Work Scotland Act 1968, s12 [1]). The Children (Scotland) Act (1995) and The Children and Young Persons (Scotland) Act (2014) place a whole authority (corporate) responsible for children 'in need', 'looked after' or 'accommodated' because of their offending. The legislation includes provision to support and maintain young people in certain circumstances into early adulthood. In principle, this should mean that these children and young people have the highest priority for education, housing, leisure and cultural services, as well as drug and mental health services, and are not the sole responsibility of social work or police.

Fine principles do not necessarily make good practice, and for many years critics of the Scottish approach pointed to the lack of an empirical basis for the assumptions underpinning the system (Cowperthwaite, 1992). Since then, studies in this field and from other jurisdictions, such as Farrington and West (1977), Hagell and Newman (1994), Graham and Bowling (1995), Rutter et al. (1998), and Scottish studies (Jamieson et al., 1999; McAra and McVie, 2007; Whyte, 2004) continued to lend support to the view that multiple difficulties relating to social adversity, socialization and social control, particularly parental supervision, are common to many, if not most, young people who offend persistently. Contemporary data support attempts to synthesize key elements of existing criminological theories, for example, the idea that social structure, including the socio-economic status of the family and the ecology of the neighbourhood, can have an influence on the social control processes of family and school, on peer groups, and hence directly or indirectly on the young person's development. While delinquency in youth can lead to adult offending through the acquisition of criminal habits, skills and associates, formal labelling as an offender can also have the effect of weakening social bonds and increasing the risk of adult offending (Braithwaite, 1989; Sampson and Laub, 1993). Commentaries on desistence from crime support approaches in which narrative, self-efficacy and supporting maturation are key to changing lives (Ward and Maruna, 2007).

In many respects Scotland's Children's Hearing system sits comfortably within the UNCRC framework of principles. Further information and discussion of its origins and the early workings of the Hearing system can be found in Martin et al. (1981), Cowperthwaite (1992), Kearney (1991), Moore and Whyte (1997) and Norrie (2000).

Getting it right: a whole systems approach

International and European developments have impacted on Scotland, particularly since 2007. The overarching assumption underlying the Scottish system is that acting in the best interest of the young person and reducing offending will, in the long run, be in the best interests of young people, victims and the public at large. While 'no child under the age of 16 years shall be prosecuted for any offence except on the instructions of the Lord Advocate', nonetheless the criminal courts do deal with children. Relatively few young people up to the age of 18 are dealt with on solemn proceedings (very serious charges), and this number declined from 556 in 2007–2008 to 250 in 2011–2012. Nonetheless, the critical age of transition to adult criminal courts in Scotland remains around 16, which is low by European standards.

The report, *It's a Criminal Waste: Stop Youth Crime Now* (Scottish Executive, 2000) provided a full review of youth justice provision. The Scottish review concluded that while the principles underpinning the Children's Hearing system were fundamentally sound and in line with UNCRC principles, practices and the resources to support them had fallen behind the times and change was overdue. To some extent the detailed findings of Audit Scotland's report (2002) confirmed this conclusion, highlighting inconsistencies in decision-making and resources across the country and expressing concern that two-thirds of financial resources were being used up in legal and administrative processes rather than on direct provision for young people. The review acknowledged that any jurisdiction seriously attempting to bring about positive change in youth crime in line with international standards requires a range of responses under the key UNCRC headings:

- **Prevention:** to increase effective progressive universal provision for all children and their families, reducing or compensating for conditions which expose children to harmful behaviours of all kinds; with particular attention to drug- and alcohol-related risks for those below 16 and to school exclusion.
- **Early Intervention:** quick, targeted assistance for individual children whose behaviour or family circumstances indicate vulnerability towards offending and other problems.
- **Diversion:** from formal processes (both Hearings and criminal courts) to allow immediate action to address problems and re-equip children and young people for more positive citizenship.
- **Intervention:** only when necessary and at the right time and right level.
- **Participation:** of young people and families; more joint action between voluntary and statutory agencies, communities and the commercial and business sectors to create safer communities in which individual needs, responsibilities and rights are respected and in which restorative justice features; better information on factors which contribute to youth crime and its reduction.

The review report acknowledged a paradox in research evidence that those most likely to make the transition to the adult court under the age of 18 are also those who are most likely to:

- be immature and impulsive risk-takers;
- re-offend on deferred sentence if not given support, default on fines, fail to keep appointments for supervised attendance orders and breach their probation, and find themselves in custody;
- lead chaotic lives which lack constructive home supports;
- be at greatest risk of substance abuse and violence;
- have been victims of offences themselves; and
- have had limited education.

(Scottish Executive, 2000: Annex C)

The review raised questions about the meaning, in practice, of the existing statutory duty placing responsibility on the whole local authority system for children in need under the Children (Scotland) Act 1995, particularly those who offend. The corporate responsibility of education, housing, leisure and recreation, cultural and other community services in assisting the most difficult young people in desistance did not seem to feature strongly in this work. The review suggested that the whole person or whole systems approach needed to be renewed and is 'no less valid for the 16 or 17 year old offender than it is for the 15 year old' (para. 13). It stressed the need for 'a unified approach at a practical level, combining care and protection with the public's concerns over the need to address offending behaviour' (para. 14).

The Scottish Government embarked on a major 'whole systems' change programme in 2010 to improve the early identification and effective response to the needs of all children, putting well-being at the heart of practice, both for children and young people and for victims. The programme aimed to achieve national outcomes identified in key policy documents since 2007, including the following:

- **Getting it Right for Every Child (GIRFEC)** articulates the need for a nationally consistent approach to supporting and working with all children and young people in Scotland to get the help they need when they need it. GIRFEC requires that all services for children and young people – social work, health, education, police, housing and voluntary organizations – adapt and streamline their systems and practices to improve how they work together.
- **Protecting Scotland's Communities: Fair, Fast and Flexible Justice** (2008) provides a blueprint for a modern, coherent approach to the management of offenders, aimed at reducing offending and repeat offending and improving public safety, including focusing on children and young people.
- **Preventing Offending by Young People: A Framework for Action** (2008) aimed at delivering real improvements in standard practice by improving the range, quality and effectiveness of provision, particularly regarding prevention and early intervention for the 8–16 age

group, and successful transitions into adulthood for young people aged 15–18.

- **Securing Our Future Initiative (SOFI) (2009)** established a vision that no children should be in locked (secure) institutions; rather they should be supported by the provision of effective community-based interventions, by informed decision making by Children's Hearings, local authorities and courts, as alternatives to the use of secure care.

The *Getting it Right* practice model promotes rights- and strengths-based approaches around eight well-being indicators (SHANARRI – safe, healthy, achieving, nurtured, active, respected, responsible, included) consistent with the UNCRC and the Scottish Children's Charter of 2004. The resulting common framework is intended to support integrated and co-ordinated systemic practice with young people and their families at the centre of multidisciplinary planning. Key features include a single multidisciplinary plan focused on outcomes, a named person as a key point of contact and a lead professional with overall responsibility for a wrap-around plan, making sure that the different agencies act as a team in partnership with young people and their family network.

Getting it Right stresses the role of proportionate and timely help from universal services, particularly health and education for all children, as this is where early identification of problems is most likely to be noted and effective early intervention most likely to be provided. The model is no less relevant for older young people who are at risk or present risks to others; the assumption being that protection and prevention should be twin aims at any level of help.

The theory behind *Getting it Right* is rooted in developmental research and contemporary theory (Whyte, 2009), which stresses that what happens to a child in one part of his or her life will have an impact on other areas, so it is important to look at the child's whole system in building resilience to help them overcome adversity and vulnerabilities. The importance of services working together to provide integrated wrap-around and coordinated family-based help, so that young people are not passed around from one agency to another, remains the focus of and challenge for practice. Assessing and managing risk and need are part of the same system, identifying immediate risk and the impact of those risks on a child's well-being in the broader sense. As a consequence the practice model has been re-cast as a Whole Systems Approach (WSA).

Key aims of the WSA are to promote work with all stakeholders that accomplishes the following:

- provides a consistent and sustainable approach for all young people under age 18, delivering the right service, to the right young person, at the right time (appropriate, proportionate and timely);
- ensures that services are responsive to the needs of all young people, whatever the risk, offending type or system they are in;

- develops integrated processes and services across children's and adults systems;
- diverts young people from formal measures (Children's Hearing and prosecution) where possible; and
- increases opportunities for community alternatives to secure care and custody designed for young people.

These aims are to be achieved through the implementation of a streamlined and effective framework for all partners that focuses on early and effective action, e.g. by using pre-referral screening (PRS), diversion, and effective risk management and intensive support for the most challenging to improve outcomes without the need for compulsory measures or removal from the community. Key elements of intensive support services should include the following:

- offence and family-focused intervention;
- life skills and recreational activities;
- evening and weekend support;
- 24/7 crisis response service;
- respite and time out;
- mentoring;
- one-to-one learning;
- counselling and mental health support.

Young people at high risk of serious offending and out-of-home placement, particularly secure accommodation and detention, are notoriously difficult to work with effectively, and the return rate to institutional provision is high and costly. This group is a priority for Preventing Offending by Young People: A Framework for Action (2008, 2012) and the WSA.

The change programme has been further strengthened by the Framework for Risk Assessment Management and Evaluation (FRAME): Planning for Local Authorities and Partners; For Children and Young People under 18 (2011) which identified five overarching national standards relating to the following:

- risk assessment;
- risk management measures;
- planning and responding to change;
- partnership working;
- quality assurance.

The five FRAME standards attempt to establish a common language and approach to the issues of risk and need, information sharing and the links between child care and adult justice practices, for example in Multi-Agency Public Protection Arrangements (MAPPA). At the same time new National

Guidance for Child Protection in Scotland (Scottish Government, 2014) stresses that young people up to 18 at self-risk or who place others at risk should come within the concerns of child protection practice and not simply be abandoned to criminal justice.

The challenge facing Scottish practitioners is to translate this change programme and whole systems approach into consistent delivery aimed at achieving desistence, restoration and social integration through reductions in the following:

- the number of young people referred to the Children's Hearing System on offending grounds;
- the number of 16- and 17-year-olds being dealt with by criminal court;
- the number of young people being placed in residential institutions including secure accommodation and detention.

Scotland's distinctive approach to dealing with young people in trouble with the law has been modernized with the aim of bringing social work practice closer in line with international standards and consistent with international research on effective approaches aimed at desistence, restoration and social integration. A number of research projects are underway evaluating the impact of this renewed approach. It remains to be seen how effective it will be in reducing the number of young people involved in formal systems and in particular in criminal processes.

References

Anderson, S., Kinsey, R., Loader, I. and Smith, C.G. (1994) *Cautionary Tales: Young People, Crime and Policing in Edinburgh*, Aldershot: Avebury.

Audit Scotland (2002) *Dealing with Offending by Young People*, Edinburgh: Audit Scotland.

Braithwaite, J. (1989) *Crime, Shame and Reintegration*, Cambridge: Cambridge University Press.

Brown, S. (1998) *Understanding Youth and Crime*, Buckingham: Open University.

Buist, M. and Whyte, B. (2004) *International Research Evidence for Scotland's Children's Hearing Review: A Report for the Scottish Executive CRU*, Edinburgh: Scottish Executive.

Capgemini Consulting (2011) *Aberdeen Youth Justice Development Programme: Interim Evaluation*, Aberdeen: Author. Online. Available at: www.scotland.gov. uk/Resource/Doc/925/0121352.pdf (retrieved 21 January 2015).

Children's Hearings Act (2011). Online. Available at: www.legislation.gov.uk/ asp/2011/1/pdfs/asp_20110001_en.pdf (retrieved 21 January 2015).

Children (Scotland) Act (1995). Online. Available at: www.opsi.gov.uk/acts/ acts1995/ukpga_19950036_en_1 (retrieved 21 January 2015).

CoE (European Commission) (2005) *Report by MR Alvarao Gil-Robles Commissioner for Human Rights on his visit to the United Kingdom*, Geneva:

European Commission. Online. Available at: https://wcd.coe.int/ViewDoc.jsp?id=948043&Site=COE. (retrieved 21 January 2015).

Cowperthwaite, D. (1992) *The Emergence of the Scottish Children's Hearings System*, Southampton: Institute of Criminal Justice University of Southampton.

Farrington, D. and West, D. (1977) *The Delinquent Way of Life*, London: Heinemann.

Graham, J. and Bowling, B. (1995) *Young People and Crime*, Home Office Research Study 145, London: HMSO.

Hagell, A. and Newman, T. (1994) *Persistent Young Offenders*, London: Policy Studies Institute.

Harvey, R. (2002) 'The UK before the UN Committee on the Rights of the Child', *ChildRIGHT*, 10(190): 9–11.

Jamieson, J., McIvor, G. and Murray, C. (1999) *Understanding Offending among Young People*, Edinburgh: HMSO.

Kearney, B. (1991) *Children's Hearings and the Sheriff Court*, 2nd edn, London: Butterworths.

Lockyer, A. and Stone, F.H. (eds) (1998) *Juvenile Justice in Scotland: 25 Years of the Welfare Approach*, Edinburgh: T & T Clark.

McAra, L. and McVie, S. (2007) 'Youth justice? The impact of system contact on patterns of desistance from offending', *European Journal of Criminology*, 4(3): 315–45.

Martin, F., Fox, S.J. and Murray, K. (1981) *Children Out of Court*, Edinburgh: Scottish Academic Press.

Moore, G. and Whyte, B. (1997) *Social Work and Criminal Law in Scotland*, Edinburgh: Mercat Press.

Norrie, K. (2000) *Children's Hearings in Scotland*, Edinburgh: W. Green.

Rutter, M., Giller, H. and Hagell, A. (1998) *Anti-Social Behaviour by Young People*, Cambridge: Cambridge University Press.

Sampson, R. and Laub, J. (1993) *Crime in the Making: Pathways and Turning Points through Life*, Cambridge, MA: Harvard University.

Schur, E. (1973) *Radical Non-intervention: Rethinking the Delinquency Problem*, Englewood Cliffs: Prentice-Hall.

Scottish Executive (2000) *It's a Criminal Waste: Stop Youth Crime Now*, Edinburgh: Scottish Executive.

The Scottish Government (2014) *National Guidance for Child Protection in Scotland*, Edinburgh: HMSO

SHHD (1964) *Children and Young Persons (Scotland)*, London: HMSO.

Smith, M. and Whyte, B. (2008) 'Social education and social pedagogy: reclaiming a Scottish tradition in social work', *European Journal of Social Work*, 11(1): 15–28.

Social Work Scotland Act (1968) Online. Available at: www.opsi.gov.uk/RevisedStatutes/Acts/ukpga/1968/cukpga_19680049_en_4#pt2-pb1-l1g16 (retrieved 21 January 2015).

Stone, F.H. (2003) *The Kilbrandon Report*. Online. Available at: www.scotland.gov.uk/Publications/2003/10/18259/26878 (retrieved 21 January 2015).

Ward, T. and Maruna, S. (2007) *Rehabilitation Beyond the Risk-Paradigm*, London: Routledge

Whyte, B. (2004) 'Responding to youth crime in Scotland', *British Journal of Social Work*, 34(4): 395–411.

Whyte, B. (2009) *Youth Justice in Practice: Making a Difference*, Bristol: The Policy Press.

Chapter 17

Australian social work in the twenty-first century

Workforce trends, challenges and opportunities

Bob Lonne

Introduction

The Australian community services, as in other countries, have undergone rapid and profound change since the 1980s, with transformation of the sector at the organizational, practice and labour force levels. As a result of the increasing domination of neo-liberal ideologies and the impacts of globalization, the role and nature of government altered, as did the broad mandate of social welfare, often through the increased use of market-based policies (McDonald 2006). In what has become known as the human services, significant modifications occurred to the ways in which programmes and services were configured, structured and delivered. New Public Management (NPM – usually termed managerialism) arrived with its associated programme management approaches and an attendant impact on professional practice, often via case management (Lonne *et al.* 2009). As a traditional professional group charged with delivering community and social services, social work has also altered, with faith in professional wisdom and discretion increasingly supplanted by reliance on highly bureaucratic and interventionist NPM approaches to management (Yeatman *et al.* 2009).

Because this chapter deals with similar problems to those being experienced elsewhere, despite contextual differences, in many senses Australia can be used as a case study for international events. In this chapter I describe these significant change processes and the underpinning ideological and policy drivers. In particular, I focus on the current directions for the profession with respect to altered social functions, practice roles and approaches to work, and then examine a range of workforce sector data trends, such as labour force diversification, rapid sector growth, and the relatively modest increases in the social work labour force. The major shortage of social workers is explored, along with problems faced in recruiting appropriately qualified staff, including international migration of social work practitioners and ensuring a sustainable sector labour force. The implications for curriculum development and social work education are outlined, along with the need to promote ethical practice and compassionate approaches to addressing social exclusion and human rights.

The Australian context

Australia is widely recognized as a wealthy and stable nation. Its British colonial history as a convict settlement established a foundation for a robust democracy, classified as a liberal state within Esping-Andersen's (1999) typology of welfare states. It was rated second highest of all nations in the 2012 United Nations Development Index (UN 2012), a composite index of health, education and income levels. It was one of a few nations which did not go into economic recession during the Global Financial Crisis in 2008–2009. Perhaps more importantly, its currency is well valued, reflecting strong economic prospects through its mining and construction industries riding on the back of the economic expansion of Asia, particularly China and India, notwithstanding a recent lowering of economic growth rates. Its workforce continues to grow rapidly, and there is a long-standing and significant programme of migration to meet labour shortfalls, including social workers.

Despite its economic, social and cultural wealth, there remains significant inequity with the distribution of incomes in Australia (Australian Bureau of Statistics [ABS] 2011a), and the federal government's treasurer has argued that the mining boom has increased income inequality (Janda 2012). Despite what is generally seen as a comprehensive community services sector, economic policy drivers dominate political debate and decision-making regarding social policy (McDonald 2006). For example, the numbers and rate of people who are on Disability Support Pensions has been increasing steadily over the past two decades, and national governments have progressively introduced restrictive definitions, policies and procedures to tighten eligibility and encourage people with disabilities into the workforce, particularly in lower paid jobs. Similarly, single parents have had their eligibility for pensions significantly reduced in a move to push them into the workforce.

Australia, with 23 million people (ABS 2012), has a long history of migration, with the rate of net migration being one of the highest in the world for the 2005–2010 period; rates are expected to decrease into the medium term but remain relatively high (ABS 2011b). Australia is a successful multicultural society, and in 2010, 27 per cent of people were born overseas, mostly in European countries but increasingly in Asia (ABS 2011b). However, like many Western nations, Australia's population is rapidly aging, and family structures have altered substantially from the past. Roughly one in three Australians resides outside the metropolitan areas and generally has poorer economic, health and social outcomes (Cheers et al. 2007). The inter-generational effects of colonization have had disastrous impacts upon the 2.5 per cent of Australians who are Aborigines and Torres Strait Islanders. They suffer profound economic and social disadvantage evidenced across a range of economic, health and social indicators, including being grossly over-represented in the justice and child protection systems

(Cheers *et al.* 2007; SCRGSP 2009). This continues despite a range of policy and practice measures designed to reduce over-representation.

Australia has a national government, six state and two territory governments, and local government councils, with regular disputes ensuing about responsibility for funding services. The Australian government provides national programmes including income support and funding for health, education and welfare, with the state and territory governments being the primary service providers for these, as well as the major funder, while local governments provide utilities such as garbage collection. Although the states deliver most social welfare programmes, which are residually oriented, community-based non-government organizations (NGOs) also play significant roles (Harris and McDonald 2000).

Over the past two decades, there has been a generalized social and political conservatism by governments of the Left and Right. Government services, and public welfare programmes in particular, have been substantially re-organized and structured within policy frameworks that have promoted market-based systems and neo-liberal ideologies (McDonald *et al.* 2003). Services have been increasingly targeted and restricted through means testing of eligibility requirements and user-pays systems, introduced in order to share the financial cost of a broad range of social programmes. Nevertheless, compared to many other nations, Australia is relatively generous and has a universal health care system and a generally high-quality public hospital system; provides income support through a broad-based system of pensions and benefits, including a national 18-week paid parental leave scheme; gives significant support to the higher education system; and funds compulsory education up to grade 10 (although many children attend private, mostly faith-based, schools with their parents paying a substantial proportion of the costs). However, as the dominance of economics has emerged (McDonald 2006), there has been decreasing concern for equity and social justice as key policy drivers (Harris and McDonald 2000; Kalisch 2000).

Globalization has affected Australia in a range of ways, including increasing exposure to the world economy and the rapid transference of ideas and technology. As a nation economically dependent upon commodity prices, Australia has had to be responsive to world trade conditions. Hence, the Australian dollar was floated in 1983 and is now one of the most highly traded currencies in the world. Since then, a raft of economically successful deregulation efforts has occurred for financial markets and the economy overall, albeit with sectors such as manufacturing shrinking in the face of increased competition. With a high take-up of new technologies by the Australian people (Department of Broad Band, Communication and the Digital Economy 2008), technological change has been rapid and its social impacts profound.

Globalization has influenced the ways governments approach governance, and the arrangements for programme and service delivery. For example, policy settings have led to the higher education system in Australia becoming marketized, corporatized and managerialized, with students paying ever increasing proportions of the cost of their education through government levies, albeit with loans being made available (Bradley *et al.* 2008; Cain and Hewitt 2004). In addition, as a result of higher education initiatives such as the Bologna Agreement (Cardoso *et al.* 2008), a major review of the Australian Qualifications Framework (AQF 2011), and the creation of a new regulatory body for the tertiary sector, the Tertiary Education Quality and Standards Agency (TEQSA), there is both rapid change and enhanced accountability in this sector, all within an increasingly competitive environment for education providers. Australia remains a major destination for international students seeking to undertake quality tertiary and higher educational courses. Other social issues affecting higher education students include the increased career choice available nowadays, particularly for women; the troubling issue of student poverty and their need to balance work, study and life on low budgets; and the rapid emergence of blended learning approaches which utilize online learning opportunities and digital simulated learning environments. Social work education operates within this context, and it has to compete with a range of other attractive course options in order to secure sufficient students to effectively redress the growing shortage of professional social workers.

The Australian community services sector

In February 2010, the federal Department of Employment, Education and Workplace Relations (DEEWR) identified the health care and social assistance industry as the largest single labour force, with 1,193,900 workers (10.9 per cent). Its categories include hospitals (368,300); residential care services (202,300); other social assistance services (166,500); allied health services (135,900); child care services (104,700); medical services (97,300); and pathology and diagnostic imaging services (37,000). The median weekly earnings for the industry was AUD$900 per week, compared to all Australian industries at AUD$1,000 per week (although hospital workers earned AUD$1,031).The community services component of the industry entails around 500,000 workers (Martin and Healy 2010).The industry had experienced strong workforce growth in the previous decade (44.2 per cent) and this is predicted to continue at an annualized rate of 3.3 per cent per annum over the five-year period to 2015, compared to average growth rate of 1.8 per cent for all industries (DEEWR 2010). Growth is driven by factors such as a growing and aging population and the expansion of community and home-based services.

The issue of ongoing workforce shortages in this industry, particularly the health-related ones, has been recognized by governments, and in 2008 the Council of Australian Governments committed AUD$1,800,000 over four

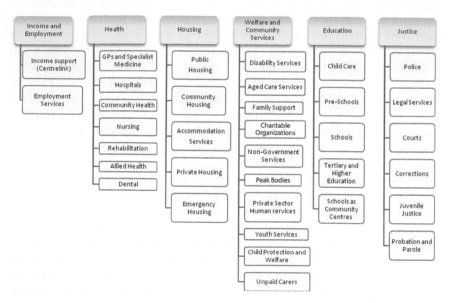

Figure 17.1 The ABS ANZSIC human services categories.

years to address them by establishing Health Workforce Australia (HWA). Its immediate predecessor, the National Health Workforce Taskforce (NHWT), reported in 2009 (NHWT 2009a, 2009b) that a range of demographic, health and systemic factors was at play (e.g. aging population, chronic disease, infrastructure depletion, etc.) and contributing to a looming health workforce crisis. Social work was identified as having a long-term disciplinary shortage (NHWT 2009b), and to address this the country required an additional 1,300 graduates per annum until 2030, equivalent to an annual increase of 83 per cent of 2012 graduates.

Within this industry, Australia's community services sector is well established, multi-faceted and broad in scope, with significant complexity evident in its structures, policies, funding arrangements and organizational relationships. It is a pluralist 'mixed economy' of structures and services consisting of national and state/territory government agencies (the primary funding sources), for-profit organizations and not-for-profit organizations, or NGOs, which operate at a community-based level and frequently utilize volunteer labour (McDonald *et al.* 2003). Despite all governments replacing their grants-based systems with a contract regime, both for-profit and not-for-profit organizations' services are heavily subsidized by the public purse. Organizational mandates include government statute, philanthropic pursuit, faith-based religious social care, and local groups addressing specific community needs.

The ABS uses the Australian and New Zealand Standard Industrial Classification (ANZSIC) for the production and analysis of industry statistics. Mel Gray (2010) researched the human services sector and concluded that there appeared to be no logical organization in the way community services are structured or the categories used for data collection, with people employed in these sectors coming from a range of occupations with various levels of qualification and professionals comprising a relatively small percentage of the community services workforce. Figure 17.1 depicts the broad categories Gray found in programmes and services, with particular practice fields such as disability, mental health and child protection spread within and across the sector. For example, although a social worker may be employed in a correctional facility, he or she would nevertheless have to provide services to people who had issues arising from mental illness and disability, as well as addressing offending.

Social work: altered circumstances

Social work in Australia had its genesis in the 1930s with the advent of hospital almoners, and the first university social work courses commenced in the 1940s. After the Second World War, in tandem with a huge influx of refugees and immigrants, the national government developed a range of policy responses to systemic poverty, and areas such as wage regulation and income support, housing, education and welfare saw the development of a social welfare system that in many instances led the world. Social work was viewed as the preferred qualification to deliver welfare services and received institutional legitimacy, albeit within the confines of a sector that was resource constrained. For women in particular, a social work degree led to a career with status like nursing and teaching, and the profession grew steadily. In 1946 the Australian Association of Social Workers (AASW) was founded with Norma Parker as the foundation President (1946–1954), and subsequently as the Vice President (1954–1958). Today the AASW has approximately 8,000 members and is responsible for setting the profession's ethics and practice standards, as well as being the accrediting body for all social work educational programmes, undertaking social policy advocacy, and accrediting mental health social workers whose clients are eligible to receive rebates for treatment services from the national government's universal Medicare scheme.

Despite a long-standing campaign by the AASW, the social work profession in Australia is not government regulated (Lonne and Duke 2008), and there appears to be little appetite from federal and state health ministers to consider this. There are various types of government regulation around the world for the social work profession, although in most countries it is not registered (Lonne and Duke 2008). But in those jurisdictions where regulation is in place, there is generally regulatory control of the education curriculum and training for the profession. In places like England, this has been done with a clear political agenda to improve practice standards and thereby address public concerns following tragedies and scandals (HM Government 2010). One of the down sides to state regulation is that the profession can lose control over key aspects of the professional curriculum to regulators who are not social workers and who, arguably, have a limited grasp of the role, functions and attributes of sound social work practice. Australia's approach to the development of a robust professional qualification and its underpinning curriculum has clearly been at the behest of the practitioner-led professional association, albeit in collaboration with educators and universities. The advent of legislated registration of social workers would place new stresses and challenges on social work educators within what is already a complex array of dynamic changes occurring within the Australian higher education sector.

Australian social work has not been immune from the ideological and other changes outlined in this book, nor tensions within the profession, including rivalries concerning macro and micro methods and focus to practice (Midgley 2001), and the pursuit of the 'professional project' (McDonald 2006). Social work has changed as neo-liberal influences on policy and programmes have progressed. Social surveillance of 'troublesome' groups, increased emphasis on risk and legalism, along with ever more restrictive eligibility for services have seen social work practice altered to have more of a social control mandate and less of a social care one, particularly in income support and child protection. Managerialism and case management have been primary tools for this change (Lonne *et al.* 2009; McDonald 2006).

The AASW accredits all Australian social work educational programmes and has, over time, altered the entry requirements for membership, originally commencing with a two-year diploma, then requiring a three-year bachelor's degree through the 1960s, and subsequently moving to a four-year Bachelor of Social Work (BSW). In 2008, it also allowed membership through a two-year master's qualification (MSW) that provided entry level into the profession, and this has attracted a strong demand from mature age people often seeking a career change (AASW 2008). However, because change has been so rapid in both higher education and the community services, the AASW (2012) commenced another review of its Australian Education and Accreditation Standards (ASWEAS) and recently completed this. This review identified a range of issues confronting social work education, including: flat demand for the BSW and growth for the MSW; promoting practitioner's reflection and critical thinking; alignment to the revised Australian Qualifications Framework (AQF) for the BSW honours degree and MSW; the degree structures; balancing generic courses and specialist ones for specific practice fields; and the nature and demands of the 1,000 hours of field education. It was surprising, therefore that the new ASWEAS (2012) did not proactively address these in the revised requirements but instead opted for the implementation of an onerous audit regime upon the social work programmes at a time when many are struggling to compete in a highly dynamic and competitive marketized environment. The advice of the Australian Heads of Schools of Social Work to allow more room to innovate and respond to the trends and pressures in higher education was not heeded.

The review entailed a detailed examination of the workforce and professional trends at play but largely ignored the several recent studies that have identified significant workforce trends and issues, including the NHWT and HWA work outlined earlier, and research reports by Healy and Lonne (2010) on workforce and curriculum for social work and the human services, and Martin and Healy (2010) on the broad community services workforce.

Healy and Lonne's 2010 research examined data from both the community services workforce and tertiary education students, and also compared the higher education curriculum across a range of relevant social and behavioural science-type qualifications. They found that an ad hoc alignment existed between employer needs and curriculum design, and that articulation arrangements between vocational training and higher education were haphazard. Overall, they concluded that the marketization of higher education had been problematic for BSWs, which have experienced overall flat student demand, while a host of social and behavioural courses, including psychology, are booming. Their conclusion was that social worker shortages would continue to be filled by people, mostly women, with generic qualifications from courses that were less capable of adequately preparing graduates with the required knowledge and skills to practice competently and ethically with vulnerable groups across a range of practice fields. Low salaries and limited career structures were identified as harming recruitment and retention, and they advocated for national workforce planning.

Martin and Healy's (2010) important research addresses some critical workforce areas that cannot be examined through the ABS and DEEWR data. They used a representative survey methodology to access data from 3,789 community services workers working across 1,040 service outlets in the fields of child protection, juvenile justice, disability services and general community services. While a high degree of staff commitment was found, satisfaction with pay levels was not particularly high in general, and this appeared related to retention and recruitment issues. All the fields had more than 80 per cent female workers except juvenile justice, which had 55 per cent. There were some important differences among the field cohorts including child protection workers tending to be young (58 per cent younger than 40 years of age), with roughly two-thirds being professionally qualified and 72 per cent employed less than five years, whereas 49 per cent of the juvenile justice workers were professionally qualified, and they tended to enter earlier but not stay long, with 57 per cent being employed less than five years. On the other hand, the disability services workers tended to be older (64 per cent older than 40 years of age) and 62 per cent did not have

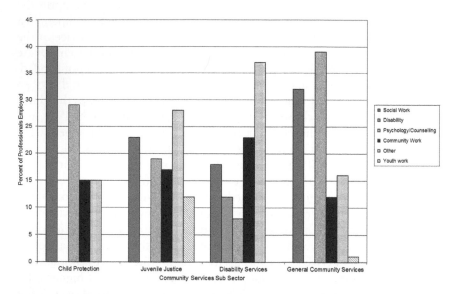

Figure 17.2 Disciplinary groups of professionals employed in the community services.

professional qualifications, while in the general community services cohort 65 per cent had professional qualifications but were also generally older (64 per cent older than 40 years of age). Figure 17.2 illustrates Martin and Healy's data on the respective disciplinary qualifications for professional staff employed in the community services sector, with the proportion of social workers among professional staff varying, and being the largest only in child protection.

Community service workforce trends and developments

There has been sustained growth in the sector over the past 20 years, as revealed in Figure 17.3, which depicts the ABS quarterly workforce survey data to compare the trends for workers with a variety of qualifications. The major growth area has been in the Welfare Support Workers category, which includes people holding a diversity of qualifications from none at all to Vocational Employment and Training (VET) certificates and diplomas, and a range of social and behavioural science degrees. It is clear that there are good job prospects for the range of helping professions broadly, with an almost organic growth in the sector. Social workers (22,000) and psychologists (23,000) have grown steadily in their numbers since 1996. It is clear that in order to address sector growth, employers have decided that they wish to select from a variety of qualification types, and that the historical role that social work has had as a disciplinary leader can no longer be taken

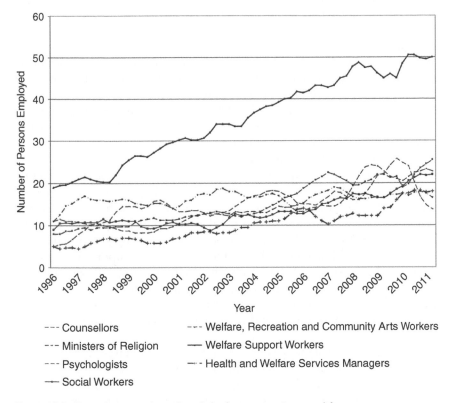

Figure 17.3 Growth in social work and the human services workforce.

for granted. DEEWR 2011 job prospects and projection summaries indicate that the medium-term anticipated employment growth for community service disciplines is higher for psychologists, social workers and welfare support workers compared to welfare, recreation and community arts worker and counsellor categories (DEEWR 2011). Around 10 to 12 per cent of the staff in each of these categories leave their occupations each year (DEEWR 2012), although in some areas, such as child protection, the rates are much higher (Martin and Healy 2010).

These data demonstrate that the workforce qualifications continue to diversify, and as the sector continues to grow this will likely continue, raising serious questions about the knowledge and skill set needed to undertake work with vulnerable populations. In their report, Healy and Lonne (2010) identified both deprofessionalization and reprofessionalization processes, with the former indicating a trend of meeting strong workforce growth through reclassifying positions so that people with lower-level qualifications can attain them, and the latter signifying a decreasing proportion overall of the workforce holding no formal qualifications. These workforce changes mean that social workers are increasingly taking up higher level supervisory and management positions, with frontline roles being filled by people with other qualifications.

Examining the VET student data indicates that numbers of students undertaking the Community Services Training Package (CSTP; National Centre for Vocational Education Research [NCVER] 2012) have continued to also grow rapidly in the 2002–2010 period, but this has primarily been in the lower Certificate III level rather than Certificate IV or Diplomas. Further, from 2008 to 2010, the numbers of CSTP students graduating doubled for most VET qualifications. Demand for workers in the sector is clearly being met by the 30,000 per annum VET graduates with Certificate III and higher qualifications. This overall trend is a positive one, because it means that the long-term trend of a decreasing proportion of people in the sector holding no formal qualifications appears to be likely to continue. However, it may also mean that the workforce pressures resulting in deprofessionalization may also persist. Nonetheless, VET graduates are an important source of labour for the sector, particularly for frontline direct care staff, with over 80 per cent gaining jobs, but in addition, a material proportion (16.6 per cent) of the Diploma level graduates proceed to university study (NCVER 2011), despite the ad hoc educational and career pathways in the sector (Healy and Lonne 2010).

Another important labour source is university graduates, and an examination of DEEWR (2012) higher education data indicates similar patterns to the sector workforce data, namely, that while numbers of BSW graduates have plateaued over the last decade at around 1,250 per annum, both psychology and the aggregated social and behavioural science degrees, here called 'other helping professions', have experienced significant growth over the past two decades and are now significantly larger and growing faster, with an upward spike from 2008–2010 (Figure 17.4). It is the case that most psychology graduates (68 per cent) in Australia do not work within the health and community services industry, whereas a majority of social workers do, but the continued growth of psychology student numbers is an established trend affecting the workforce composition.

For more than a decade, about 2,200 students each year have enrolled in BSW courses and approximately 1,250 have graduated, but there was a 26 per cent growth in total enrolled BSW students during the 2001–2010 period, indicating that students are increasingly taking longer than four years to complete their course, possibly due to the difficulties of completing the two 500-hour placements that usually take around 14 weeks. Generally speaking, there has also been a significant decrease in social work student numbers in the more established programmes, the shortfall being taken up by the newly established programmes. In addition, there has been a gradual decrease in the tertiary entrance cut-off scores for social workers and psychologists since

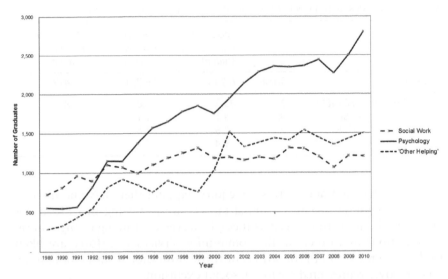

Figure 17.4 Number of bachelor-level helping profession graduates 1989–2010.

2004, and both are at relatively low levels, a trend experienced by many non-'pinnacle' type professions during a period of economic growth.

The growth in the other helping professions has been largely driven by student and workforce demand for undergraduate counselling courses, and reflects the success by one large private education provider in supplying quality programmes that are accessible to students – in essence, a niche market. When combined with social work's rapidly aging labour force, the growth in numbers of psychology and other helping profession graduates has significant implications for meeting the social worker shortages (NHWT 2009a, 2009b) and foreshadows a continuing decline in the social work proportion of the sector's workforce.

Changes in the workforce composition and the respective proportions from different disciplines have implications for equity groups. Compared to workers with other qualifications, social workers have higher proportions of women, Aboriginal and Torres Strait Islander people, and those identifying as having a disability or being from non-English speaking backgrounds (NESB), groups which tend to be over-represented in disadvantaged and marginalized peoples and those who receive social services. This is also reflected in DEEWR (2012) student data, which indicates that social work, compared to psychology and the other helping professionals, has higher proportions of undergraduate students from these equity groups (Table 17.1). For several years, the federal government has been providing incentive funding to universities to widen participation of identified disadvantaged groups

Table 17.1 DEEWR 2010 university student data: membership of equity groups

2010 year			Social work bachelor-level students	Psychology bachelor-level students	Other helping bachelor-level students
Students		Total	6,935	16,731	11,417
Equity Groups	WOMEN	%	85.8	76.8	79.8
	ATSI	%	4.1	1.1	1.7
	NESB	%	2.5	1.6	1.4
	DISABILITY	%	9.4	7.3	6.9

in higher education and redress the equity gap, but there have been recent reports suggesting that the required targets are not being met (Trounson 2013). Without measures such as these, however, continuing changes in the qualifications of workers in the community services workforce are likely to decrease the overall proportions of those professional staff from groups who are over-represented regarding social exclusion.

However, the advent of the 2008 entry-level MSW programmes is playing a major part, because they are attracting a new graduate cohort to social work that had hitherto largely been uninterested in undertaking a BSW. In 2015 there are 21 entry-level MSW programmes, compared to 26 BSW programmes around the country, with 17 universities running both, and 29 of Australia's 43 universities, and one private educational provider, offering social work programmes, whereas they all have psychology courses. Many of these graduate MSW students, 60 per cent of whom are aged 30 or above, are seeking a career change to social work, having already worked as teachers, nurses, etc., or they are already working in the sector and have a social and behavioural science qualification and are seeking to 'upgrade' to an MSW. Figure 17.5 outlines the rapid growth since 2008 in MSW entry-level students over the past few years, with approximately 450 students in advanced social work master's degrees, and over 1,200 students enrolled in entry level master's, and an expected 500 graduating each year, with further growth expected. Nevertheless, despite the overall growth, these figures still fall well short of the NHWT estimate of 1,300 additional graduates per annum to meet workforce needs.

Australia has been attracting many overseas social workers as immigrants and, despite also having them emigrate to take up overseas opportunities, this is likely to continue, with employers, particularly child protection agencies, having international recruitment programmes. Social work is on the Australian government's skilled migration list as a labour force shortage. However, there is a shortage of social workers in many countries, and, in this competitive international environment, recruitment of overseas qualified staff can be difficult. Many challenges confront newly arrived social

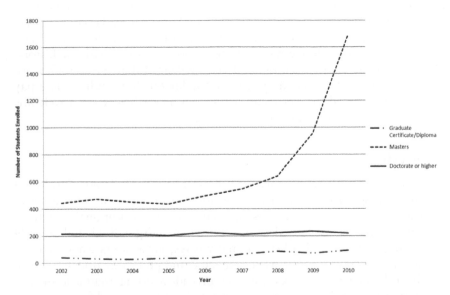

Figure 17.5 Number of enrolled students in Australian social work postgraduate programmes 2002–2010.

workers, including adjusting to the broader cultural context and understanding the new structural and professional environment. Depending on the precise nature of their existing qualification, they may have to do a bridging course if they wish to practise in a position where eligibility for membership of the AASW is a requirement, but otherwise this is not necessary. Employer support to aid the transition process and necessary adjustments is not guaranteed and can be quite variable. There are also significant issues concerning the ability of many new migrant social workers to practise in culturally safe ways with Australia's Indigenous peoples. New Zealand's national registration system, however, requires social workers to demonstrate competency in working with Maori people (Lonne and Duke 2008).

Starting salaries for social work graduates have traditionally been quite good (in the top third of all graduates), but as people progress in their careers they are quickly overtaken by graduates in other professions and parts of the economy. It is likely that the generally lower salaries paid in the community services have an impact on recruiting and retaining staff, and social workers in particular, who earn more when they work in health sector roles (Healy and Lonne 2010; Martin and Healy 2010). However, there is room for some optimism on this front. In 2009, the Queensland Industrial Relations Commission extensively cited evidence by myself and Karen Healy when determining a revaluation of the Social and Community Services Award's classification structures, position descriptors and salaries that equated with 15–37 per cent wage increases. Perhaps more important, in February 2012 the national regulator Fair Work Australia handed down a decision that aligned the national Social, Community, Home Care and Disability Services Industry Award 2010 (modern Award) with the historic Queensland pay equity decision, and acknowledged that the sector's work had been undervalued based on gender for far too long. While these pay rises will be phased in over eight years, they nevertheless are a welcome boost for recruitment and retention.

Conclusion

Social work and the community services sector have undergone profound systemic change over the past two decades, resulting in an altered social mandate and function, and a restructuring of the institutional structures and arrangements used to deliver services to marginalized and socially excluded groups and individuals. In many ways, social welfare assistance to those in need is now harsher, more restricted and punitively oriented. These neo-liberal policy frameworks, however, provide a strong argument for why we need more social workers in the community services workforce, because their ethical framework, embracing of social justice and human rights, and their compassion and humanity are critical if we are to remain a caring civil society. In this tough policy and organizational environment for social workers to operate in, the tensions around dominant policy values and discourses may well be contributing to staff turnover and retention problems experienced in some sectors, such as child protection.

The long-standing workforce shortages stand in the way of a sustainable sector labour force and contribute to the ongoing diversification of labour force qualifications and the trend for fewer social workers to be on the front line. Social work is under significant threat on a range of fronts. If social work's traditional primary role in providing the theoretical knowledge, skills and values framework for social welfare practice is to continue, we need to address the significant structural, organizational, professional and practice issues which impede growth of the social work labour force.

Addressing the impacts of neo-liberalism is a difficult task given its almost ubiquitous spread and dominance as a discourse. It cannot be ignored and must be critically engaged by the profession through its professional association, practitioners and academics. Its values and assumptions need to be exposed and critiqued, and the outcomes of programmes, both intended and unintended, need to be comprehensively evaluated through detailed research. Stronger public advocacy by social workers in social policy and programme debates is necessary, along with involvement within internal organizational processes and forums, although this needs to be done in ways that are savvy and not naive regarding the possible consequences of speaking up.

Attracting more students is essential, but while the growth of the MSW graduates is an important factor, far more than incremental change is needed to ensure the long-term sustainability of the BSW, a major educational pathway for key equity groups. The AASW's 2012 ASWEAS is disappointing because its imposition of a bureaucratic administrative compliance regime does not help programmes to innovate and to grow and meet the challenges posed by other qualifications within a highly competitive educational environment. Essentially, as the accrediting authority for social work education, the AASW has failed to address pressing curriculum and systemic issues in order to make it more attractive to students, who are predominantly female and seek a satisfying and well paid career. Time will tell the extent to which programmes are unduly affected by these developments.

The forthcoming salary increases will help but are not the sole answer to workforce shortages. Employers and educators also have critically important roles to play here, including building the social work health workforce capacity and facilitating curriculum development, such as the development of virtual simulated learning programmes available through the Internet. Without a collaborative, sector-wide approach, the ongoing impacts of globalization and competitive forces will likely ensure that the community services remain fragmented, and its workforce highly diversified. National leadership by the professional association is critical here, as are local initiatives.

Perhaps more importantly, national workforce planning for the sector is urgently required, like that taking place in the United Kingdom (HM Government 2010), to address the range of issues outlined in this chapter and text. The workforce data outlined here demonstrate many sector strengths and predict long-term growth, but this will, on current indications, also entail further qualification diversification, and deprofessionalization and reprofessionalization processes. The data indicate the size and scope of the trends and issues that are forcing social work to operate within a competitive professional environment that is growing overall, but where the scope for social work to build its human resource capacity is constrained. While increased skilled immigration is needed to address the short- to medium-term social work labour force shortages, it is imperative that recruitment strategies entail proper support and assistance to help practitioners make the many adjustments required to successfully operate in their professional, organizational and personal spheres.

While there are many challenges facing the social work profession, there are also emerging opportunities to strengthen the quality and professionalism of practitioners through a broad embracing of professional development strategies that are linked to career progression and higher salaries.

Within the complex and dynamic environment outlined in this chapter and text, social work leadership should not be about 'protecting turf' but, rather, about ensuring that effective practice frameworks and approaches to helping the most vulnerable and marginalized people are maintained within the professional armoury that the sector has at its disposal. Social work has proved to be remarkably resilient and adaptable in the past, and these same attributes are needed now, because there is much at stake. A civil society requires equity, social justice and income distribution to provide the glue necessary to bind the social fabric. Well-functioning health and community services are essential institutions for social harmony, and we must therefore ensure that there is a properly educated, trained and prepared social work labour force to ensure a sustainable sector workforce. Perhaps more importantly, social work needs to take charge of its own destiny and seize available opportunities, just as it has done in the past when facing threats and challenges to its role and standing.

References

Australian Association of Social Workers (2008) *Australian Social Work Education And Accreditation Standards*, Canberra: AASW.

Australian Association of Social Workers (2012) *Australian Social Work Education and Accreditation Standards*, Canberra: AASW.

Australian Bureau of Statistics (2011a) *Household Income and Income Distribution, Australia 2009–10*. Online. Available at: www.abs.gov.au/AUSSTATS/abs@.nsf/DetailsPage/6523.02009-10?OpenDocument (accessed 15 January 2015).

Australian Bureau of Statistics (2011b) *Migration Australia 2009–10*. Online. Available at: www.abs.gov.au/ausstats/abs@.nsf/Products/2265A45B0BA62770CA2578B00011956C?opendocument (accessed 10 March 2012).

Australian Bureau of Statistics (2012) *Population Clock*. Online. Available at: www.abs.gov.au/ausstats/abs%40.nsf/94713ad445ff1425ca25682000192af2/1647509ef7e25faaca2568a900154b63?OpenDocument (accessed 10 March 2012).

Australian Qualifications Framework Council (2011) *Australian Qualifications Framework*. Online. Available at: www.aqf.edu.au/ (accessed 12 March 2012).

Bradley, D., Noonan, P., Nugent, H. and Scales, B. (2008) *Review of Australian Higher Education, Final Report (the Bradley Report)*, Canberra: Department of Education, Employment and Workplace Relations. Online. Available at: http://gellen.org.au/wp-content/uploads/2011/04/Higher_Educatio_Review.pdf (accessed 15 January 2015).

Cain, J. and Hewitt, J. (2004). *Off Course: From Public Place to Marketplace at Melbourne University*, Melbourne: Scribe Publications.

Cardoso, A.R., Portela, M., Sa, C. and Alexandre, F. (2008) 'Demand for higher education programmes: the impact of the Bologna process', *CESifo Economic Studies*, 54(2): 229–47.

Cheers, B., Darracott, R. and Lonne, B. (2007) *Social Care Practice in Rural Communities*, Annandale: Federation Press.

Department of Broad Band, Communication and the Digital Economy (2008) *Online Statistics*. Online. Available at: www.archive.dbcde.gov.au/2008/01/statistical_benchmarking/online_statistics (accessed 10 March 2012).

Department of Employment, Education and Workplace Relations (DEEWR) (2010) *Employment Outlook for Health Care and Social Assistance*, Canberra: DEEWR.

Department of Employment, Education and Workplace Relations (DEEWR) (2011) *Job Outlook*. Online. Available at: http://joboutlook.gov.au/pages/occupation.asp x?search=category&cluster=41&code=4117 (accessed 14 March 2012).

Department of Employment, Education and Workplace Relations (DEEWR) (2012) *University and Bachelor Level Graduate Data*, Canberra: DEEWR.

Esping-Andersen, G. (1999) *Social Foundations of Postindustrial Economies*, Oxford: Oxford University Press.

Gray, M. (2010) *Mapping the Human Services in Australia*, paper presented to the Australian Council of Heads of Schools of Social Work, University of Tasmania, Launceston, Tasmania, 2–4 February.

Harris, J. and McDonald, C. (2000) 'Post-Fordism, the welfare state and the personal social services: a comparison of Australia and Great Britain', *British Journal of Social Work*, 30: 51–70.

Healy, K. and Lonne, B. (2010) *The Social Work and Human Service Workforce: Report from a National Study of Education, Training and Workforce Needs*, Sydney: Australian Learning and Teaching Council.

HM Government (2010) *Building a Safe and Confident Future: Implementing the Recommendations of the Social Work Taskforce – A Joint Implementation Plan from the Department for Children, Schools and Families, the Department of Health and the Department for Business, Innovation and Skills in Partnership with the Social Work Reform Board*, London: HM Government.

Janda, M. (2012) 'Swan's inequality warnings reflected in statistics', *Seven News*, 5 March. Online. Available at: http://au.news.yahoo.com/latest/a/-/latest/13091562/ swans-inequality-warning-reflected-in-statistics/ (accessed 10 March 2012).

Kalisch, D.W. (2000) *Social Policy Directions across the OECD Region: Reflections on a Decade of Change*, Canberra: Department of Family and Community Services, Commonwealth of Australia.

Lonne, B. and Duke, J. (2008) 'Social work registration: the Holy Grail or fool's gold?', in M. Connelly and L. Harms (eds) *Social Work: Contexts and Practice*, Oxford: Oxford University Press.

Lonne, B., Parton, N., Thomson, J. and Harries, M. (2009) *Reforming Child Protection*, London: Routledge.

McDonald, C. (2006) *Challenging Social Work: The Context of Practice*, Basingstoke: Palgrave Macmillan.

McDonald, C., Harris, J. and Wintersteen, R. (2003) 'Contingent on context? Social work and the state in Australia, Britain, and the USA', *British Journal of Social Work*, 33(2): 191–208.

Martin, B. and Healy, J. (2010) *Who Works in Community Services? A Profile of Australian Workforces in Child Protection, Juvenile Justice, Disability Services and General Community Services*. Report prepared for the Community and Disability Services Ministerial Advisory Council, Adelaide, South Australia: National Institute of Labour Studies, Flinders University.

Midgley, J. (2001) 'Issues in international social work: resolving critical debates in the profession', *Journal of Social Work*, 1(1): 21–35.

National Health Workforce Taskforce (NHWT) (2009a) *Health Workforce in Australia and Factors for Current Shortages*, Melbourne: NHWT.

National Health Workforce Taskforce (NHWT) (2009b) *Health Professional Entry Requirements 2009–2025, Macro Supply and Demand Report*, Melbourne: NHWT.

NCVER (2011) *Student Outcomes Survey 2011*. Online. Available at: www.ncver. edu.au/publications/2442.html (accessed 31 March 2012).

NCVER (2012) *Vocstats*. Online. Available at: www.ncver.edu.au/resources/voc-stats/intro.html (accessed 24 March 2012).

Steering Committee for the Review of Government Service Provision (SCRGSP) (2009) *Overcoming Indigenous Disadvantage: Key Indicators 2009*, Canberra: Productivity Commission.

Trounson, A. (2013) 'Diversity goals fall far short', *The Australian*, Higher Education Supplement, 16 January, p. 27. Online. Available at: www.theaustralian.com.au/ higher-education/diversity-goals-fall-far-short/story-e6frgcjx-1226554593974 (accessed 18 January 2013).

United Nations (2012) *International Human Development Indicators*. Online. Available at: http://hdrstats.undp.org/en/countries/profiles/AUS.html (accessed 10 March 2012).

Yeatman, A. with Dowsett, G.W., Fine, M. and Gursansky, D. (2009) *Individualisation and the Delivery of Welfare Services: Contestation and Complexity*, Basingstoke: Palgrave Macmillan.

Conclusion

Social work: a unique profession in a diverse context

Dina Sidhva, George Palattiyil and Mono Chakrabarti

An important issue that emerges from the various chapters in this edited volume is that social work has become a global profession; one that is underpinned by a commitment to promote social justice, human rights and equality (IFSW, 2001; Hare, 2004; Sewpaul and Jones, 2004). Over the last couple of centuries, social work has evolved into a unique profession, practised in diverse contexts through a multitude of approaches (Dominelli, 2010). The Directory of Schools of Social Work compiled by the International Association of Schools of Social Work suggests that there are around 3,000 schools of social work and IFSW's website indicates that there are 1.5 million professional social workers practising in at least eighty-four countries (Dominelli, 2010). One thing that clearly emerges from this data is the sheer diversity that social work encompasses, making it a profession that is global in nature, yet responding to local needs. However, no matter how diverse social work is, the core of the social work profession is embedded in the universal values of equality, worth and dignity of all people; is motivated by the aspirations for human rights and social justice; and strives to alleviate poverty and empower marginalised and oppressed people in order to realise their true potential (Palattiyil and Sidhva, 2012). In that sense, social work can be described as an empowering and emancipatory practice.

We live in a globalised world – a global village, where geographical distance has been narrowed by the technological developments which have advanced the condition of many of us. Yet, the world is also witnessing heightened inequality (Jones and Truell, 2012), poverty, human rights violations, forced migration and such like. With access to the Internet and social media and the ever increasing rich–poor divide, the world is becoming increasingly complex (Dominelli, 2010). The net impact of all these developments is increasingly exacerbating inequality and further marginalising sections of populations, denying them the ability to achieve their full potential. Terrorism, natural disasters, new pandemics and new forms of conflict and their catastrophic impact on people (in Syria, Iraq, Nigeria and Darfur, to name a few) place tremendous responsibility on social work and social development practitioners across the world to respond to these challenges.

Social work needs to reflect on these global challenges and find newer ways of addressing these issues, which means perhaps more of the same may not be appropriate or even desirable. The Global Agenda for Social Work and Social Development agreed by IASSW, IFSW and ICSW (2014) endorsed four priority themes to promote (1) social and economic equalities; (2) the dignity and worth of people; (3) environmental and community sustainability; and (4) the importance of human relationships; thus identifying a shared commitment and a renewed determination to promote social work and social justice globally (Jones and Truell, 2012).

Social work: a profession in myriad shades

Social workers operate at the point where social forces and individual behaviour meet (IFSW/IASSW, 2000). Nonetheless, the contexts in which contemporary social work operates are multi-faceted and cover the global, the regional, the national and the local (Dominelli, 2010: 26). In most Western nation states, social work assumes a statutory welfare role with legal powers for assessment and intervention in situations of need, while in developing countries social work is concerned more with issues of poverty, education and development and is linked to humanitarianism, activism and empowerment. For example, social work in the UK is more formalised and has a statutory status with the title of social work given protection in the law. Social work education is underpinned by standards laid down by the regulatory bodies and social workers have the powers to intervene in times of crisis where the welfare of a service user (child neglect or abuse of older people, for example) is at risk. Social work's primary role is to intervene early, minimise risks and promote welfare; in most of the European countries, thus social work has come to be recognised as an important public service and can be said to be an element within the European social model (Lorenz, 1994; Jones, 2013).

On the other hand, social work operates to effect structural changes through social and political action in some of the developing countries of the Global South. Social workers in such contexts have been working to eradicate poverty and promote health and education, efforts which gained further impetus with the launch of the Millennium Development Goals by the United Nations (2000). The formal training and practice of social workers is also less regulated in these contexts. For example, the First Report of the Global Agenda for Social Work and Social Development (2014) indicates that social work is an established, but mostly unregulated, profession across the African continent, although some national governments are discussing formal regulations of qualifications and title, as has been implemented in South Africa (Osei-Hwedie, 2013). In the Asian region, especially in China and India, there has been a rapid growth in the number of schools of social work, and India continues to produce a large number of social workers

(Tan, 2013) who operate at the grassroots level. For example, in India, globalisation and its overwhelming impact on India's masses have led to a more radical and activist type of intervention with mass movements, such as mass agitation in support of the poor displaced by multi-national hydro-electric projects, or supporting the victims of industrial accidents (the Bhopal Gas tragedy) or advocacy movements promoting the equality of Dalits (Palattiyil and Sidhva, 2012). In these situations, it is fair to say that social work is no longer seen as being confined to the narrow realms of statutory interventions mandated by the state; rather it strives to effect social and economic changes by radical actions aimed at social and community development. For example, some schools of social work in India have social action projects that advocate for and improve the conditions of unorganised construction workers; marginalised fishing communities; trafficked women and children; informal education for street children; and people living with HIV (Kuruvilla, 2004; Alphonse et al., 2008). What is noteworthy is the fact that while risk and vulnerability of marginalised people are the driving force behind social work interventions, many of the interventions take place without the statutory powers as understood in the Western social work context (Palattiyil and Sidhva, 2012).

An emerging field of operation for social workers in some of the developing countries of the world is organising poverty alleviation programmes through micro-finance (Hulme and Moore, 2006; Ali and Hatta, 2010). Participation, self-reliance, sustainability and empowerment are the key principles often applied by social workers in the design of poverty reduction strategies (IFSW, 2012a), which seek to involve other stakeholders including civil society and community organizations. Moreover, industrial corporations are a key destination for qualified social workers, who are tasked with promoting the virtues of large business corporations in the name of 'corporate social responsibility'. Interestingly, one of the most life-changing spheres that social workers operate in is in managing the after-effects of natural disasters (for example, tsunami or earthquake) and supporting efforts at rehabilitation (Palattiyil and Sidhva, 2012).

The growing impact of globalisation, cross-border human mobility and natural disasters poses new challenges for social workers (Dominelli, 2010). With climate change, the emergence of new pandemics and the increasing threat of terrorism, there is an ever greater need for social work to champion and uphold our basic human rights; these global issues hamper social and economic development, which are central to social work involvement at the global level.

Social work: a global profession

We are living in a period of globalisation (Kuruvilla, 2004; Alphonse et al., 2008) that is impacting almost every country in the world. The social work profession worldwide has been increasingly influenced by globalisation (Midgley, 2001; Lalayants *et al.*, 2014) and it has begun to recognise the impact of globalisation on almost every problem that social work practitioners deal with (Kendall, 2008). Social workers are frequently called upon to deal with global social problems such as asylum seekers and refugees (Palattiyil and Sidhva, 2011), street children, alcohol and substance abuse, HIV and AIDS, human trafficking, cross-border adoption and so on. The field of international social work holds significant potential in this context as a response to globalisation (Cox, 2000; Caragata and Sanchez, 2002). Social workers use diverse approaches, ranging from culturally sensitive and cross-cultural practices to advocacy and campaigns to work with asylum seekers and refugees and in diverse contexts such as aid/humanitarian settings, social development and human rights organisations; these diverse approaches across different cultural settings have now been broadly labelled as international social work (Midgley, 2001; Dominelli, 2005; Healy, 2008; Cox and Pawar, 2013).

The recent past has seen a considerable increase in the coverage of international social work in the wider literature (Midgley, 2001; Caragata and Sanchez, 2002; Healy, 2008; Mohan, 2008; Razack, 2009; Cox and Pawar, 2013). The Global Agenda for Social Work and Social Development (IFSW, 2012b), along with the global demand for social workers, international placements for qualifying social work students, social workers without borders, role of social workers in humanitarian and aid agencies and so on have further contributed to this debate.

While globalisation has led to increased economic independence for many, it has also exacerbated the rich–poor divide and inequalities and other social problems experienced by large sections of the population. The world is witnessing complex emergencies, creating major global challenges. The question is whether social work practitioners are adequately trained to understand the global forces driving these problems or are in a position to respond to them effectively (Lalayants *et al.*, 2014). More precisely, how can contemporary social work respond to these complex and emerging needs; how can social work educators prepare a workforce fit to respond to the Global Agenda (IFSW, 2012b), how can we find commonalities and shared commitments from across the more established Western models of social work and more humanitarian/development oriented social work as practised in many of the developing countries of the world?

As social work globally moves towards realising the Global Agenda, there are a number of challenges that need to be addressed in ensuring a shared commitment and common platform for promoting social justice, equality and human rights. Cox and Pawar (2013) examine these challenges in depth in their latest book (*International Social Work: Issues, Strategies and Problems*). Some of these challenges however are briefly summarised below:

- Social work and social development: social work education needs to reflect on the wider social and structural issues of poverty, inequality and the impact of conflict on forced migration and enable social work practitioners to develop knowledge and skills to work in global social work and social development settings responding to complex emergencies.

- Standards of social work education: while the regulatory frameworks that inform social work in many of the Western social work contexts are formal and attuned to local needs, a deeper understanding of global issues and challenges would enable students to gain a wider perspective. Similarly, there is an imperative on social work education and training in developing countries to regulate the profession with professional accreditation with a view to driving up standards.

- International social work as a core element of social work curricula: while the concept of international social work has gained momentum in the recent past, particularly in some parts of the world, a commitment to incorporating international social work into the teaching curriculum would enable students to be better prepared for dealing with global challenges and cross-cultural issues in practice. Increasingly, there is a growing interest in international placements for social work students as part of degree programmes; a step in the right direction. The success of creating a workforce that is equipped to deal with the global challenges of the twenty-first century depends on acquiring the skills and knowledge to respond to them effectively; the more international exchanges and work experience a practitioner has, the better.

- Social work as a human rights discipline: reviewing the various chapters incorporated in this book and evidence from elsewhere indicates that social work is a discipline that strives to deal with local problems and challenges rather than a grand human rights endeavour (Stark, 2014). However, central to social work is a commitment to respond to poverty, inequality and to promote social justice; a commitment to empower marginalised individuals and communities. If this is the core identity of social work, then there is a need to understand social work as an important social justice effort and human rights as a core principle underlying social work education.

- Collective action and social movements: social work in more formal settings such as in the West has become rather oblivious to the global challenges, such as climate change, disaster management, forced displacement or migration, food and water scarcity and so on. Collective action and social movements are pivotal to challenging institutions and multi-national corporations to understand the impact of these challenges on the global poor in such a way that action can be taken to address these issues.

- The Global Agenda: while the three international bodies representing social work and social welfare (namely, IFSW, IASSW and ICSW) reached a commitment to promote the core themes identified in the Global Agenda for Social Work and Social Development, the success depends on the extent to which these aspirations are embedded in social work curriculum and practice – locally and globally.

Social work in much of the Western world benefits from formally recognised standards, regulatory powers and protected title, however, the field of social work in developing countries and particularly in the least developed countries of the world is being diluted by other allied professions. Conversations with academics and practitioners in such contexts point to an emerging paradigm where new applied courses such as international development and development studies, human rights, law and community management programmes are edging social work practitioners onto the margins. The number of non-governmental organisations (NGOs) is on the rise, but they operate with shrinking funds and their survival is uncertain. This can be challenging not only for the people social work exists to serve, but also for those who are qualifying as social workers with fewer job opportunities (Palattiyil and Sidhva, 2012). Interestingly, many of the International Development and comparable degrees offered in the West equip their students for work in NGOs in developing countries, while what these NGOs are engaged in doing is social work or, more precisely, international social work.

In conclusion, social work both locally and globally needs to embark on bold and innovative approaches, such as social development and community engagement, collective action and social movements, reflecting the conscientisation approach of Paulo Freire (1972), with a commitment to revolutionary change (Kendall, 2000) to realise equality, human rights and social justice. While honouring the diversity of social work practice and the increasing role of allied professionals in NGOs, there is a clear need for reclaiming international social work with a view to realising the Global Agenda for Social Work and Social Development. Does this mean a new consortium for international social work is called for? Or are the existing set-ups, such as the Katherine A. Kendall Institute for International Social Work or the International Consortium for Social Development, equipped to provide the leadership and direction for international social work for global action?

The need of the hour is to have the courage, vision and fortitude to be open to local as well as global challenges, to realise the transformative power of social work and to stand united to promote social justice, equality and human rights for all. For, when we stand united, we can challenge oppression, discrimination and inequality, as embodied in the following quote:

> I will never forget that the only reason that I'm standing here today is because somebody, somewhere stood up for me when it was risky. Stood

up when it was hard. Stood up when it wasn't popular. And because that somebody stood up, a few more stood up. And then a few thousand stood up. And then a few million stood up. And standing up, with courage and clear purpose, they somehow managed to change the world.

(Barack Obama. Remarks at the Democratic National Committee Fall Meeting in Washington, DC. 30 November 2007. Retrieved from www.presidency.ucsb.edu/ws/?pid=77023 on 19 February 2015)

References

Ali, I. and Hatta, Z.A. (2010). Microfinance and Poverty Alleviation in Bangladesh: Perspective from Social Work. *Hong Kong J. Social Work*, 44: 121.

Alphonse, M., George, P. and Moffat, K. (2008). Redefining Social Work Standards in the Context of Globalisation: Lessons from India. *International Social Work*, 51(2): 145–58.

Caragata, L. and Sanchez, M. (2002). Globalisation and Global Need: New Imperatives for Expanding International Social Work Education in North America. *International Social Work*, 45(2): 217–38.

Cox, D. (2000). Internationalizing Social Work Education. *Indian Journal of Social Work*, 61(2): 157–73.

Cox, D. and Pawar, M. (2013). *International Social Work: Issues, Strategies and Problems*. London: Sage.

Dominelli, L. (2005). International Social Work: Themes and Issues for the 21st Century. *International Social Work*, 48(4): 504–7.

Dominelli, L. (2010). *Social Work in a Globalizing World*. Cambridge: Polity Press.

Freire, P. (1972). *Pedagogy of the Oppressed*. Harmondsworth: Penguin.

Hare, I. (2004). Defining Social Work for the 21st Century: The International Federation of Social Workers' Revised Definition of Social Work. *International Social Work*, 47(3): 407–24.

Healy, L.M. (2008). *International Social Work: Professional Action in an Interdependent World*. New York: Oxford University Press.

Hulme, D. and Moore, K. (2006). Why Has Microfinance Been a Policy Success in Bangladesh (and Beyond)? Global Poverty Research Group Working Paper Series, Paper No-041. Available at: www.gprg.org/pubs/workingpapers/pdfs/gprg-wps-041.pdf.

International Association of Schools of Social Work, International Council on Social Welfare and International Federation of Social Workers (2014). Global Agenda for Social Work and Social Development: First Report. *International Social Work*, 57(S4): 3–16.

International Federation of Social Workers (2001). Global Standards. Available at: http://ifsw.org/policies/global-standards/.

International Federation of Social Workers (2012a). Poverty Eradication and the Role for Social Workers. Available at: http://ifsw.org/policies/poverty-eradication-and-the-role-for-social-workers.

International Federation of Social Workers (2012b). The Global Agenda for Social Work and Social Development – Commitment to Action. Available at: http://cdn.ifsw.org/assets/globalagenda2012.pdf.

International Federation of Social Workers/International Association of Schools of Social Work (2000). *Definition of Social Work*. In International Association of Schools of Social Work, International Council on Social Welfare and International Federation of Social Workers (2014). Global Agenda for Social Work and Social Development: First Report. *International Social Work*, 57(S4): 3–16.

Jones, D. (2013). *International Social Work and Social Welfare: Europe*. In *Encyclopaedia of Social Work*. New York: Oxford University Press.

Jones, D. and Truell, R. (2012). The Global Agenda for Social Work and Social Development: A Place to Link Together and be Effective in a Globalised World. *International Social Work*, 55(4): 544–72.

Kendall, K. (2000). *Social Work Education: Its Origins in Europe*. Washington, DC: Council on Social Work Education.

Kendall, K. (2008). Foreword. In Lynne M. Healy, *International Social Work: Professional Action in an Independent World*. New York: Oxford University Press.

Kuruvilla, S. (2004). Social Work and Social Development in India. In I. Ferguson, M. Lavalette and E. Whitmore, *Globalisation, Global Justice and Social Work*. London: Routledge.

Lalayants, M., Doel, M. and Kachkachishvili, I. (2014). Pedagogy of International Social Work: A Comparative study in the USA, UK, and Georgia. *European Journal of Social Work*, 17(4): 455–74.

Lorenz, W. (1994). *Social Work in a Changing Europe*. London: Routlege.

Midgley, J. (2001). Issues in International Social Work: Resolving Critical Debates in the Profession. *Journal of Social Work*, 1(1): 21–35.

Mohan, B. (2008). Rethinking International Social Work. *International Social Work*, 51(1): 11–24.

Osei-Hwedie, K. (2013). International Social Work and Social Welfare: Africa (Sub-Sahara). In *Encyclopaedia of Social Work* (online). Oxford: Oxford University Press.

Palattiyil, G. and Sidhva, D. (2011). *They Call Me 'You are AIDS': A Report on HIV, Human Rights and Asylum Seekers in Scotland*. Edinburgh: University of Edinburgh.

Palattiyil, G. and Sidhva, D. (2012). Guest Editorial – Social Work in India. *Practice: Social Work in Action*, 24(2): 75–8.

Razack, R. (2009). Decolonizing the Pedagogy and Practice of International Social Work. *International Social Work*, 52(1): 9–21.

Sewpaul, V. and Jones, D. (2004). Global Standards for Social Work Education and Training. *Social Work Education: The International Journal*, 23(5): 493–513.

Stark, R. (2014). Social Work is a Human Rights Discipline. Available at: www.communitycare.co.uk/2014/07/23/social-work-human-rights-discipline-ifsw-president-speaks-profession/.

Tan, N.T. (2013). International Social Work and Social Welfare: Asia. In *Encyclopaedia of Social Work* (online). Oxford: Oxford University Press.

United Nations (2000). Millennium Development Goals. Available at: www.unmillenniumproject.org/goals/.

Index

AASW (Australian Association of Social Workers) 45, 273, 274
Aboriginal peoples 15, 16–17, 19, 58, 70, 269, 270 *see also* Canada, First Nation peoples; Maori peoples
Abram, F.Y. and Cruce, A. 3
Access to Medicine Campaign 182
adult protection and safeguarding *see* vulnerability
Adult Support and Protection (Scotland) Act *see* ASPA
advocacy: approaches 36; evidence-based practice 49; for Indigenous peoples 19; global role 4; MSM in India 175; natural disasters 248; and neo-liberalism 282; post 9/11 128, 131, 134; and professionalization 34; user-led 201; and vulnerable people 113, 119
Africa 12, 288
Ager, W. *et al.* 197
Aghabakhshi, H. and Gregor, C. 239
Akiyama, K. and Buchanan, A. 47
Alanen, L. 145
Allain, L. *et al.* 197
Allen, T. and Heald, S. 153, 154
Anghel, R. and Ramon, S. 196, 197
antiretroviral therapy, HIV/AIDS *see* ART/ARV
ANZASW (Aotearoa New Zealand Association of Social Workers) 27, 33
AOP/ADP (anti-oppressive and anti-discriminatory practice considerations) 22, 24
Aotearoa New Zealand *see* New Zealand
Arnstein, Sherry R. 196

ART/ARV (antiretroviral therapy) 153, 155, 159, 170, 182, 184; and behaviour change 164, 165; bridge population 176; children 163; and gender 174
ASPA (Adult Support and Protection (Scotland) Act) 2007 114–15
asylum seekers and refugees 3, 105, 106, 290
Attlee, C.R. 93
'audit culture' 29
Australia 15, 25; assimilation policy 24n2; *Closing the Gap* initiative 16; colonization 269; community services sector 271–3; 276–81 ; Community Services Training Package 278; context 269–71; contextual paradigm 16–17; disability 19, 20–2, 23; Disability Discrimination Act 15, 19; disadvantaged groups employed in social work 279, 280t; effect of globalization 270–1; employment and social inclusion 24; government pressure for effectiveness 43; higher education 271; Indigenous Australians 15, 16–17, 19, 269, 270; inequalities 269, 270; lack of regulation 273, 274; life expectancy 16; Medicare and health insurance 19; mental health 17–19, 22, 23; migration 269; National Disability Insurance Scheme 21–2; neo-liberalism 270; origins of social work 273; policy into practice 22–4; remuneration 281; social work education 274–5, 277–81; shortage of social workers 272; social orientations 22, 23;